Computational Approaches in Biomaterials and Biomedical Engineering Applications

Computational Approaches in Bioengineering, Volume 2—*Computational Approaches in Biomaterials and Biomedical Engineering Applications* is a comprehensive and up-to-date resource that provides a broad overview of the use of computational methods in the fields of biomaterials and biomedical engineering. Written by a team of experts in the field of biomaterials and biomedical engineering, it provides a wealth of information on the use of computational methods in these fields. Furthermore, it explores emerging trends and discusses future directions and associated limitations in the field. Through thorough exploration and explanation, it showcases the latest research and advancements, offering valuable insights into how computational methods are utilized to design and optimize biomaterials, simulate biological processes, and develop innovative medical devices.

FEATURES

- Provides practical guidance and real-world examples to help readers apply computational approaches effectively in their work.
- Explores the diverse computational approaches employed in biomaterials and biomedical engineering applications, offering a comprehensive view of the field.
- Introduces emerging topics and cutting-edge techniques, keeping wide range of readers at the forefront of advancements in computational bioengineering.
- Discusses the integration of computational methods in biomaterials and biomedical engineering, fostering a deeper understanding of their synergistic potential.
- Provides a valuable resource for researchers, practitioners, and students alike, serving as a comprehensive guide to computational approaches in biomaterials and biomedical engineering applications.

The book is well-organized and easy to read. The chapters are written in a clear and concise style, and they provide a comprehensive overview of the topics covered. The book is also well-illustrated with figures and tables that help to explain the concepts discussed in the text. With its comprehensive coverage, practical examples, and expert insights, this book serves as a valuable resource for researchers, students, and professionals in the fields of biomaterials and biomedical engineering.

Emerging Trends in Biomedical Technologies and Health Informatics Series

Series Editors:

Subhendu Kumar Pani
Orissa Engineering College, Bhubaneswar, Orissa, India

Sujata Dash
North Orissa University, Baripada, India

Sunil Vadera
University of Salford, Salford, UK

Everyday Technologies in Healthcare
Chhabi Rani Panigrahi, Bibudhendu Pati, Mamata Rath, Rajkumar Buyya

Biomedical Signal Processing for Healthcare Applications
Varun Bajaj, G R Sinha, Chinmay Chakraborty

Deep Learning in Biomedical and Health Informatics
M. Jabbar, Ajith Abraham, Onur Dogan, Ana Madureira, Sanju Tiwar

Computational Approaches in Biotechnology and Bioinformatics
Pranav Deepak Pathak, Roshani Raut, Sebastian Jaramillo-Isaza, Padnya Borkar and Rutvij H. Jhaveri

Computational Approaches in Biomaterials and Biomedical Engineering Applications
Pranav Deepak Pathak, Roshani Raut, Sebastian Jaramillo-Isaza, Padnya Borkar, and Rutvij H. Jhaveri

For more information about this series, please visit: www.routledge.com/Emerging-Trends-in-Biomedical-Technologies-and-Health-informatics-series/book-series/ETBTHI

Computational Approaches in Bioengineering

Volume 2: Computational Approaches in Biomaterials and Biomedical Engineering Applications

Edited by Pranav Deepak Pathak,
Roshani Raut, Sebastián Jaramillo-Isaza,
Pradnya Borkar, and Rutvij H. Jhaveri

CRC Press
Taylor & Francis Group
Boca Raton London New York

CRC Press is an imprint of the
Taylor & Francis Group, an **informa** business

Designed cover image: © iStock, Credit: Kateryna Bereziuk

First edition published 2024
by CRC Press
2385 NW Executive Center Drive, Suite 320, Boca Raton FL 33431

and by CRC Press
4 Park Square, Milton Park, Abingdon, Oxon, OX14 4RN

CRC Press is an imprint of Taylor & Francis Group, LLC

Library of Congress Cataloging-in-Publication Data
Names: Pathak, Pranav Deepak, editor. | Raut, Roshani, 1981– editor. | Jaramillo-Isaza, Sebastián, editor. | Borkar, Pradnya, editor. | Jhaveri, Rutvij, editor.
Title: Computational approaches in biomedical engineering / edited by Pranav Deepak Pathak, Roshani Raut, Sebastian Jaramillo-Isaza, Pradnya Borkar and Rutvij H. Jhaveri.
Description: First edition. | Boca Raton FL : CRC Press, 2024. | Includes bibliographical references and index. | Contents: v. 1. Computational approaches in biotechnology and bioinformatics — v. 2. Computational approaches in biomaterials and biomedical engineering applications.
Identifiers: LCCN 2023048741 (print) | LCCN 2023048742 (ebook) | ISBN 9781032406107 (v. 1 ; hardback) | ISBN 9781032407128 (v. 1 ; paperback) | ISBN 9781032635255 (v. 2 ; hardback) | ISBN 9781032635279 (v. 2 ; paperback) | ISBN 9781003354437 (v. 1 ; ebook) | ISBN 9781032699882 (v. 2 ; ebook)
Subjects: MESH: Biomedical Engineering—methods | Computational Biology—methods | Biotechnology—methods | Biocompatible Materials
Classification: LCC R857.M3 (print) | LCC R857.M3 (ebook) | NLM QT 36 | DDC 610.28/4—dc23/eng/20240301
LC record available at https://lccn.loc.gov/2023048741
LC ebook record available at https://lccn.loc.gov/2023048742

ISBN: 978-1-032-63530-9 (set)
ISBN: 978-1-032-63525-5 (hbk)
ISBN: 978-1-032-63527-9 (pbk)
ISBN: 978-1-032-69988-2 (ebk)

DOI: 10.1201/9781032699882

Typeset in Times
by Apex CoVantage, LLC

Contents

Preface

This book, *Computational Approaches in Biomaterials and Biomedical Engineering Applications*, is a comprehensive guide to understanding and exploring the cutting-edge applications of computational methods in these interdisciplinary domains. This book is Volume 2 of the *Computational Approaches in Bioengineering* set.

Biomaterials and biomedical engineering are undergoing a profound transformation due to the integration of computational approaches and techniques. This book, *Computational Approaches in Biomaterials and Biomedical Engineering Applications*, aims to give a thorough overview of the most recent developments and applications of computational methods in these dynamic and interdisciplinary domains.

In order to offer their expertise and ideas on various themes, this book brings together eminent experts and researchers from academia, business, and healthcare facilities. The chapters covered in this book discuss a variety of topics like drug delivery, challenges of biomaterials in ophthalmology, machine learning for cancer diagnosis, genetic diagnosis, etc.

The book chapters include theoretical and real-world examples to give readers a thorough and current understanding of the subject. This book brings together leading experts and researchers from academia, industry, and healthcare institutions to share their knowledge and insights on various topics.

This book comprises twelve chapters.

Chapter 1 presents current trends, challenges, and opportunities in biomaterial implementations in biomedical engineering. Metals are favoured in almost all constant stream applications due to their greater structural rigidity and high flexibility. The requirement for advanced implanted biomaterials that can manage unique problems in the cardiovascular system, orthotics, shock, backbone, dental, and wound care has developed into a common concern. Enzymes and proteases can change most natural biomaterials and are biodegradable. Using this characteristic, unique medical devices and therapies can be created that only temporarily change the implant site or are resorbable. Future research projects may be possible to integrate supramolecular, injectable, and immunomodulation biomaterials and develop a self-sufficient power source. This chapter also explains modern set trends and opportunities in biomedical engineering with their novel applications in the biomedical field and other imperative domains.

Chapter 2 explains the applications of biomaterials in advanced drug delivery systems. It explains how the best strategy to reduce the adverse effects of medications is to increase the effectiveness of drug nano-carriers in delivering drugs to the targeted areas. The medication administration process becomes more challenging due to high activation barriers for drug adsorption and unfavourable thermodynamic properties. In this regard, the use of advanced biomaterials, such as synthetic polymeric and self-assembled materials, for the implementation of drug transportation systems has been expanding quickly due to their increased biocompatibility, ability to cross biological membranes easily, and ability to deliver controlled and sustainable drug release to the target sites. Regarding applications of cutting-edge drug transportation networks and the rehabilitation of health-related concerns, this chapter also discusses the synthesis and properties of relevant biomaterials.

Chapter 3 explains the advantages and challenges of biomaterials in ophthalmology. Biomaterials are polymers (synthetic or modified) or other substances (metals, glasses, and ceramics) used to prepare implants or other medical devices to interact with biological systems. The use of synthetic polymers as biomaterials has been pioneered by ophthalmology more than by other medical specialties. Biomaterials are used in or around the eye for various applications. Applications of biomaterials in ophthalmology include several eye implants used to repair and restore the function of the cornea, lens, vitreous fluid, etc., when they are diseased or damaged. Different biomaterials are available to manufacture intraocular and contact lenses to correct vision. Biomaterials are applied during surgical operations, allowing for corneal curvature correction and a detached retina indentation. Biomaterial solutions are used as replacements in tears and vitreous liquids. Corneal tissue engineering uses silk as a biomaterial and collagen in eye shields for corneal protection, opening the application of biomaterial in ocular drug delivery systems to treat various microbial infections.

Chapter 4 explains using artificial intelligence and machine learning to analyse cellular images in breast cancer. By enabling early diagnosis and treatment, using artificial intelligence and machine learning efficiently in identifying and treating numerous fatal diseases has raised patient survival rates. Deep knowledge has been developed to explore the critical factors affecting the diagnosis and treatment of serious illnesses. It will be covered in detail how previous studies have examined the early detection and treatment of breast cancer using genetic sequencing or histopathological imaging. Convolutional neural networks (CNNs), support vector machines (SVMs), Bayesian techniques, and other semisupervised and unsupervised techniques have been used to categorise breast images.

Chapter 5 presents genetic diagnosis, classification, and risk prediction in cancer using next-generation sequencing in oncology. Identifying and extracting these biomarkers and genetic signs of various cancers from among the thousands of genes appears complex and challenging. This research aims to create an algorithm to assist with next-generation sequencing data gene extraction, identification, and prediction. Three folds compose the proposed technique: a filtering fold using minimum redundancy maximum relevance (mRMR), a wrapper fold using the Boruta algorithm, and a final fold using deep learning (DL). Using five RNA-seq datasets from a cancer patient, a comparative assessment between the suggested algorithm and the current approaches has been carried out. The final results show that the proposed algorithm significantly outperformed the existing techniques.

Chapter 6 covers how artificial intelligence and machine learning treat cardiovascular diseases. Various applications in cardiovascular risk assessment, imaging, and emerging therapeutic targets in cardiovascular therapy are based on AI. This chapter aims to discuss various AI applications, such as ML and DL, and how they are used in cardiovascular care. AI-based solutions have improved knowledge of heart failure and congenital heart disease phenotypes. These applications have produced newer approaches to cardiovascular drug therapy, more unique treatment techniques for various types of cardiovascular illnesses, and post-marketing analyses of pharmaceuticals. Data privacy, poorly chosen/outdated data, selection bias, and inadvertent perpetuation of historical biases/stereotypes in the data are some of the difficulties in the clinical application of AI-based applications and interpretation of the results, which might result in incorrect conclusions. However, AI is a revolutionary technology with enormous potential for the healthcare industry.

Chapter 7 explains the role of big data, AI, and machine learning in decision making for disease diagnosis and treatment. This chapter describes the emerging field of big data analytics in healthcare, provides an overview of artificial intelligence (AI) and machine learning (ML), discusses the subsets of AI, outlines the benefits of AI and ML in disease diagnosis, describes examples reported in the literature, briefly discusses the challenges, provides few open-source distributed data analytics software platform, and offers conclusions and future directions. The chapter makes it easy for readers to recognise potential technologies like big data, AI, and ML that provide creative solutions for processing patient data. It generates patient reports, helps grade patient illness conditions based on molecular changes in their bodies, and allows immediate medication actions for revolutionary AI-based precision medicine for all patients.

The application of artificial intelligence to drug research is discussed in Chapter 8. This chapter demonstrates current and historical data interactions, including access to new or enhanced biological and chemical processes, higher success rates, and more efficient and cost-effective discovery techniques. Identifying specific known genes associated with diseases and selecting new therapy targets is feasible based on analysing databases with gene–disease correlations. This chapter presents a complete overview of network pharmacology based on current research, highlighting numerous active ingredients, accompanying techniques, tools, databases, and use in efficient drug development and discovery.

The importance of artificial intelligence is discussed in Chapter 9, which present the identification, classification, and prognosis of hepatocellular carcinoma. The relevance of artificial intelligence to hepatocellular carcinoma (HCC) research is updated in this chapter. For the detection of HCC, AI algorithms that analyse and incorporate massive datasets are used. AI can help interconnect various data variables to predict survival chances after HCC treatment. Benign tumours, malignant tumours, and HCC can now be classified or recognised better by using AI.

Artificial intelligence for neuromotor rehabilitation engineering is discussed in Chapter 10. This chapter discusses the developments and issues that currently affect the field of rehabilitation engineering for neuromotor disabilities from the perspective of artificial intelligence and how this allows for improving the performance of systems for adequate accessibility of this population in daily activities. In light of the planned 2030 Sustainable Development Goals for Health and Welfare, it is possible to highlight specific solutions and future work that will benefit people with disabilities.

Chapter 11 discusses innovative computational techniques for recovering motor functions in brain–computer interface (BCI) systems. Electroencephalogram (EEG)-based BCI systems use EEG data to determine the user's intention, which requires different computational methods to interpret the electrical activity of the EEG. The number of mental states that can be classified, the interference from other signals (artefacts) that contaminate the EEG, the effectiveness of the EEG in generating commands, and the slow rate of information transfer are some of the significant restrictions that still apply to using EEG signals for BCI applications at the moment. Several processes are involved in processing EEG signals, including trial/artefact rejection, eye tracking, filtering, feature extraction, and classification/regression. This chapter explains the EEG signal processing pipelines utilised in the scientific literature and introduces novel methods for analysing EEG data utilising advanced computing techniques used in BCI applications.

Using wearable sensors and AI-based machine learning methods, Chapter 12 describes how to improve telerehabilitation. In addition to highlighting potential applications of AI to enhance the delivery of telerehabilitation, this chapter gives an overview of the obstacles, facilitators, and challenges associated with telerehabilitation. Also included are cutting-edge technologies that can provide pertinent information during rehabilitation, such as wearable sensors, the Internet of Things, sensor-based devices, and video applications.

The material collected in this book has been edited to provide knowledge about the current research achievements and challenges in biomaterial and biomedical engineering applications. The book targets senior and junior engineers, undergraduate and postgraduate students, researchers, and anyone interested in these concept trends, development, and opportunities.

The editors would like to acknowledge and appreciate the contributions of all the authors who have submitted the chapter manuscripts to this book.

Editors

About the Editors

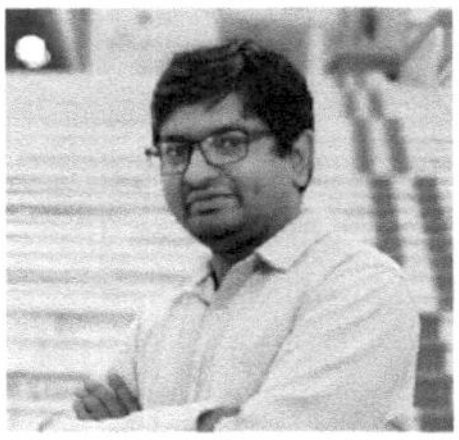

Dr. Pranav Deepak Pathak is an associate professor at the MIT School of Bioengineering Sciences & Research, MIT Art, Design and Technology University, Pune. He has more than 14 years of teaching experience in Fundamentals of Biochemical Engineering, metabolic engineering, Biotransport, Mass transfer, Heat Transfer, and Reaction Engineering. He received his undergraduate and postgraduate degrees in chemical engineering from Sant Gadge Baba Amravati University, India, and a doctoral degree in chemical engineering from Visveswaraya National Institute of Technology, Nagpur, India. His research specializations are bio-refinery, biomass and waste utilization, microbial engineering and fermentation & extraction technology. He has published more than 40 research articles in peer-reviewed international journals/book chapters and has three edited books on his credit. He has also filed several patents to his credit. He participated in various national/international conferences, workshops, and training. His research interests include bioengineering, biorefinery, and wastewater treatment.

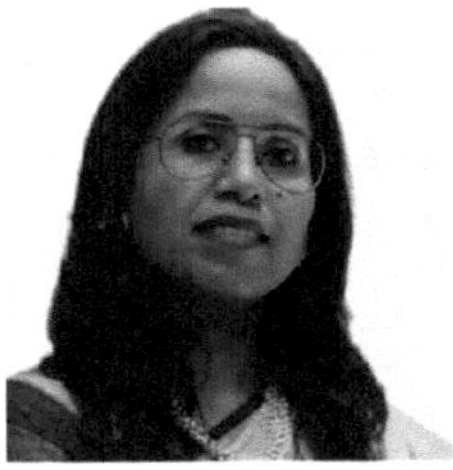

Dr. Roshani Raut obtained her PhD degree in computer science and engineering and ME and BE degrees in computer science and engineering. She has more than 20 years of experience and currently she is working as a professor in the Department of Information Technology and Dean International Relations at Pimpri Chinchwad College of Engineering, Pune, India. She is guiding a PhD research scholar in the University of Technology, Petronas, Malaysia.

She is a member of IEEE and ISTE. She has availed research and workshop grants from BCUD, Pune University. She has presented more than 125 research communications in national and international conferences and journals. She has published 15 patents and has received grants for 10 patents. She worked as a convener for national and international conferences. She has published 10 books, where she worked as an author or editor, of various national and international publications like IGI Global, CRC/Taylor & Francis, and Scrivener Wiley. Her research area includes artificial intelligence, machine learning, data mining, and deep learning, among other areas.

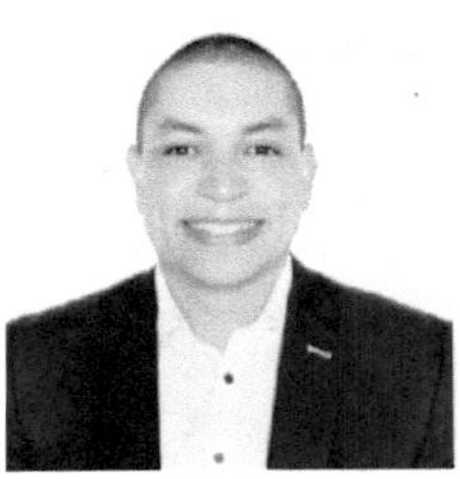

Sebastián Jaramillo-Isaza is a skilled, rigorous, and highly motivated bioengineer. He holds an MSc in mechanics and materials and a doctoral degree in biomechanics, biomaterials, and bioengineering. In addition, he has substantial experience researching and teaching in motion capture and analysis, biomaterials, rehabilitation, bioinstrumentation, and materials characterization. Furthermore, he has participated in and organized national/international conferences and workshops.

Currently, he is working as Associate Professor in Biomedical Engineering at Antonio Nariño University in Bogotá, Colombia.

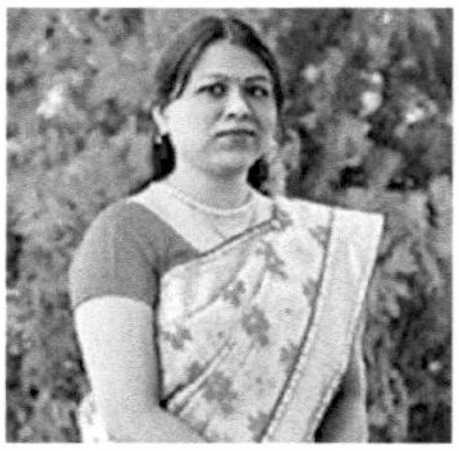

Dr. Pradnya Borkar is Assistant Professor in the Department of Computer Science and Engineering at the Symbiosis Institute of Technology, Nagpur (Constituent of Symbiosis International University, Pune). She earned her BE in computer technology in 2002, her MTech in computer science and engineering in 2008, and her PhD in computer science and engineering in 2018 from Rashtrasant Tukdoji Maharaj Nagpur University (formerly Nagpur University). She has worked with many reputed organizations and has an overall teaching experience of around 19 years. One patent has been granted to her account, and she has filed two more patents. She had handled major responsibilities at the time of accreditation. Her areas of interest are high-performance computing, bioinformatics, parallel computing, database management systems, compilers and theory of computation, etc. She has presented and published many papers in national/international conferences as well as journals. She has published nine book chapters. She is a reviewer of two international journals and has reviewed book chapters for various publishers of repute. She has chaired sessions at international and national conferences. She is a member of professional societies such as the ISTE, CSI, SDIWC, etc. She worked as a committee member in various capacities at the institute and university levels.

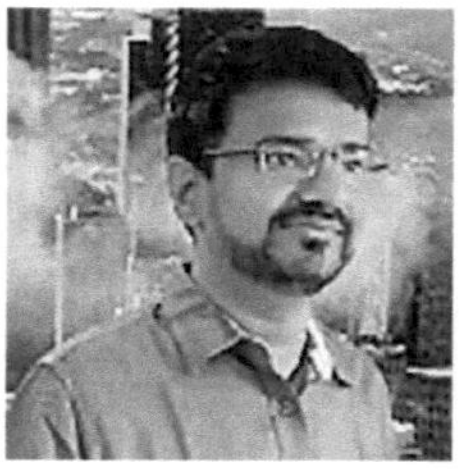

Dr. Rutvij H. Jhaveri (Senior Member, IEEE) is an experienced educator and researcher working in the Department of Computer Science & Engineering, Pandit Deendayal Energy University, Gandhinagar, India. He conducted his postdoctoral research at Delta-NTU Corporate Lab for Cyber-Physical Systems, Nanyang Technological University, Singapore. He completed his PhD in computer engineering in 2016. In 2017, he was awarded with the prestigious Pedagogical Innovation Award by Gujarat Technological University. Currently, he is co-investigating a funded project from GUJCOST. He was ranked among top 2% scientists around the world in 2022 and 2021. He has 3000+ Google Scholar citations with an H-index of 29. He is an editorial board member of various journals of repute, including IEEE Transactions on Industrial Informatics and Scientific Reports. He also serves as a reviewer in several international journals and as an advisory/TPC member at renowned international conferences. He authored 145+ articles including the IEEE/ACM Transactions and flagship IEEE/ACM conferences. Moreover, he has several national and international patents and copyrights to his name. He also possesses memberships in various technical bodies such as the ACM, CSI, ISTE, and others. He is the coordinator of the SCAN—Smart Cities Air Quality Network. Moreover, he has been a member of the advisory board of the Symbiosis Institute of Digital and Telecom Management and other reputed universities since 2022. He is an editorial board member in several Springer and Hindawi journals. He also served as a committee member in the "Smart Village Project"—Government of Gujarat at the district level during the year 2017. His research interests are Cyber Security, IoT systems, SDN, and smart healthcare.

Contributors

Antelis Javier M.
Tecnologico de Monterrey
Escuela de Ingeniería y Ciencias
Monterrey, Mexico

Aruna S.
Department of Master of Computer Applications
Sona College of Technology
Salem, Tamil Nadu, India

Ayipo Yusuf O.
Kwara State University
Malete, Kwara, Nigeria

Baildya Nabajyoti
Department of Chemistry
Milki High School
Milki, Malda, West Bengal, India

Banjoko Alabi W.
University of Ilorin
Kwara State University
Malete, Kwara, Nigeria

Bastos-Filho Teodiano Freire
Federal University of Espírito Santo
Postgraduate Program in Electrical Engineering
Vitoria, Brazil

Bhanarkar Parul
Jhulelal Institute of Technology
Nagpur, India

Blanco-Díaz Cristian Felipe
Federal University of Espírito Santo
Postgraduate Program in Electrical Engineering
Vitoria, Brazil

Borkar Pradnya S.
Symbiosis Institute of Technology
Symbiosis International (Deemed University)
Pune, India

Cerquera Alexander
Department of Engineering
Neuro Wave Systems
Beachwood, OH, USA

Choudhury Prosenjit
Department of Physics
Dr. Meghnad Saha College
Itahar, India

Choudhury Subhankar
Department of Chemistry
Malda College
Malda, India

Dauda Kazeem A.
Kwara State University
Malete, Kwara, Nigeria

Delis Alberto López
Centrode Biofísica Médica
Universidad de Oriente
Cuba

Duraiswamy Basavan
Department of Pharmacology
JSS College of Pharmacy
JSS Academy of Higher Education & Research
Ooty, Nilgiris, Tamil Nadu, India

Elayaperumal Sumitha
Department of Biotechnology and Bioinformatics
JSS Academy of Higher Education and Research
Mysore, Karnataka, India

Gaddigal Anjana Thatesh
P. G. Department of Studies in Biochemistry
Karnataka University
Dharwad, India

Ganeshkar Madhu Prakash
P. G. Department of Studies in Biochemistry
Karnataka University
Dharwad, India

Gautam Rupesh K.
Department of Pharmacology
Indore Institute of Pharmacy
Rau-Indore, India

Ghosh Narendra Nath
Pakuahat A. N. M. High School
Malda, West Bengal, India

Ghosh Puja
Department of Pharmacology
JSS College of Pharmacy
JSS Academy of Higher Education & Research
Ooty, Nilgiris, Tamil Nadu, India

Goder Premakshi Hucharayappa
P. G. Department of Studies in Biochemistry
Karnataka University
Dharwad, India

Guerrero-Mendez Cristian David
Federal University of Espírito Santo
Postgraduate Program in Electrical Engineering
Vitoria, Brazil

Herrera Edith Pulido
Escuela Militar de Cadetes General "José María Córdova", Engineering and Simulation Research Group (GINSI)
Bogotá, Colombia

Jana Poulami
Department of Chemistry
Kaliachak College Sultanganj
Malda, West Bengal, India

Jaramillo-Isaza Sebastián
Antonio Nariño University
Faculty of Mechanical, Electronic and Biomedical Engineering
Bogotá, Colombia

Justin Antony
Department of Pharmacology
JSS College of Pharmacy
JSS Academy of Higher Education & Research
Ooty, Nilgiris, Tamil Nadu, India

K. M. Muhasina
Department of Pharmacology
JSS College of Pharmacy
JSS Academy of Higher Education & Research
Ooty, Nilgiris, Tamil Nadu, India

Kamanavalli Chandrappa Mukappa
P. G. Department of Studies in Biochemistry
Karnataka University
Dharwad, India

M. Esakkimuthukumar
Department of Pharmaceutical Chemistry
JSS College of Pharmacy
JSS Academy of Higher Education & Research
Ooty, Nilgiris, Tamil Nadu, India

Mirjankar Manisha Rajendra
P. G. Department of Studies in Biochemistry
Karnataka University
Dharwad, India
Olorede Kabir O., Kwara State University
Malete, Kwara, Nigeria

Panse Prashant
Department of IT
Medi-Caps University
Indore, India

Parashar Smriti
Vedic Institute of Pharmaceutical Education and Research
Sagar, India

Pattar Shridhar Veeresh
P. G. Department of Studies in Biochemistry
Karnataka University
Dharwad, India

Poojari Paramanna Bhagappa
P. G. Department of Studies in Biochemistry
Karnataka University
Dharwad, India

Rangaswamy Ramyakrishna A.
Department of Biotechnology and Bioinformatics
JSS Academy of Higher Education and Research
Mysore, Karnataka, India

Ruiz-Olaya Andrés Felipe
Antonio Nariño University
Faculty of Mechanical, Electronic and Biomedical Engineering
Bogotá, Colombia

Sajal Harshit
Department of Biotechnology and Bioinformatics
JSS Academy of Higher Education and Research
Mysore, Karnataka, India

Sarulatha R.
Department of Master of Computer Applications
Sona College of Technology
Salem, Tamil Nadu, India

Selvaraj Jubie
Department of Pharmaceutical Chemistry
JSS College of Pharmacy
JSS Academy of Higher Education & Research
Ooty, Nilgiris, Tamil Nadu, India

Shivappa Parashuram
P. G. Department of Studies in Biochemistry
Karnataka University
Dharwad, India

Singh Ramveer
Department of Botany and Microbiology
Gurukula Kangri University
Haridwar, India

Singh Rana Pratap
Department of Pharmaceutical Regulatory Affairs
JSS College of Pharmacy
JSS Academy of Higher Education & Research
Ooty, Nilgiris, Tamil Nadu, India

Sivamani Yuvaraj
Department of Pharmaceutical Chemistry
Cauvery College of Pharmacy
Mysore, India

Suji priya J.
Department of Master of Computer Applications
Sona College of Technology
Salem, Tamil Nadu, India

Swaroop Akey Krishna
Department of Pharmaceutical Chemistry
JSS College of Pharmacy
JSS Academy of Higher Education & Research
Ooty, Nilgiris, Tamil Nadu, India

Thakur Reena
Jhulelal Institute of Technology
Nagpur, India

Thirumalaisamy R.
Department of Biotechnology
Sona College Arts and Science
Salem, Tamil Nadu, India

Venkatesh Apoorva M.
Department of Biotechnology and Bioinformatics
JSS Academy of Higher Education and Research
Mysore, Karnataka, India

Wairagade Madhavi
Jhulelal Institute of Technology
Nagpur, India

Yahya Waheed B.
University of Ilorin
Kwara State University
Malete, Kwara, Nigeria

1 Use of Biomaterials in the Field of Biomedical Engineering

Current Trends, Challenges, and Opportunities in Implementations

Manisha Rajendra Mirjankar, Madhu Prakash Ganeshkar*, Anjana Thatesh Gaddigal*, Parashuram Shivappa*, Paramanna Bhagappa Poojari*, Shridhar Veeresh Pattar*, Premakshi Hucharayappa Goder**, and Chandrappa Mukappa Kamanavalli*,†*

*P. G. Department of Studies in Biochemistry, Karnataka University, Dharwad, India; **P. G. Department of Studies in Chemistry, Karnatak University, Dharwad, India.
†Corresponding Author: cmkamanavalli@gmail.com

ABBREVIATIONS

3D	Three-dimensional
Ag	Argentum (silver)
Au	Arum (gold)
BMG	Bulk metallic glass
CAR-T	Chimeric antigen receptor T-cells
Ce	Cerium
CRT	Cardiac resynchronization therapy
Cu	Copper
DB	Droplet-based
DBS	Deep brain stimulation
EB	Extrusion-based
EBM	Electron beam melting
ECM	Extracellular matrix

DOI: 10.1201/9781032699882-1

EM	Electromechanical
FDM	Fused deposition modelling
Fe^{+3}	Ferric cation
GF	Growth factor
ICD	Implantable cardioverter defibrillator
iPSCs	Induced pluripotent stem cell
LB	Laser-based
m	Metre
Mb	Methylene blue
MESW	Melt electrospinning writing
Mg	Magnesium
Mn	Manganese
MRI	Magnetic resonance imaging
MRSA	Methicillin-resistant staphylococci
N	Nitrogen
Ni	Nickel
NK	Natural killer cell
O	Oxygen
P	Phosphorus
PCL	Polycaprolactone
PGA	Poly glycolic acid
PHA	Polyhydroxy alkenoate
PHB	Polyhydroxy butyrate
PLA	Polylactic acid
PLGA	Poly lactic-co-glycolic acid
PVA	Polyvinyl alcohol
S	Sulphur
SLA	Stereolithography
SLM	Selective laser melting
SLS	Selective laser sintering
TE	Tissue engineering
Ti	Titanium
Zn	Zinc

1.1 INTRODUCTION

Biomaterials play an important role in modern medicine since they aid in patients' recuperation from disease or injury by restoring function. According to National Institute of Health (NIH),

> any substance or association of chemical compounds, other than drugs, that maybe exploited for any event momentary and that can improve or entirely supplant any tissue, organ, or bodily function so that preserve or embellish an individual's value of life are refer to as biomaterials.
>
> (Farag, 2023)

In therapeutic applications, biomaterials may be either organic or synthetic and are intended to sustain, enhance, or replace damaged tissue or a biological function.

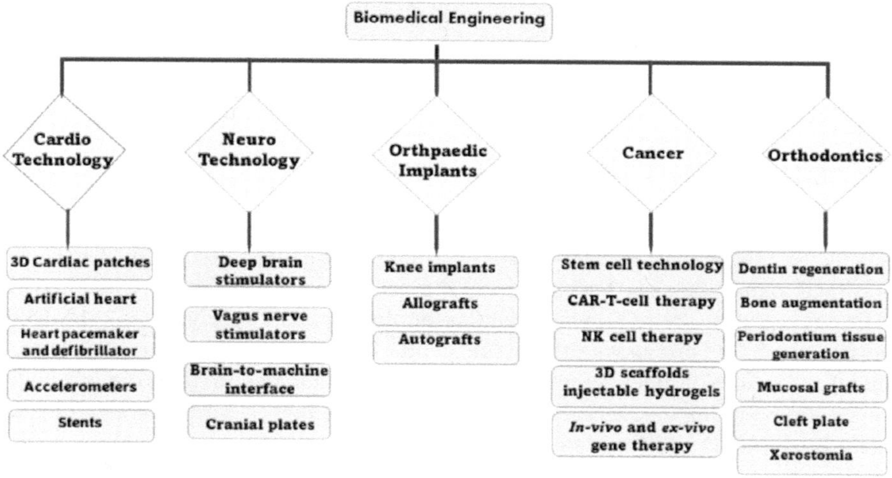

FIGURE 1.1 Subdisciplines of biomedical engineering.

Biomaterials were first employed historically by ancient Egyptians, who used sutures constructed from animal tendons. The modern field of biomaterials integrates medicine, any branch of natural science, physics, chemistry, and recent influences from tissue manufacturing and material technologies. The discipline has extended considerably over the past decade on account of advancements in constructive medication, tissue design, and additional areas (Figure 1.1). Biomedical engineering is a much broader field, despite the fact that biomaterials can also be considered a larger field than materials used in medical applications (Ha et al., 2013). The discipline of bioengineering has made numerous strides, these developments are directly reliant on the availability of biomaterials, or suitable materials, without which bioengineering would be severely constrained. Biomaterials, for instance, are used in disposable plastics and other things. From a medical perspective, biomaterials are substances found in therapeutic or diagnostic systems that come into contact with biological fluids but are not foods or medications (Zargar et al., 2015). Biomaterials have had, and will continue to have, a significant influence on biomedical engineering. Studying materials for use in medicine is the specific emphasis of this chapter (Ahsan et al., 2018). Despite the fact that numerous synthetic polymers are used in biomaterials, many polymers that are naturally generated are also in use. Naturally derived polymers have the possibility to be used in drug delivery systems and medical devices because they can help cells function more efficiently than many synthetic alternatives for adhesion, migration, proliferation, and differentiation (Gutiérrez, 2017). The development and improvement of biomaterials are primarily motivated by the need to satisfy the physical and biological needs of injured tissues (Firdous et al., 2013; Ali and Ahmed, 2018).

This, in turn, increases the demand for biomaterial qualities such as biocompatibility, biodegradability, non-antigenicity, and cost-effectiveness. The development of biomaterials such films, foams, gels, scaffolds for implants, and microporous particles has been made possible by the capacity to improve the aforementioned qualities. However, problems with biocompatibility limit the use of biomaterials manufactured from synthetic polymers; this is driving research into biomaterials made from naturally occurring polymers. This chapter focuses on the uses of naturally occurring polymers as biomaterials in cutting-edge research, including chitosan, collagen, hyaluronic acid, and silk fibroin (Rodrigues et al., 2012).

1.2 MULTI-FUNCTIONAL BIOMATERIALS FOR ADVANCED THERAPIES

The interaction of engineered tissues and materials with their surroundings and cells is critical to their success. Various levels of material integration and interaction with their environment are required depending on the application (Figure 1.2). Bioinert substances should merge with the tissue as little as possible, whereas materials that are bioactive or biomimetic are intended to directly interact with their organic environment by altering, encouraging, and stimulating cellular reactions (Pacelli et al., 2016; Kyziol et al., 2017). Materials with active or preliminary characteristics can be surface-altered to produce bio interfaces that must be specifically functionalized for the intended tissue or use in the body (Aamodt et al., 2016; Hinderer et al., 2016; Zhang et al., 2018; Ganeshkar et al., 2022). The majority of tissues is composed of gradients or various distributions rather than containing an established extracellular matrix (ECM) and growth factor composition, a single topographical feature, or a distinct mechanical value. It is well known that cellular migration and differentiation are led by biophysical and biochemical gradients during organogenesis, tissue renovation and conversion, inflammation, and diseases (Hale et al., 2010).

The surface coarseness (bulk and size of conferred geological surface patterns) of biomaterials also considerably influences the cell behaviour (Fiedler et al., 2013). A complex interaction of biochemical and mechanobiological processes manages how cells communicate with the ECM. Transmembrane proteins (integrins), for instance, arbitrate adhesion to ECM proteins by identifying particular amino acid sequences (adhesion peptides) (Kim et al., 2011; Xiang et al., 2022). Tissues make up intricate and incredibly vital systems. The multi-functional microenvironments coordinate cellular behaviour through a dynamic interplay of biochemical and material patterns from the ECM accompanying soluble determinants like tumour factors, cell–cell contacts, and hydrostatic pressure.

1.2.1 Biomaterials for 3D Scaffolds

Implantable three-dimensional (3D) scaffolds are designed to repair and reorganize anatomical imperfections in intricate organs and functional tissues. These scaffolds represent a model for the restoration and reconstruction of defects while advancing cell connection, expansion, ECM creation, and the reestablishment of vessels, nerves, muscles, cartilage, etc. Scaffolds with the least amount of toxicity and inflammation, stringy, or penetrable biomaterials created to elevate ECM deposition, cell synergy, and viability. Moreover, they biodegrade steadily as well. At the same time, 3D scaffolds may be used to form tissue models that mimic the sophisticated skeletal structure of living tissues (Chen et al., 2022). The macro-, micro-, and nano-architecture of the scaffolds, in addition to the biomaterial employed, are therefore crucial (Nikolova and Chavali, 2019).

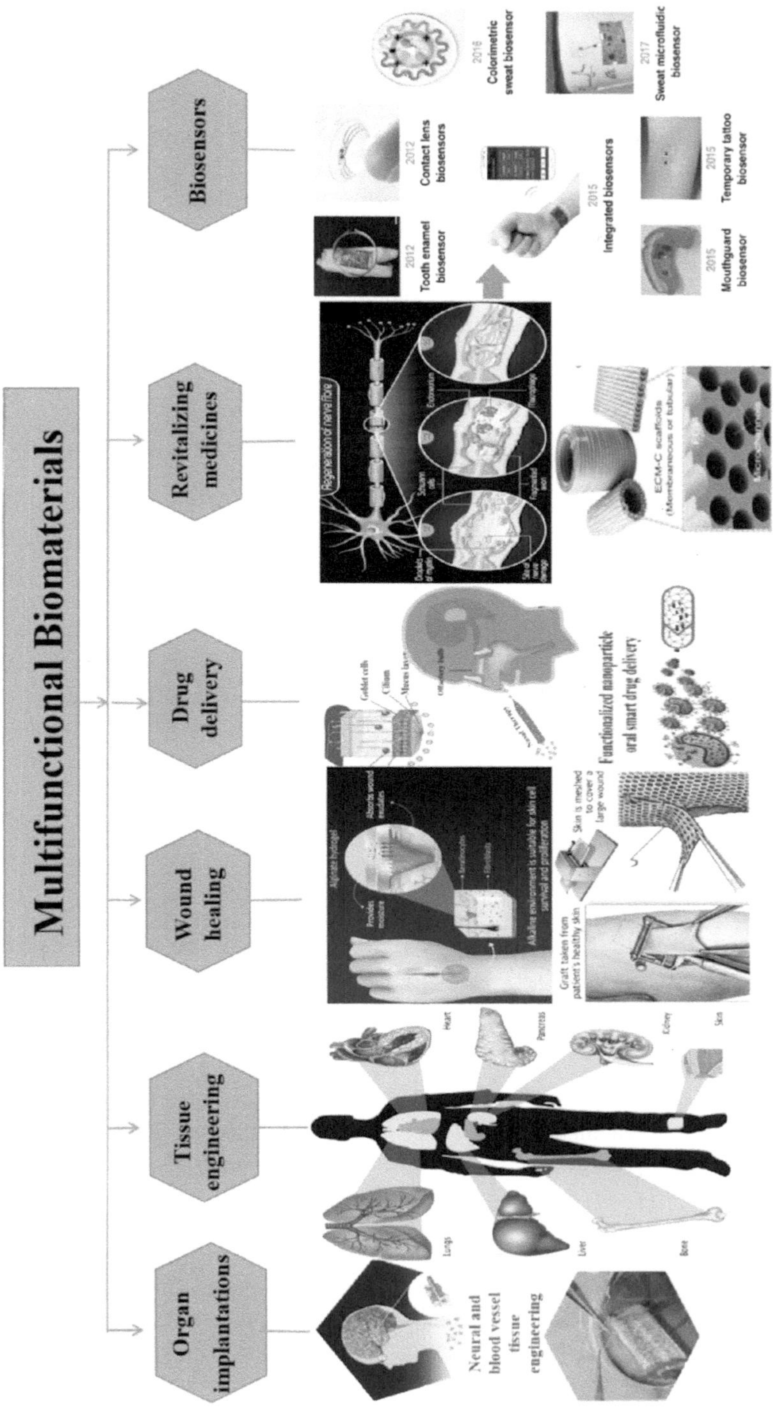

FIGURE 1.2 Applications of multi-functional biomaterials.

Biomaterials may degrade in bulk or on the surface. Bulk deterioration devastates the material's internal structure rather than the surface, maintaining the majority of the structure. Without the partition of lethal byproducts, the rate of degradation is presumed to be effectively equal to the rate of tissue progress. Physical, chemical organic, or connected processes may be used to degrade a biomaterial, facilitating the biocompatibility of the 3D platform. Permanent (nondegradable) or semi-constant scaffolds, for instance, may be used to repair articular cartilage when it is not essential for the scaffolds to degrade entirely. Nanostructured surfaces have a greater surface energy than refined substances, which improves hydrophilicity and, thus, improves protein adhesiveness and cell attachment. Not merely because it boosts mechanical strength, the smaller grain size was found to be more beneficial for osteogenic cell adhesion and proliferation in metal and ceramic scaffolds (Saiz et al., 2013).

1.2.2 Sponge or Foam Porous Scaffolds

In order to promote cartilage regrowth, arterialization, and ECM deposition, sponge scaffolds often have an inter-linked pore construction (either organized or random). These scaffolds increase the flow of nutrients and gas across the channel network on account of the extreme physical surface, improving external nerve and artery development. However, the automated properties of the scaffold must be maintained while increasing pore interconnectivity. If not, nourishment flow and cell in-growth will be restricted. Cellular penetration, ECM deposition, and neovascularization might not occur if the pores are extremely narrow. The interconnected porous structure should ideally have 90% porosity (Feng and others, 2015), which could have a serious influence the final mechanical properties. But various cells and tissues have diverse optimum pore sizes (Marrella et al., 2018).

1.2.3 Fibrous Scaffolds

An assortment of environmentally friendly polymers made up of polylactic acid (PLA) (Rampichová et al., 2014), polycaprolactone (PCL) (Ren et al., 2013), poly lactic-co-glycolic acid (PLGA) (Wang et al., 2011), gelatine (Loordhuswamy et al., 2014), cellulose (Xu et al., 2016), and silk fibroin (Melke et al., 2016) has been employed to build fibrous scaffolds. The standard characteristics of these fibres make them exemplary carriers of drugs, DNA, and proteins in addition to scaffolds for skin, cartilage, ligaments, bone, tissue, and veins (Vasita et al., 2006). Nanofibres as scaffolds are demonstrated to be more promising biomaterials than microfibres because the nanosize encourages cells to gain a normal form *in vivo*. By demonstrating topographical signifiers impacting cell differentiation and fate, nanofibres have the competence to offer leading arrangements for neurite formation (Xia et al., 2014). These nanofibres are more successful at inducing basic affinity than microfibres cause they closely simulate the makeup and aspects of the ECM (Hejazian et al., 2012). They also have a more advanced feature arrangement, greater porosity, and higher surface-to-volume arrangement. When compared to the features of individual scaffolds, assorted fibre–mesh scaffolds offer the chance to build structures with upgraded biomechanical, physico-synthetic, and biological traits (Wade et al., 2014). The management of nanofibre reinforced composites, for instance, shall result in substances with higher mechanical energy than typical unfilled composites (Subbiah et al., 2005). But there are various drawbacks to emblematic fibre scaffolds, including their restricted width and tiny pore capacity. These scaffolds exhibit a definite level of site-specific targeting while being widely used in splitting applications including DNA therapy, regulated medication, and tumour growth factor administration (Cai et al., 2018).

The bioactive moiety release refers to a scaffold's capacity to prudently regulate and switch on the element release by interacting with bio-microscopic cues (Yin et al., 2015). High-molecular-weight microspheres produce a more sluggish release of the medication than low molecular weight polymers (Frohbergh et al., 2012). Microspheres are capable of release optimized bioactive compounds gradually when included in 3D scaffolds as construction blocks (Repanas et al., 2016). Oil-in-water dispersion, solvent/non-solvent sintering, solvent vapour analysis, and selective laser sintering (SLS) are a few of the methods created utilizing microspheres and microsphere based 3D scaffolds (Christopherson et al., 2009).

1.2.4 Cellular 3D Printing

Selective laser melting (SLM), electron beam melting (EBM), fused deposition modelling (FDM), and melt electrospinning writing (MESW) are subcategories of acellular distribution, and extrusion-based (EB), droplet-based (DB), laser-based (LB), and stereolithographic approaches are subcategories of cellular 3D printing (Datta et al., 2017; Deng et al., 2019). A photoreactive adhesive is selectively treated at the same time as the stereolithography (SLA), or vat polymerization process, which shifts the scaffold following the establishment of each new layer. With tremendous preciseness and resolution, the approach is utilized to amalgamate polymer, ceramic, and polymer–ceramic composite scaffolds (Algardh et al., 2016; Yang et al., 2019).

1.2.5 Resorbable Biomaterials

Bioresorbable materials have advantages over permanent biostable implants due to the latter's risk of immunological reactions and biocompatible issues. Natural qualities like mechanical strength and steady growth are restored as the bioresorbable material degrades over time (Ulery et al., 2011). The non-toxic, non-inflammatory, non-carcinogenic, and non-immunogenic properties of biocompatible resorbable materials make them suitable for bone graft alternatives and other biomedical applications.

Chitosan is a flexible biopolymer that has been widely used in tissue architecture due to its biocompatibility, biodegradability, and antibacterial characteristics. When combined with different natural components like calcium hydroxide, hydroxyapatite, etc., chitosan scaffolds' bioresorbability and mechanical energy increase, making them the ideal material for cartilage implants (Chaya et al., 2015). Moreover, chitosan's reciprocal action with DNA fragments reinforces its potential for use in genetic code remedy for orthopaedic anomalies. Bioresorbable biomaterials' chemical, material, mechanical, and biological traits change as they diminish gradually. In comparison to the source material, these alterations bring about distinct host responses (Bhatnagar et al., 2013).

The number of artificial bioresorbable polymers that are realistic for use is constrained on account of the complicatedness of the criteria. Given the complications and restraints of shaped bioresorbable polymers, individuals may favour normal polymers that share structural correspondences with components in host tissues. Natural polymers have many basic benefits, including bioactivity, the ability to administer receptor binding ligands to cells, susceptibility to cell-prompted proteolytic breakdown, and unrefined renovation (Avila et al., 2010). The critical deep-rooted bioactivity of these natural polymers does, however, have drawbacks, in conjunction with a harsh immune response and the chance of rejection. External drawbacks involve missing mechanical substance, trouble obtaining compatible features, the need for purification, and the chance of disease transmission (Balani et al., 2015). In contrast, artificial biomaterials typically lack biological action and have more consistent features from cluster to cluster in addition to certain properties. Their traits maybe modified for certain uses (Bender et al., 2012).

1.3 SUSTAINABLE APPROACH TO BIOPOLYMERS

Biopolymers are characterized as polymers that can degrade biologically (Yadav et al., 2015; Bala et al., 2017; Udayakumar et al., 2021) and are produced by living things. A thriving interest in promoting tangible sustainability make them potential replacements for fabricated plastics (Pattanashetti et al., 2017). Biopolymers are effortlessly environmentally safe because of their fundamental basis of carbon, oxygen, and nitrogen atoms. Biodegradation converts these components into carbon dioxide, water, humic matter (organic macromolecular material), biomass, and different instinctive compounds, allowing them to be consistently reused (Rendón-Villalobos et al., 2016). The natural biological origins of biopolymers include plants, animals, microorganisms, and land waste. Rice, maize, wheat (Kumar et al., 2017), sorghum (Nath et al., 2020), yams (Arora, 2018), cassava (Díez-Pascual, 2019), potatoes (Qasim at al., 2021), banana (Hamouda, 2021), tapioca (Shivam, 2016), corn (Chen, Xie et al., 2019), cotton (Swain et al., 2018), and barley (Varma and Gopi, 2021) biopolymers can be chemically synthesised from monomeric components such as oils, sugars, and amino acids. Cattle are the common animal origin, whereas corals, sponges, fish, invertebrates, and shrimp are the most frequent aquatic sources. Algae, fungi, and yeasts constitute the majority of microbiological origins (Baranwal et al., 2022). Table 1.1 depicts the source, types, extraction methods, advantages, and disadvantages of natural and synthetic biopolymers.

1.3.1 Applications of Biopolymers

Studies from several fields have explained the potential of using biopolymers as elements in the production of medical instruments (Wróblewska-Krepsztul et al., 2019). Other enterprises that utilize biopolymers involve those in the foodstuff industry (edible film wrap and emulsifiers), pharmaceuticals (encapsulation), the cosmetic

TABLE 1.1
Advantages and Disadvantages of Natural and Synthetic Biopolymers

Bio-Derived Polymers	Polymers	Extracted From	Advantages	Disadvantages	References
Synthetic biodegradable polymers	Biomass	Polylactic acid (PLA)	Improved cell viability	High water solubility; low tensile strength	Wu, 2016; Singh et al., 2020
	Petrochemicals	Polycaprolactone (PCL)	Biodegradable, non-toxic, low melting point	Hydrophobicity, slow degradation	Asti and Gioglio, 2014
		Polyvinyl alcohol (PVA)	Good architectural accuracy, desired drug loading, and quick melting	Random shapes and sizes of pores, generating in homogeneity and low structural strength	Diaz et al., 2018; Cernencu et al., 2019; Musazzi et al., 2018
		Poly (glycolic acid) (PGA)	Biocompatible, non-toxic, biodegradable, low solubility in organic solvents	High degradation rate, poor solubility	Sanko et al., 2019
Natural biopolymers extracted from biomass	Polysaccharides	Starch	Shear-thinning behaviour; good geometries, structural homogeneity, and deposition; high gelation temperature; thixotropic behaviour	Low structural strength, adhesion between layers, spreading after printing, and some of thermal instability	Lille et al., 2018; Zheng et al., 2019; Maniglia et al., 2020; Theagarajan et al., 2020; Liu, Bhandari et al., 2019; Paggi et al., 2019; Chen et al., 2019
		Cellulose	Good printing accuracy and resolution, shear-thinning behaviour, high yield stress	Spreading after printing, limitation of layer number, continuous deformation until spreading	Lille et al., 2018; Holland et al., 2018
		Alginate	Biocompatible, non-toxic, biodegradable, non-thrombogenic, non-antigenic, cost effective	High hydrophilicity, low protein adsorption	Sun and Tan, 2013; Ruvinov and Cohen, 2016

(Continued)

TABLE 1.1 (*Continued*)
Advantages and Disadvantages of Natural and Synthetic Biopolymers

Bio-Derived Polymers	Polymers	Extracted From	Advantages	Disadvantages	References
		Carrageenan	Desired rheological parameters, increased gelling temperature, enhanced mechanical performance	Poor structural strength	Warner et al., 2019; Caroway et al., 2020
		Chitosan	Non-toxic, non-immunogenic, biocompatible, biodegradable, mucoadhesive, antimicrobial, haemostatic, good cytocompatibility, processability, and renewability,	Too fragile, limited solubility at physiological pH	Sivashankari and Prabaharan, 2017; Jing et al., 2017
	Lipids	Glycerides/Waxes	Absorbable, soft, malleable, provides sealing capacity	Inherent haemostatic quality, promotes infection and induces thrombosis	Zhou et al., 2019
	Proteins	Gelatine	Excellent biocompatibility and biodegradability, non-toxic, fully absorbable	Lower melting temperature, rapid dissolution in water, lack of 3D structural integrity	Yang et al., 2016; Feyen et al., 2016; Nikkhah et al., 2016
		Casein	Thermally stable gels improve thixotropy, high-fidelity parts	Some extent of aggregation, low printability due to low gelation temperature, somewhat heterogeneous matrix	Daffner et al., 2021; Schutyser et al., 2018; Liu et al., 2019
		Whey protein	Desired shape fidelity inducing a homogeneous matrix, shear-thinning behaviour, high fidelity	Low hardness and solid-gel structure due to the increase in particle size	Liu and Ciftci, 2021; Oliveira et al., 2020; Liu et al., 2018

		Soy protein	Enhanced geometric accuracy, shear-thinning behaviour, proper flow properties	Limited cell proliferation, low hardness, and low cohesiveness	Chen et al., 2019; Phuhongsung et al., 2020; Chien et al., 2013
		Zein	Improved printability, enhanced mechanical strength, improved convexity index	Lower mechanical properties, some extent of macroscopic contraction, slow sintering kinetics	Jing et al., 2018; Chaunier et al., 2017; Chaunier et al., 2019
		Wheat flour	Improved printability, enhanced flow properties	Collapsing the uppermost layer	Pulatsu et al., 2020; Fahmy et al., 2020
		Gluten	Improved rheological properties	Poor mechanical strength	Liu et al., 2020
Polymers produced by microorganisms	Microbial products	Bacterial cellulose	Versatility, moldability *in situ*, biocompatibility, used as a wound dressing composite, in the production of scaffolds, transdermal applications, as a pharmaceutical excipient	Bacterial cellulose production requires efficient and stable bacterial strains	Gorgieva and Trcek, 2019
		Polyhydroxyalkanoates (PHA)/ Polyhydroxybutyrate (PHB)	Biocompatible and biodegradable, potentially ideal alternatives to synthetic polymers, degradation products can be excluded from the body	Degradation by bulk erosion, poor mechanical properties, hydrophobic polymer surface	McAdam et al., 2020
		Poly(3-hydroxybutyrate-co-3-hydroxyvalerate) (PHBV)	Supports cell growth, delivery of drugs or growth factors	Lacks mechanical strength, water sorption and diffusion	Rivera-Briso, and Serrano-Aroca, 2018

industry (especially hydrogels), water treatment, biosensor manufacturing, and even data storage (Ezeoha and Ezenwanne, 2013). Biopolymer composites are galvanized biopolymers. They can be supported with fillers that considerably reinforce these features to make them more acceptable for particular applications. In order to maximize the influence of bioactive particles, drug delivery approaches are still passed down, and progress in this field has significant advancements have been made in this field. Natural and semi-artificial polymers are repeatedly employed in the incorporation of drug delivery methods in this framework (Redondo-Gómez et al., 2020). Bio-based polymers still account for a very small percentage of the global plastic market. Due to their unusual conditions, biopolymer-based nanocomposites are suitable to be accepted to a greater extent. An appropriate matrices were preferred, such as aliphatic polyesters, polypeptides, proteins, polysaccharides, and polynucleic acids, and their chemistry and design were altered to match the target field in order to produce bionanocomposite. Due to their extraordinary eco-friendly properties, biopolymers like polyhydroxyalkanoates (PHAs) and polyhydroxybutyrates (PHBs) are common in a variety of enterprises. PHAs are compelling biopolymers with a growing manufacturing demand. PHAs are a class of polyesters that may be constructed through bacterial fermentation and have the potential to replace usual hydrocarbon-based polymers (Nezakati et al., 2018). They are found naturally in many species, but bacteria may be used to manage their fabrication in cells. Biomedical implants commonly use PHA and its copolymers as their material. These include tissue repair patches, cardiovascular patches, arched repair gadgets, rivets, bone plates, surgical mesh, and stem cell growth. PHAs' controlled degradability and biocompatibility make them suitable for use in drug delivery. PHBs are biopolymers with short chains of polyhydroxyalkanoates (3–5 carbons) and are created naturally by microorganisms fermenting sugars and lipids. These polyesters are hoarded as carbon and energy sources inside microbial cells and are produced in ecosystems with reduced nutrient availability (P, S, N, and O).

PHBs are mostly present in *Alcaligenes eutrophus*, and they build up inside of cells as granules. Biomedical applications include sutures, bond substitution, wound dressings, medication delivery, and tissue engineering (Martău et al., 2019). A growing class of biomaterials, chitosan-based nanocomposites, has the potential to support and promote cell development for the controlled administration of drugs in addition to forming a part of biosensors to label levels of glucose in the blood. Sensors are important in diagnosing molecular changes and may be used to check ailments such as carcinogenic epigenetic changes (Gonçalves et al., 2022). Biopolymers' internal structure-dependent are dependent functional qualities such as microstructure, permeability, and chargeability and can be obtained by modifying the composition and matrix of the polymer. The ability of particles to aggregate and form bonds inside the biopolymer matrix is influenced by their electrical properties. The biopolymer fractions with a high electrical charge are those that inhibit aggregation (Wróblewska-Krepsztul et al., 2019). The class of biopolymers called polysaccharides is the one that is most frequently used to supplement or replace synthetic materials, either alone or in combination with other biopolymers. Biopolymers are propitiously used to constitute nanoparticles, nanoemulsions, nanogels, or hydrogels that are recycled as carrier structures in the biomedical field (Severino et al., 2019).

1.3.2 Biocompatibility and Biodegradability of Biopolymers

Polymeric components for medical equipment that may come into contact with blood should be able to withstand protein adsorption and blood cell adhesion without setting off the body's defensive mechanisms. The term "biocompatibility" is used broadly and emphasized to describe the property of materials to not cause harm when they come in contact with biological cells, tissues, or proteins. Three distinct types of biocompatible polymer surfaces have been devised, including hydrophilic surfaces, surfaces with micro-point-separated realms, and surfaces with zwitter ionic groups that resemble biomembranes. Physical and synthetic characteristics include moistening, texture, stiffness, flexibility, and strength. Extrusion, electrospinning, grafting, diversified shape techniques (Velu et al., 2019), solvent casting, liquefied mixing, intercalation, filament bending, stage separation (Chaitanya and Singh, 2017), radiation printing, and film stacking (Udayakumar et al., 2021) are just some of the approaches that can be used to design biopolymer composites. In order to improve physical, chemical, electrical, and mechanical properties and increase resistance to humid, warm, or cold storage conditions, biopolymers are currently being constructed and optimized using mathematical models. This is advantageous for applications that call for specialized features (Ncube et al., 2020). Even though plenty of research has been performed on the use of an array of biopolymers, the majority of studies have been hinged on polysaccharides due to their superior features when compared to different materials like proteins or lipids.

Therefore, a research focus is on biopolymers' potential for efficient encapsulating agents in pharmaceutical manufacturing, especially for the transfer of pharmaceuticals and probiotics. By uncovering their benefits over chemically produced polymers, the use of cellulose, starch, agar, chitosan, and alginate makes them viable options for product distribution (Idumah, 2016).

Natural polymers exhibit a number of advantages and disadvantages. Similarity to the host tissue, interaction with biological systems, compatibility with host metabolism, lack of toxicity and inflammation, enzyme degradability, and use of their degradation products in cellular metabolism are a few potential benefits (Tiwari et al., 2023). However, due to their sensitivity to temperature, natural polymers are destroyed before they melt, and their intricate structure makes processing them challenging. One of the known drawbacks of these polymers is the potential for disease transfer from other species to humans as a result of the production of various natural polymers using plant and animal resources (Sonia and Sharma, 2012). The biopolymers are made to be biocompatible and biodegradable, which helps them in a variety of utilizations, such as edible films, emulsions, packing materials, and therapeutic implants for organs, wounds, tissue scaffolds, and dressing materials in the pharmaceutical industry (Abraham and Venkatesan, 2023). The most accepted macromolecules are biopolymers, which comprise large, non-polymeric particles like macrocycles and lipids in addition to nucleic acids, proteins, carbohydrates, and lipids. Plastics, artificial fibres, and scientific necessities like carbon nanotubes are few examples of fabricated macromolecules. PHA and polylactic acid (PLA) are two types of biopolymers that have been discovered in bacteria or genetically mutated organisms utilizing traditional synthetic procedures. These are made up of hydrogen-derivative carbohydrates and milk or collagen proteins (Rouchi and Mahdavi-Mazdeh, 2015). Microorganisms could be genetically altered to produce biopolymers with distinguishing characteristics that are suitable for extremely valuable medicinal uses like tissue design and drug release. The supramolecular methods used to produce innovative biocompatible polymers are advancing towards highly efficient methods. All grading levels of cell behaviour are significantly influenced by surfaces constructed of biocompatible and biodegradable polymers. A few scientific articles have illustrated that biopolymers derived from plant-based and organic materials are superior for packaging products. Biopolymers are more biocompatible and biodegradable than plastics, which benefits both human health and the conservation of ecosystems. These precisely designed polymeric biomaterials might be useful in the era of customized medicine (Fang et al., 2013).

1.4 TISSUE ENGINEERING IN BIOMEDICINE

The first line of treatment for maintaining or restoring an organ or tissue's function is transplantation (Tonelli et al., 2012). The classical implants used for organ or tissue transplantation are autografts, allografts, and xenografts. Even though autografts are more commonly employed to treat tissue abnormalities, donor sites are frequently limited. As a result, a new remedy that can get around the drawbacks of traditional therapy is required.

Biomedicine is the scientific application of biology and physiology. A possible biomedical engineering field of tissue engineering (TE) combines biology and engineering for treating damaged tissues or replacing them with healthy tissue or organs (Figure 1.3). The three critical fundamentals of TE are cells, scaffolds (3D polymeric models), and growth determinants (signalling molecules). The scaffold is the most influential of these three units because it accommodates the cells and creates an environment where they can reproduce and differentiate into a particular tissue by discharging nutrients and development components (Krishnan et al., 2012; Li et al., 2013). TE primarily entails performing the *ex vivo* culture of living human cells, usually in a biocompatible polymer scaffold, and then allowing them to grow into a 3D tissue. TE could thereby avoid the issues related to tissue deterioration, which are currently managed *via* transplants, mechanical devices, or surgical reconstruction (De Peppo et al., 2013).

1.4.1 Use of Scaffolds and Cells for Tissue Engineering

The development of scaffolds that can mimic the *in vivo* microenvironment, which is primarily provided by the ECM, is a fundamental aim of TE. Therefore, these structures should include the appropriate biophysical, biomechanical, and pharmacological inputs that control cell proliferation, differentiation, maintenance, and function (Sah and Pramanik, 2012). Scaffolds must be mechanically consistent with natural tissue and must be biocompatible, non-immunogenic, biodegradable, and non-toxic. Additionally, they must be simple to produce, sterilize, and implant (Bhardwaj and Kundu, 2010). Most significantly, scaffolds should rarely or never result in immunological or foreign-body reactions. Cells should be guided by scaffolds as they

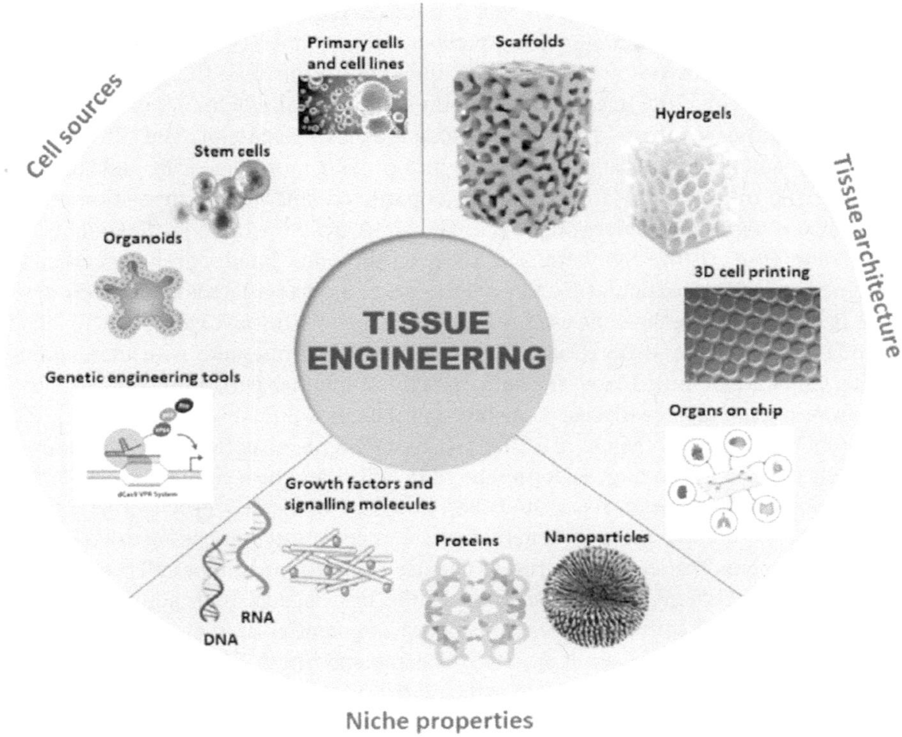

FIGURE 1.3 Tissue engineering in biomedicine.

develop into 3D tissues. Cell adherence, endurance, proliferation, differentiation, movement, and organization should be likely under both *in vitro* and *in vivo* conditions. Additionally, they should result in optimal cell shape and ECM composition by cells. Cell arrangement and adjustment are particularly important in the architecture of neuronal, cardiac, and ocular tissues because exact cell alignment is necessary for active tissue function (Ranakoti et al., 2023). The separation, expansion, and neurite offshoot of cells are necessary for productive nerve regeneration in neurological fabric design. Many recent studies have focused on the use of scaffolds to specify contact guidance for better cell adjustment. By electrospinning, a coordinated PLA nanofibrous scaffold was generated that addresses cell extension and neurite projection *in vitro* along the scaffold's fibre aspect (Zarekhalili et al., 2017).

The positioning of rooted cells and the regeneration of exterior nerves were supported in an investigation by adapting collagen-based nerve guide channels (Yang et al., 2018). An imperative capacity of the ECM in biophysical communication is to determine anchoring for cells. They are given a suitable 3D environment by the highly porous ECM nanostructure, which also transmits biochemical signalling *via* two mechanisms: (i) the binding of diverse dissolved growth factors (GF) and enzymes, which manages their local concentrations and dissipation; and (ii) the identification of particular patterns that cellular attachment receptors can perceive. Therefore, the intracellular signalling pathways that control gene verbalization and influence cell phenotypes are dynamically integrated amidst the ECM (Khorshidi et al., 2016; Wu et al., 2017). According to their source, scaffolds for TE can be classified as natural or synthetic. Natural scaffolds are easily accessible and offer a wide variety of signals that assist various cell types in their morphogenesis and function *in vivo*. The *in vivo* assay's reliability is jeopardized since the composition of the substance is highly dependent on the animal origin, isolation, and purification methods (Yang et al., 2018). Synthetic scaffolds, on the other hand, can be specifically designed to imitate particular ECM properties and offer regulated cellular settings.

It is important that the cells used to regenerate new tissue have the ability to adapt to their surroundings, differentiate into new tissue, and integrate with the existing tissue. Cells are obtained from the same patient or another person to heal damaged tissues or regenerate new tissue. The choice of the cell source is crucial when developing methods for TE (Ma et al., 2023). If tissue engineering technique was to be used in a therapeutic setting, selecting the right cell would be a significant challenge. Integration into the target tissue and the release of numerous growth factors and cytokines that promote the body's natural tissue regeneration process are two important requirements that cells must fulfil. The use of native precursor cells constitutes the first cell-occupying order procedure. In the last decade, both adult stem cells and immature stem cells have been considered as potential sources to rejuvenate or repair damaged tissues (Kaur et al., 2017; Sharma and Sinha, 2018).

Pre-implantation embryonic stem cells are the origin of immature stem cells and can eventually become tissue or organ cells (Logith Kumar et al., 2016). Adult stem cells, like mesenchymal stem cells (MSCs), are very attractive and a promising origin for TE applications, as they can differentiate into a variety of tissues, including osseous matter, cartilage, muscle, ligaments, fat, and connective tissue. Similarly, these cells present fewer ethical challenges (Kadner et al., 2012). Induced pluripotent stem cells (iPSCs) are another cell type being studied for their applicability in TE that were first obtained from rodent fibroblasts (Zhu and Huangfu, 2013) and thereafter derived from adult human cells (Alves et al., 2014). In general, iPSCs are somatic cells that have been treated with a specific set of transcription factors to retrain them into a pluripotent state. These cells' primary benefits include their autologous nature, ability to differentiate, robustness, and ease of reprogramming (Bose et al., 2012).

1.4.2 Tissue Engineering in Regenerative Medicine

Regenerative medicine is a multidisciplinary field of research that offers novel methods for preserving healthy human tissues and organs, particularly when some form of impairment occurs in them (Stoltz et al., 2015). An example of this includes tissue loss followed by injury, which necessitates support to enable tissue regeneration in order to return to normal function. In addition to regenerating damaged or ill tissue, TE also influences the mechanisms that determine cell fate and looks for promising diagnostic tools (Sallustio et al., 2015). The terms "tissue engineering" and "regenerative medicine" have been broadly used in opposition to one another in an attempt to concentrate on remedies rather than therapies for complex and chronic ailments (Diez-Pascual and Rahdar, 2022). By studying how individual cells respond to signals, engage with their environment, and arrange into tissues and organisms, researchers have endured to control these processes to replace damaged tissues or even produce new ones (Jayarama et al., 2013). The construction of a scaffold from an array of potential sources, including proteins and polymers, is a prevailing beginning in the procedure. Cells may expand the scaffolds either with or without a "cocktail" of development forces. In some instances, the growth determinants, scaffolds, and cells are all linked directly, enabling the tissue to "self-assemble". Making convenience of an existing scaffold is another approach to produce new tissue (Linh and Lee, 2012). The collagen scaffold that is left behind after discarding the cells from a donor organ is therefore used to develop new tissue. A tissue can evolve if the circumstances are conducive.

The bioengineering of internal organs like kidney, alveolus, liver, and heart tissue has been performed by applying this arrangement. By utilizing scaffolds from human tissue that was left over after abscission and merging it with a patient's own cells, this approach has the potential to produce made-to-order organs that will not be refused by the immune system. Figure 1.4 provides a diagrammatic summary of

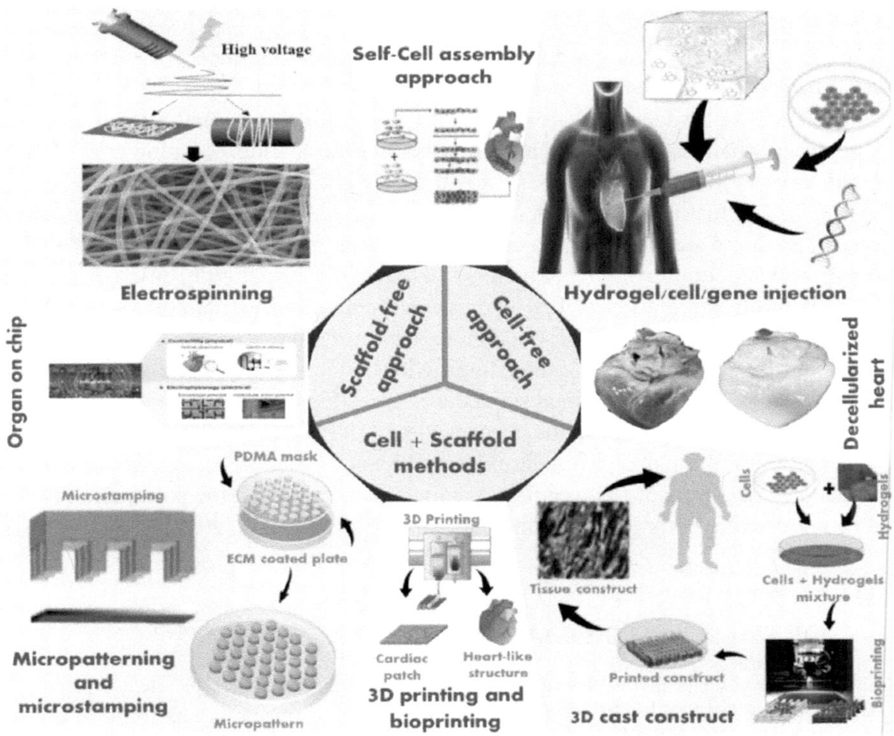

FIGURE 1.4 Schematic summary of cardiovascular tissue engineering.

cardiovascular tissue design. Tissue architecture is currently used to treat patients, even though its impact continues to be restricted. In patients, extra bladders, miniature arteries, skin grafts, ossein, and even an entire oesophagus have been implanted, but the medications are still in the exploratory stage and are very expensive (Huang et al., 2012). Although more complex organ tissues, for instance heart, lung, and liver tissues, have been strongly reconstructed in the laboratory, they are still far from being completely reproducible and ready for implantation into a patient. However, these tissues have enough potential for research, specifically in the area of drug advancement.

Utilizing active human tissue for drug screening research could expedite development, provide critical and essential tools for facilitating individualized care, save money, and minimize the need for animal testing (Zhang et al., 2012).

1.5 BIOMEDICAL DEVICES

A device with combined mechanical and electronic functions is referred to as a biomedical device. Typically, the device uses a charged signal to drive an automated motion or a mechanical motion to propel an electrical signal (Khakbaz et al., 2014). The essential fields of biomedical equipment experimental approach include gene therapeutics (Pattar et al., 2020; Pattar et al., 2021) and regenerative therapy. Electromechanical (EM) systems can be used in medical devices to improve control over the device's operation, support sustainable energy use, produce clean and hygienic equipment, develop compact and potent tools, reduce costs for all parties involved, and adhere to regulatory requirements. Few EM devices are being designed with a tendency towards miniaturization in order to make them as small as possible, whether for use in healthcare or as wearable units (Lyndon et al., 2014). Healthcare practitioners would benefit from having a system that can identify even the smallest actuation of a medication delivery mechanism, for instance, as drug delivery systems are indeed a major focus (Saharan et al., 2017). The various beneficial devices contain micro actuators for cochlear stimulation, microelectrodes for deep brain stimulation (DBS) and nerve reclamation, ocular micro prosthetic devices, and microneedles. These technologies limit the instability and inefficiency of human processes, providing the patient with better serenity and a greater opportunity for an outstanding medical procedure. Transducers are low-cost, lightweight, and reliable sensors that sense the acceleration of the body parts causing tremors, so they can be used in place of accelerometers, piezoelectric, piezoresistive, or capacitive sensors (Figure 1.5) that regulate tremor limits by feeling the stimulation of the vibration-causing body part (Sutton et al., 2016; Sharma et al., 2017).

1.6 FUTURE PROSPECTS AND LIMITATIONS OF EMERGING BIOMATERIALS

Due to the ageing populations in developed countries and patients' desire to maintain their standard of health and wellbeing, the use of implants has increased considerably over the past few years. The need for high-performance implantable biomaterials that can deal with unique difficulties in cardiology, vascular therapy,

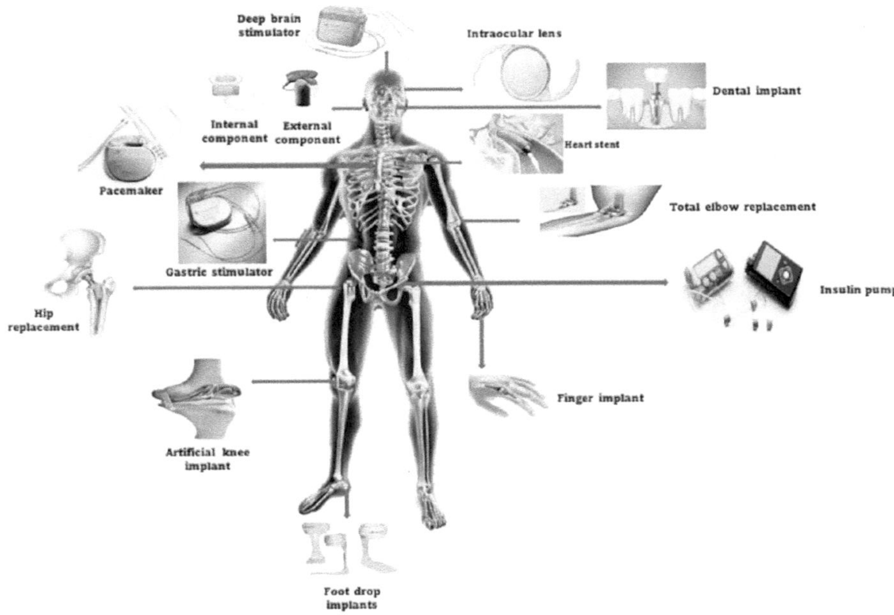

FIGURE 1.5 Various biomedical devices for implantation in different body parts.

orthopaedics, trauma, spine (vertebrae), dentistry, and wound care has thus been steadily increasing. According to Wang et al. (2022), advancements in the study of biomaterials have been used in contraception, TE, prosthetic ovaries, and follicle culture (Peng et al., 2023). The most accepted resorbable biomaterials are presumably sutures for intramural stitching, which use biopolymers like PLA/PGA with regulated deterioration rates (Bhat and Kumar, 2013). The key benefit of utilizing resorbable components is that it removes the need for additional surgery to eliminate the material. Apart from compositional differences, porosity plays an important role in the achievement of these structures since tissue in-development and scaffold disruption are critical components. Although 100 μm is the minimum hole size required for vascularization, 300–600 μm size have been shown to be more effective in these scaffolds. However, there are still great challenges in devising absorbent scaffolds with interconnected porosity that are potent enough automatically *in vivo* for tissue assimilation and growth with healing. An even more challenging task is making compositional changes to the demands of the patient. Although resorbable materials are attractive and have full potential for treating cartilage complications, some challenges include: product degradation, automated strength, processing competence, and tissue component intercommunication. To date, the majority of medical apparatuses are inactive, favouring persons being treated for medical problems to live more healthily (Henkel et al., 2013).

Controlling infections is one of the main limitations of bone condition treatments. Frequently used procedures that typically have a high success rate can still cause infection and seriously traumatize the patients. The majority of treatment methods include using antibiotics, which is effective for the first 12 weeks. One such example is MRSA, which can lay dormant for several months but then, even after three or six months, still develop into a biofilm. Unfortunately, the only course of action if a biofilm develops is to remove the implant and clean the area to stop infection before another implant is placed (Hallab and Jacobs, 2017). Better and more dependable therapy solutions, however, remain elusive and require invention. A key challenge that must be addressed in the use of naturally derived materials for implantable medical devices is the consistency and integrity of the materials' features and properties. It is possible to anticipate a natural variation in the qualities and traits of such materials due to the sources' uniqueness. When it comes to collagen made from animals (e.g., bovine or porcine), the procedures used to manufacture animal-derived biomaterials for use in medical devices and treatments must, therefore, be continually improved (Wang et al., 2016). The fact that the human body is typically ready to detect these biomaterials and to respond negatively to their implantation presents a significant challenge for the development of biomaterials derived from natural sources. While some biomaterials, like collagen, exhibit immunogenic tolerance, the majority of natural materials need to be customized to reduce the host response after implantation. Combining with other, more tolerable biomaterials is one approach that might be taken to address this problem.

Certainly, the use of computer-assisted design and modelling is responsible for 3D printing to ensure the high-quality 3D representation of the fundamental results procured from the patient utilizing computer tomography (CT) and produce a model that portrays the anatomic surfaces and corrects any disparities (Ortolani et al., 2016). Nevertheless, the improvement of 3D printing is still impeded by a variety of technological concerns. The integration of a vascular network is the biggest biological barrier in 3D printing because without it, the built 3D tissue or organ will not receive enough nutrients, undergo the right amount of gas exchange, or exhibit the right amount of waste elimination, all of which are crucial for maturation during perfusion (Zhao et al., 2017) and would have a direct impact on cell viability and artificial organ performance. Economic concerns regarding 3D-printed parts must likewise be taken into account. Currently, printing customized surgical implements and implants is substantially more expensive than using standard equivalents, and there are supplementary costs, including the supplementary scans required to amass the essential facts. Stainless steel used in biomedical appeals is usually categorized as either conventional stainless steels or Ni-free stainless steel. As the name implies, Ni-free stainless steels are free of Ni, as Ni not only increases oxidation resistance but also lowers stress corrosion and biocompatibility (Vaithilingam et al., 2015). An exemplification of a typical hypersensitivity connected to the use of Ni-containing gird implants is shown in Figure 1.2. In order to ensure low Ni aggregation, nitrogen is repeatedly alloyed with Ni-free stainless steel. Nitrogen's nonmagnetic property has no influence on the MRI technology that is widely used in the biomedical field. In contrast to ecological ceramics and polymers, dormant golden scaffolds cannot be easily introduced *in situ* with bioactive chemicals or cells, restricting their application for thorough tissue transformation.

The functionalization of pharmaceutically relevant biomolecules, like paracetamol (Kruzic, 2016), coupled onto phosphonic acid-based self-assembled monolayers is therefore necessary to control surface chemistry. Thus, there is a chance that metal ions from stainless steel, Ti, and Co–Cr, and Ti alloys will be extracted into the peri-implant environment on the grounds that the significantly heightened surface-to-quantity ratio causes the individual inclusion of filling pores. Given that surface oxide films are known to restrict ion release *in vivo*, this may be especially important when applied to environments with low levels of dissolved oxygen. Ion release could be hastened even more by inorganic ions, proteins, and cells found in bodily fluids. The plethora of unknown natural biomaterials that can play a significant part in cutting-edge biomedical applications and therapies is one of the most obvious potentials in investigating natural biomaterials for biomedical applications. The biomaterials starch and silk fibroin, which have previously demonstrated a variety of desirable qualities for the biomedical industry, are two notable examples. Utilizing high-throughput approaches to screen biomaterial libraries and assess biological performance in a subject newly designated materiomics is a prominent area of study in this regard. These procedures appear to influence an extending body of research specifically proclaimed in the literature, providing a more deeper understanding of the real design intercommunication between living things and organic biomaterials. Bulk metallic glass (BMG) alloys may utilize bioinert metals like Ti and bioresorbable metals like Zn and Fe. These alloys have better characteristics than current biometals, including high strength, reduced deformability, and an extreme flexural strain limit when compared to traditional alloys. When selected in hard-tissue prosthetic devices, these qualities offer a better fit to cortical osseous matter and, thus, a decrease in stress guarding.

Devices made of bioinert BMG offer controlled surface topography and resistance to corrosion. They could be utilized in flexible vascular stents, surgical scalpels, and orthopaedic prostheses (Kim et al., 2017; Shen et al., 2017). Stress shielding is weaker because the strength degradation has an inverse relationship with bone formation and fracture healing. These actions result in the release of non-toxic ions. Once the procedure is finished, no surgery is required to remove the device because it has been absorbed. Bioresorbable BMGs have the potential to be employed as temporary vascular stents, intramedullary nails, bone screws, or surgical plates. A biomaterial with a Ti basis and 50% atomic Ni concentration is called nitinol. Nitinol possesses mechanical resistance, decreased rigidity, thermal resilience, and biodegradation and corrosion resistance, making it one of the most anticipated shape-memory alloys. Materials based on titanium have these characteristics. The promising properties of nitinol allow it to potentially replace stainless steel implants. In addition to these, wires, palatal arches, intramedullary nails, staples, intraspinal implants, and scoliosis therapy devices like self-augmenting vascular stents and spinal vertebrae spacers all contain nitinol (Moghaddam et al., 2016).

Advanced-age implant patients frequently exhibit functional dependency, systemic health issues (comorbidities), and frailty. Additionally, immunosenescence, the term for the ageing immune system, may lead to a weakened host defence against a bacterial challenge at dental implants, which is harmful to the health of the surrounding tissue. In comparison to younger patients, older recipients of conventional and cardiac resynchronization therapy (CRT) defibrillators experience higher mortality but require fewer cardioverter defibrillator (ICD) shocks and/or therapies.

There may be a need to conduct randomized controlled studies to assess the role of defibrillator therapy in elderly individuals. Despite the fact that other technological challenges remain to be solved, innumerable opportunities exist for researchers and industries to augment biomedical devices with the ideal conductivity and strength for widespread use.

1.7 CONCLUSION

Demand for environmentally friendly biomaterials has increased amidst concerns over the usage of non-renewable resources. The biomedical and pharmaceutical industries have been completely transformed by this research, but there is still a lot of work to be done if we want to focus on making changes that affect not only the individual but also the environment and are environmentally sustainable and approachable. The mechanical, thermodynamic, environmental, and biocompatible properties of the biomaterials have been significantly improved. However, there are still challenges in developing carriers that are specific to the target and biocompatible with different transfer patterns in order to offer a maintained release at the target site. Applications that are based on biomaterials are extremely advantageous for transferring small compounds that are highly efficient, biopotent, and secure.

REFERENCES

Aamodt, J. M., and Grainger, D. W. (2016). Extracellular matrix-based biomaterial scaffolds and the host response. *Biomaterials*, *86*, 68–82.

Abraham, A. M., and Venkatesan, S. (2023). A review on application of biomaterials for medical and dental implants. *Proceedings of the Institution of Mechanical Engineers, Part L: Journal of Materials: Design and Applications*, *237*(2), 249–273.

Ahsan, S. M., Thomas, M., Reddy, K. K., Sooraparaju, S. G., Asthana, A., and Bhatnagar, I. (2018). Chitosan as biomaterial in drug delivery and tissue engineering. *International Journal of Biological Macromolecules*, *110*, 97–109.

Algardh, J. K., Horn, T., West, H., Aman, R., Snis, A., Engqvist, H., and Harrysson, O. (2016). Thickness dependency of mechanical properties for thin walled titanium parts manufactured by electron beam melting (EBM)®. *Additive Manufacturing*, *12*, 45–50.

Ali, A., and Ahmed, S. (2018). A review on chitosan and its nanocomposites in drug delivery. *International Journal of Biological Macromolecules*, *109*, 273–286.

Alves Cardoso, D., Van Den Beucken, J. J. J. P., Both, L. L. H., Bender, J., Jansen, J. A., and Leeuwenburgh, S. C. G. (2014). Gelation and biocompatibility of injectable alginate–calcium phosphate gels for bone regeneration. *Journal of Biomedical Materials Research Part A*, *102*(3), 808–817.

Arora, S. (2018). Biopolymers as packaging material in food and allied industry value addition of makhana and its by-products view project. *International Journal of Chemical Studies*, *6*, 2411–2418.

Asti, A., and Gioglio, L. (2014). Natural and synthetic biodegradable polymers: Different scaffolds for cell expansion and tissue formation. *The International Journal of Artificial Organs*, *37*(3), 187–205.

Avila, G., Neiva, R., Misch, C. E., Galindo-Moreno, P., Benavides, E., Rudek, I., and Wang, H. L. (2010). Clinical and histologic outcomes after the use of a novel allograft for maxillary sinus augmentation: A case series. *Implant Dentistry*, *19*(4), 330–341.

Bala, I. A., Abdullahi, M. R., and Bashir, S. S. (2017). A review on formulation of enzymatic solution for biopolymer hydrolysis. *Journal of Chemistry*, *6*, 9–13.

Balani, K., Narayan, R., Agarwal, A., and Verma, V. (2015). Surface engineering and modification for biomedical applications. In *Biosurfaces: Materials Science and Engineering Perspective*. John Wiley, 201–238.

Baranwal, J., Barse, B., Fais, A., Delogu, G. L., and Kumar, A. (2022). Biopolymer: A sustainable material for food and medical applications. *Polymers*, *14*(5), 983.

Bender, S., Chalivendra, V., Rahbar, N., and El Wakil, S. (2012). Mechanical characterization and modeling of graded porous stainless steel specimens for possible bone implant applications. *International Journal of Engineering Science*, *53*, 67–73.

Bhardwaj, N., and Kundu, S. C. (2010). Electrospinning: A fascinating fiber fabrication technique. *Biotechnology Advances*, *28*(3), 325–347.

Bhat, S., and Kumar, A. (2013). Biomaterials and bioengineering tomorrow's healthcare. *Biomatter*, *3*(3), e24717.

Bhatnagar, A., Bansal, V., Kumar, S., and Mowar, A. (2013). Comparative analysis of osteosynthesis of mandibular anterior fractures following open reduction using 'stainless steel lag screws and mini plates'. *Journal of Maxillofacial and Oral Surgery*, *12*(2), 133–139.

Bose, S., Roy, M., and Bandyopadhyay, A. (2012). Recent advances in bone tissue engineering scaffolds. *Trends in Biotechnology*, *30*(10), 546–554.

Cai, J., Wang, J., Ye, K., Li, D., Ai, C., Sheng, D., and Chen, S. (2018). Dual-layer aligned-random nanofibrous scaffolds for improving gradient microstructure of tendon to bone healing in a rabbit extra articular model. *International Journal of Nanomedicine*, *13*, 3481.

Caroway, B., Malo, S., and Parsons, F. (2020). The effectiveness of a 3D printed hydrogel membrane to sustain algal growth. *Biological and Medicinal Chemistry*, *1*, 1–31.

Cernencu, A. I., Lungu, A., Stancu, I. C., Serafim, A., Heggset, E., Syverud, K., and Iovu, H. (2019). Bioinspired 3D printable pectin nanocellulose ink formulations. *Carbohydrate Polymers*, *220*, 12–21.

Chaitanya, S., and Singh, I. (2017). Processing of PLA/sisal fiber biocomposites using direct and extrusion injection molding. *Materials and Manufacturing Processes*, *32*(5), 468–474.

Chaunier, L., Della Valle, G., Lourdin, D., Réguerre, A. L., Cochet, K., and Leroy, E. (2019). Viscous sintering kinetics of biopolymer filaments extruded for 3D printing. *Polymer Testing*, *77*, 105873.

Chaunier, L., Leroy, E., Valle, G. D., Dalgalarrondo, M., Bakan, B., Marion, D., and Lourdin, D. (2017). 3D printing of maize protein by fused deposition modeling. In *AIP Conference Proceedings*, *1914*(1), 190003. AIP Publishing LLC.

Chaya, A., Yoshizawa, S., Verdelis, K., Noorani, S., Costello, B. J., and Sfeir, C. (2015). Fracture healing using degradable magnesium fixation plates and screws. *Journal of Oral and Maxillofacial Surgery*, *73*(2), 295–305.

Chen, H., Wang, J., Cheng, Y., Wang, C., Liu, H., Bian, H., and Han, W. (2019). Application of protein based films and coatings for food packaging: A review. *Polymers*, *11*(12), 2039.

Chen, H., Xie, F., Chen, L., and Zheng, B. (2019). Effect of rheological properties of potato, rice and corn starches on their hot-extrusion 3D printing behaviors. *Journal of Food Engineering*, *244*, 150–158.

Chen, J., Mu, T., Goffin, D., Blecker, C., Richard, G., Richel, A., and Haubruge, E. (2019). Application of soy protein isolate and hydrocolloids based mixtures as promising food material in 3D food printing. *Journal of Food Engineering*, *261*, 76–86.

Chen, Y., Dong, X., Shafiq, M., Myles, G., Radacsi, N., and Mo, X. (2022). Recent advancements on three dimensional electrospun nanofiber scaffolds for tissue engineering. *Advanced Fiber Materials*, *4*(5), 959–986.

Chien, K. B., Makridakis, E., and Shah, R. N. (2013). Three dimensional printing of soy protein scaffolds for tissue regeneration. *Tissue Engineering Part C: Methods*, *19*(6), 417–426.

Christopherson, G. T., Song, H., and Mao, H. Q. (2009). The influence of fiber diameter of electrospun substrates on neural stem cell differentiation and proliferation. *Biomaterials*, *30*(4), 556–564.

Daffner, K., Vadodaria, S., Ong, L., Nöbel, S., Gras, S., Norton, I., and Mills, T. (2021). Design and characterization of casein-whey protein suspensions via the pH–temperature-route for application in extrusion based 3D printing. *Food Hydrocolloids*, *112*, 105850.

Datta, P., Dhawan, A., Yu, Y., Hayes, D., Gudapati, H., and Ozbolat, I. T. (2017). Bioprinting of osteochondral tissues: A perspective on current gaps and future trends. *International Journal of Bioprinting*, *3*(2).

Deng, C., Chang, J., and Wu, C. (2019). Bioactive scaffolds for osteochondral regeneration. *Journal of Orthopaedic Translation*, *17*, 15–25.

De Peppo, G. M., Marcos-Campos, I., Kahler, D. J., Alsalman, D., Shang, L., Vunjak-Novakovic, G., and Marolt, D. (2013). Engineering bone tissue substitutes from human induced pluripotent stem cells. *Proceedings of the National Academy of Sciences*, *110*(21), 8680–8685.

Diaz, J. V., Van Bommel, K. J. C., Noort, M. W. J., Henket, J., and Briër, P. (2018). *U.S. Patent No. 10,092,030*. Washington, DC: U.S. Patent and Trademark Office.

Díez-Pascual, A. M. (2019). Synthesis and applications of biopolymer composites. *International Journal of Molecular Sciences*, *20*(9), 2321.

Diez-Pascual, A. M., and Rahdar, A. (2022). Functional nanomaterials in biomedicine: Current uses and potential applications. *Chemistry and Medicinal Chemistry*, *17*(16), e202200142.

Ezeoha, S. L., and Ezenwanne, J. N. (2013). Production of biodegradable plastic packaging film from cassava starch. *IOSR Journal of Engineering*, *3*(10), 14–20.

Fahmy, A. R., Becker, T., and Jekle, M. (2020). 3D printing and additive manufacturing of cereal-based materials: Quality analysis of starch-based systems using a camera-based morphological approach. *Innovative Food Science and Emerging Technologies*, *63*, 102384.

Fang, M., Goldstein, E. L., Matich, E. K., Orr, B. G., and Banaszak Holl, M. M. (2013). Type I collagen self-assembly: The roles of substrate and concentration. *Langmuir*, *29*(7), 2330–2338.

Farag, M. M. (2023). Recent trends on biomaterials for tissue regeneration applications. *Journal of Materials Science*, 1–32.

Feng, L., Lingling, E., and Liu, H. (2015). The effects of separating inferior Alveolar neurovascular bundles on osteogenesis of tissue engineered bone and vascularization. *Biomedical Papers*, *159*(4), 637–641.

Feyen, D. A., Gaetani, R., Deddens, J., van Keulen, D., van Opbergen, C., Poldervaart, M., and Sluijter, J. P. (2016). Gelatin microspheres as vehicle for cardiac progenitor cells delivery to the myocardium. *Advanced Healthcare Materials*, *5*(9), 1071–1079.

Fiedler, J., Özdemir, B., Bartholomä, J., Plettl, A., Brenner, R. E., and Ziemann, P. (2013). The effect of substrate surface nanotopography on the behavior of multipotnent mesenchymal stromal cells and osteoblasts. *Biomaterials*, *34*(35), 8851–8859.

Firdous, S., Ahmed, A., Nawaz, M., and Ikram, M. (2013). Optical characterization of chitosan for application as an engineered biomaterial. *Optik*, *124*(12), 1297–1302.

Frohbergh, M. E., Katsman, A., Botta, G. P., Lazarovici, P., Schauer, C. L., Wegst, U. G., and Lelkes, P. I. (2012). Electrospun hydroxyapatite containing chitosan nanofibers cross-linked with genipin for bone tissue engineering. *Biomaterials*, *33*(36), 9167–9178.

Ganeshkar, M. P., Goder, P. H., Mirjankar, M. R., Gaddigal, A. T., Shivappa, P., and Kamanavalli, C. M. (2022). Characterization and screening of anticancer properties of cerium oxide nanoparticles synthesized using *Averrhoa carambola* plant extract. *Inorganic and Nano-Metal Chemistry*, 1–14.

Gonçalves, I. M., Rodrigues, R. O., Moita, A. S., Hori, T., Kaji, H., Lima, R. A., and Minas, G. (2022). Recent trends of biomaterials and biosensors for organ-on-chip platforms. *Bioprinting*, e00202.

Gorgieva, S., and Trček, J. (2019). Bacterial cellulose: Production, modification and perspectives in biomedical applications. *Nanomaterials*, *9*(10), 1352.

Gutiérrez, T. J. (2017). Chitosan applications for the food industry. In *Chitosan: Derivatives, Composites and Applications*. Wiley, 183–232.

Ha, T. L. B., Quan, T. M., and Vu, D. N. (2013). Naturally derived biomaterials: Preparation and application. In *Regenerative Medicine and Tissue Engineering*. Intech Open, 248–274.

Hale, N. A., Yang, Y., and Rajagopalan, P. (2010). Cell migration at the interface of a dual chemical-mechanical gradient. *ACS Applied Materials and Interfaces*, *2*(8), 2317–2324.

Hallab, N. J., and Jacobs, J. J. (2017). Chemokines associated with pathologic responses to orthopedic implant debris. *Frontiers in Endocrinology*, *8*, 5.

Hamouda, T. (2021). Sustainable packaging from coir fibers. In *Biopolymers and Biocomposites from Agro-waste for Packaging Applications*. Woodhead Publishing, 113–126.

Hejazian, L. B., Esmaeilzade, B., Ghoroghi, F. M., Moradi, F., Hejazian, M. B., Aslani, A., and Nobakht, M. (2012). The role of biodegradable engineered nanofiber scaffolds seeded with hair follicle stem cells for tissue engineering. *Iranian Biomedical Journal*, *16*(4), 193.

Henkel, J., Woodruff, M. A., Epari, D. R., Steck, R., Glatt, V., Dickinson, I. C., and Hutmacher, D. W. (2013). Bone regeneration based on tissue engineering conceptions a 21st century perspective. *Bone Research*, *1*(1), 216–248.

Hinderer, S., Layland, S. L., and Schenke-Layland, K. (2016). ECM and ECM like materials biomaterials for applications in regenerative medicine and cancer therapy. *Advanced Drug Delivery Reviews*, *97*, 260–269.

Holland, S., Foster, T., MacNaughtan, W., and Tuck, C. (2018). Design and characterisation of food grade powders and inks for microstructure control using 3D printing. *Journal of Food Engineering*, *220*, 12–19.

Huang, C., Fu, X., Liu, J., Qi, Y., Li, S., and Wang, H. (2012). The involvement of integrin β1 signaling in the migration and myofibroblastic differentiation of skin fibroblasts on anisotropic collagen containing nanofibers. *Biomaterials*, *33*(6), 1791–1800.

Idumah, C. I. A. (2016). Emerging trends in flame retardancy of biofibers, biopolymers, biocomposites, and bionanocomposites. *Reviews in Chemical Engineering*, *32*(1), 115–148.

Jayarama, R. V., Radhakrishnan, S., Ravichandran, R., Mukherjee, S., Balamurugan, R., Sundarrajan, S., and Ramakrishna, S. (2013). Nanofibrous structured biomimetic strategies for skin tissue regeneration. *Wound Repair and Regeneration*, *21*(1), 1–16.

Jing, L., Wang, X., Liu, H., Lu, Y., Bian, J., Sun, J., and Huang, D. (2018). Zein increases the cytoaffinity and biodegradability of scaffolds 3D printed with zein and poly (ε-caprolactone) composite ink. *ACS Applied Materials and Interfaces*, *10*(22), 18551–18559.

Jing, X., Mi, H. Y., Napiwocki, B. N., Peng, X. F., and Turng, L. S. (2017). Mussel-inspired electroactive chitosan/graphene oxide composite hydrogel with rapid self healing and recovery behavior for tissue engineering. *Carbon*, *125*, 557–570.

Kadner, K., Dobner, S., Franz, T., Bezuidenhout, D., Sirry, M. S., Zilla, P., and Davies, N. H. (2012). The beneficial effects of deferred delivery on the efficiency of hydrogel therapy post myocardial infarction. *Biomaterials*, *33*(7), 2060–2066.

Kaur, M., Sharma, S., and Sinha, V. R. (2017). Polymer based microspheres of aceclofenac as sustained release parenterals for prolonged anti-inflammatory effect. *Materials Science and Engineering: C*, *72*, 492–500.

Khakbaz, H., Walter, R., Gordon, T., and Kannan, M. B. (2014). Self-dissolution assisted coating on magnesium metal for biodegradable bone fixation devices. *Materials Research Express*, *1*(4), 045406.

Khorshidi, S., Solouk, A., Mirzadeh, H., Mazinani, S., Lagaron, J. M., Sharifi, S., and Ramakrishna, S. (2016). A review of key challenges of electrospun scaffolds for tissue-engineering applications. *Journal of Tissue Engineering and Regenerative Medicine*, *10*(9), 715–738.

Kim, S. H., Turnbull, J., and Guimond, S. (2011). Extracellular matrix and cell signalling: The dynamic cooperation of integrin, proteoglycan and growth factor receptor. *The Journal of Endocrinology*, *209*(2), 139–151.

Kim, S. Y., Park, G. H., Kim, H. A., Lee, A. Y., Oh, H. R., Lee, C. W., and Lee, M. H. (2017). Micro deposition of Cu based metallic glass wire by direct laser melting process. *Materials Letters*, *202*, 1–4.

Krishnan, R., Rajeswari, R., Venugopal, J., Sundarrajan, S., Sridhar, R., Shayanti, M., and Ramakrishna, S. (2012). Polysaccharide nanofibrous scaffolds as a model for *in vitro* skin tissue regeneration. *Journal of Materials Science: Materials in Medicine*, *23*(6), 1511–1519.

Kruzic, J. J. (2016). Bulk metallic glasses as structural materials: A review. *Advanced Engineering Materials*, *18*(8), 1308–1331.

Kumar, S., and Thakur, K. S. (2017). Bioplastics classification, production and their potential food applications. *Journal of Hill Agriculture*, *8*(2), 118–129.

Kyziol, K., Kaczmarek, L., and Kyziol, A. (2017). Surface functionalization of biomaterials. In *Handbook of Composites from Renewable Materials*. Wiley, Chapter 4, 457–490.

Li, Y. C., Chen, C. R., and Young, T. H. (2013). Pearl extract enhances the migratory ability of fibroblasts in a wound healing model. *Pharmaceutical Biology*, *51*(3), 289–297.

Lille, M., Nurmela, A., Nordlund, E., Metsä-Kortelainen, S., and Sozer, N. (2018). Applicability of protein and fiber-rich food materials in extrusion based 3D printing. *Journal of Food Engineering*, *220*, 20–27.

Linh, N. T. B., and Lee, B. T. (2012). Electrospinning of polyvinyl alcohol/gelatin nanofiber composites and cross-linking for bone tissue engineering application. *Journal of Biomaterials Applications*, *27*(3), 255–266.

Liu, L., and Ciftci, O. N. (2021). Effects of high oil compositions and printing parameters on food paste properties and printability in a 3D printing food processing model. *Journal of Food Engineering*, *288*, 110135.

Liu, Y., Liu, D., Wei, G., Ma, Y., Bhandari, B., and Zhou, P. (2018). 3D printed milk protein food simulant: Improving the printing performance of milk protein concentration by incorporating whey protein isolate. *Innovative Food Science and Emerging Technologies*, *49*, 116–126.

Liu, Y., Yu, Y., Liu, C., Regenstein, J. M., Liu, X., and Zhou, P. (2019). Rheological and mechanical behavior of milk protein composite gel for extrusion based 3D food printing. *LWT-Food Science and Technology*, *102*, 338–346.

Liu, Z., Bhandari, B., Prakash, S., Mantihal, S., and Zhang, M. (2019). Linking rheology and printability of a multicomponent gel system of carrageenan-xanthan-starch in extrusion based additive manufacturing. *Food Hydrocolloids*, *87*, 413–424.

Liu, Z., Chen, H., Zheng, B., Xie, F., and Chen, L. (2020). Understanding the structure and rheological properties of potato starch induced by hot extrusion 3D printing. *Food Hydrocolloids*, *105*, 105812.

LogithKumar, R., KeshavNarayan, A., Dhivya, S., Chawla, A., Saravanan, S., and Selvamurugan, N. (2016). A review of chitosan and its derivatives in bone tissue engineering. *Carbohydrate Polymers*, *151*, 172–188.

Loordhuswamy, A. M., Krishnaswamy, V. R., Korrapati, P. S., Thinakaran, S., and Rengaswami, G. D. V. (2014). Fabrication of highly aligned fibrous scaffolds for tissue regeneration by centrifugal spinning technology. *Materials Science and Engineering: C*, *42*, 799–807.

Lyndon, J. A., Boyd, B. J., and Birbilis, N. (2014). Metallic implant drug/device combinations for controlled drug release in orthopaedic applications. *Journal of Controlled Release*, *179*, 63–75.

Ma, Y., Zhang, B., Sun, H., Liu, D., Zhu, Y., Zhu, Q., and Liu, X. (2023). The dual effect of 3D-printed biological scaffolds composed of diverse biomaterials in the treatment of bone tumors. *International Journal of Nanomedicine*, *31*, 293–305.

Maniglia, B. C., Lima, D. C., Junior, M. D. M., Le-Bail, P., Le-Bail, A., and Augusto, P. E. (2020). Preparation of cassava starch hydrogels for application in 3D printing using dry heating treatment (DHT): A prospective study on the effects of DHT and gelatinization conditions. *Food Research International*, *128*, 108803.

Marrella, A., Lee, T. Y., Lee, D. H., Karuthedom, S., Syla, D., Chawla, A., and Jang, H. L. (2018). Engineering vascularized and innervated bone biomaterials for improved skeletal tissue regeneration. *Materials Today*, *21*(4), 362–376.

Martău, G. A., Mihai, M., and Vodnar, D. C. (2019). The use of chitosan, alginate, and pectin in the biomedical and food sector biocompatibility, bioadhesiveness, and biodegradability. *Polymers*, *11*(11), 1837.

McAdam, B., Brennan Fournet, M., McDonald, P., and Mojicevic, M. (2020). Production of polyhydroxybutyrate (PHB) and factors impacting its chemical and mechanical characteristics. *Polymers*, *12*(12), 2908.

Melke, J., Midha, S., Ghosh, S., Ito, K., and Hofmann, S. (2016). Silk fibroin as biomaterial for bone tissue engineering. *Acta Biomaterialia*, *31*, 1–16.

Moghaddam, N. S., Skoracki, R., Miller, M., Elahinia, M., and Dean, D. (2016). Three dimensional printing of stiffness-tuned, nitinol skeletal fixation hardware with an example of mandibular segmental defect repair. *Procedia CIRP*, *49*, 45–50.

Musazzi, U. M., Selmin, F., Ortenzi, M. A., Mohammed, G. K., Franzé, S., Minghetti, P., and Cilurzo, F. (2018). Personalized orodispersible films by hot melt ram extrusion 3D printing. *International Journal of Pharmaceutics*, *551*(1–2), 52–59.

Nath, K., Bhattacharyya, S. K., and Das, N. C. (2020). Biodegradable polymeric materials for EMI shielding. In *Materials for Potential EMI Shielding Applications*. Elsevier, 165–178.

Ncube, L. K., Ude, A. U., Ogunmuyiwa, E. N., Zulkifli, R., and Beas, I. N. (2020). Environmental impact of food packaging materials: A review of contemporary development from conventional plastics to polylactic acid based materials. *Materials*, *13*(21), 4994.

Nezakati, T., Seifalian, A., Tan, A., and Seifalian, A. M. (2018). Conductive polymers: Opportunities and challenges in biomedical applications. *Chemical Reviews*, *118*(14), 6766–6843.

Nikkhah, M., Akbari, M., Paul, A., Memic, A., Dolatshahi Pirouz, A., and Khademhosseini, A. (2016). Gelatin-based biomaterials for tissue engineering and stem cell bioengineering. In *Biomaterials from Nature for Advanced Devices and Therapies*. Wiley, 37–62.

Nikolova, M. P., and Chavali, M. S. (2019). Recent advances in biomaterials for 3D scaffolds: A review. *Bioactive Materials*, *4*, 271–292.

Oliveira, S. M., Fasolin, L. H., Vicente, A. A., Fuciños, P., and Pastrana, L. M. (2020). Printability, microstructure, and flow dynamics of phase separated edible 3D inks. *Food Hydrocolloids*, *109*, 106120.

Ortolani, A., Bianchi, M., Mosca, M., Caravelli, S., Fuiano, M., Marcacci, M., and Russo, A. (2016). The prospective opportunities offered by magnetic scaffolds for bone tissue engineering: A review. *Joints*, *4*(4), 228–235.

Pacelli, S., Manoharan, V., Desalvo, A., Lomis, N., Jodha, K. S., Prakash, S., and Paul, A. (2016). Tailoring biomaterial surface properties to modulate host implant interactions: Implication in cardiovascular and bone therapy. *Journal of Materials Chemistry B*, *4*(9), 1586–1599.

Paggi, R. A., Salmoria, G. V., Ghizoni, G. B., de Medeiros Back, H., and de Mello Gindri, I. (2019). Structure and mechanical properties of 3D-printed cellulose tablets by fused deposition modeling. *The International Journal of Advanced Manufacturing Technology*, *100*(9), 2767–2774.

Pattanashetti, N. A., Heggannavar, G. B., and Kariduraganavar, M. Y. (2017). Smart biopolymers and their biomedical applications. *Procedia Manufacturing*, *12*, 263–279.

Pattar, S. V., Adhoni, S. A., Kamanavalli, C. M., and Kumbar, S. S. (2020). *In silico* molecular docking studies and MM/GBSA analysis of coumarin-carbonodithioate hybrid derivatives divulge the anticancer potential against breast cancer. *Beni-Suef University Journal of Basic and Applied Sciences*, *9*(1), 1–10.

Pattar, S. V., Mirjankar, M. R., Kulkarni, S., Gai, P. B., Pujar, N. K., Premakshi, H. G., Sikandar, I. M., Babu, R. L., and Kamanavalli, C. M. (2021). Analysis of human aldehyde dehydrogenases (ALDH) gene expression pattern in breast cancer tissue samples: Rutin-copper complex inhibit the breast cancer cell proliferation. *Egyptian Journal of Medical Human Genetics*, *22*(1), 1–10.

Peng, X., Cheng, C., Zhang, X., He, X., and Liu, Y. (2023). Design and application strategies of natural polymer biomaterials in artificial ovaries. *Annals of Biomedical Engineering*, *2023*, 1–8.

Phuhongsung, P., Zhang, M., and Devahastin, S. (2020). Investigation on 3D printing ability of soybean protein isolate gels and correlations with their rheological and textural properties via LF-NMR spectroscopic characteristics. *LWT-Food Science and Technology*, *122*, 109019.

Pulatsu, E., Su, J. W., Lin, J., and Lin, M. (2020). Factors affecting 3D printing and post processing capacity of cookie dough. *Innovative Food Science and Emerging Technologies*, *61*, 102316.

Qasim, U., Osman, A. I., Al-Muhtaseb, A. A. H., Farrell, C., Al-Abri, M., Ali, M., and Rooney, D. W. (2021). Renewable cellulosic nanocomposites for food packaging to avoid fossil fuel plastic pollution: A review. *Environmental Chemistry Letters*, *19*(1), 613–641.

Rampichová, M., Buzgo, M., Chvojka, J., Prosecká, E., Kofroňová, O., and Amler, E. (2014). Cell penetration to nanofibrous scaffolds: Forcespinning®, an alternative approach for fabricating 3D nanofibers. *Cell Adhesion and Migration*, *8*(1), 36–41.

Ranakoti, L., Gangil, B., Bhandari, P., Singh, T., Sharma, S., Singh, J., and Singh, S. (2023). Promising role of polylactic acid as an ingenious biomaterial in scaffolds, drug delivery, tissue engineering, and medical implants: Research developments, and prospective applications. *Molecules*, *28*(2), 485.

Redondo-Gómez, C., Rodríguez Quesada, M., Vallejo Astúa, S., Murillo Zamora, J. P., Lopretti, M., and Vega-Baudrit, J. R. (2020). Biorefinery of biomass of agro industrial banana waste to obtain high value biopolymers. *Molecules*, *25*(17), 3829.

Ren, L., Pandit, V., Elkin, J., Denman, T., Cooper, J. A., and Kotha, S. P. (2013). Large scale and highly efficient synthesis of micro and nano fibers with controlled fiber morphology by centrifugal jet spinning for tissue regeneration. *Nanoscale*, *5*(6), 2337–2345.

Rendón-Villalobos, R., Ortíz-Sánchez, A., Tovar-Sánchez, E., and Flores Huicochea, E. (2016). The role of biopolymers in obtaining environmentally friendly materials. In *Composites from Renewable and Sustainable Materials*. Intech, 151–159.

Repanas, A., Andriopoulou, S., and Glasmacher, B. (2016). The significance of electrospinning as a method to create fibrous scaffolds for biomedical engineering and drug delivery applications. *Journal of Drug Delivery Science and Technology*, *31*, 137–146.

Rivera-Briso, A. L., and Serrano-Aroca, Á. (2018). Poly (3-Hydroxybutyrate-co-3-Hydroxyvalerate): Enhancement strategies for advanced applications. *Polymers*, *10*(7), 732.

Rodrigues, A. I., Gomes, M. E., Leonor, I. B., and Reis, R. L. (2012). Bioactive starch-based scaffolds and human adipose stem cells are a good combination for bone tissue engineering. *Acta Biomaterialia*, *8*(10), 3765–3776.

Rouchi, A. H., and Mahdavi-Mazdeh, M. (2015). Regenerative medicine in organ and tissue transplantation: Shortly and practically achievable? *International Journal of Organ Transplantation Medicine*, *6*(3), 93.

Ruvinov, E., and Cohen, S. (2016). Alginate biomaterial for the treatment of myocardial infarction: Progress, translational strategies, and clinical outlook: From ocean algae to patient bedside. *Advanced Drug Delivery Reviews*, *96*, 54–76.

Sah, M. K., and Pramanik, K. (2012). Surface modification and characterisation of natural polymers for orthopaedic tissue engineering: A review. *International Journal of Biomedical Engineering and Technology*, *9*(2), 101–121.

Saharan, L., de Andrade, M. J., Saleem, W., Baughman, R. H., and Tadesse, Y. (2017). iGrab: Hand orthosis powered by twisted and coiled polymer muscles. *Smart Materials and Structures*, *26*(10), 105048.

Saiz, E., Zimmermann, E. A., Lee, J. S., Wegst, U. G., and Tomsia, A. P. (2013). Perspectives on the role of nanotechnology in bone tissue engineering. *Dental Materials*, *29*(1), 103–115.

Sallustio, F., Serino, G., and Schena, F. P. (2015). Potential reparative role of resident adult renal stem/progenitor cells in acute kidney injury. *BioResearch Open Access*, *4*(1), 326–333.

Sanko, V., Sahin, I., Aydemir Sezer, U., and Sezer, S. (2019). A versatile method for the synthesis of poly (glycolic acid): High solubility and tunable molecular weights. *Polymer Journal*, *51*(7), 637–647.

Schutyser, M. A. I., Houlder, S., de Wit, M., Buijsse, C. A. P., and Alting, A. C. (2018). Fused deposition modelling of sodium caseinate dispersions. *Journal of Food Engineering*, *220*, 49–55.

Severino, P., da Silva, C. F., Andrade, L. N., de Lima Oliveira, D., Campos, J., and Souto, E. B. (2019). Alginate nanoparticles for drug delivery and targeting. *Current Pharmaceutical Design*, *25*(11), 1312–1334.

Sharma, A., Saharan, L., and Tadesse, Y. (2017). 3-D printed orthotic hand with wrist mechanism using twisted and coiled polymeric muscles. In *ASME International Mechanical Engineering Congress and Exposition* (58363, V003T04A057). American Society of Mechanical Engineers.

Sharma, S., and Sinha, V. R. (2018). Current pharmaceutical strategies for efficient site specific delivery in inflamed distal intestinal mucosa. *Journal of Controlled Release*, *272*, 97–106.

Shen, Y., Li, Y., Chen, C., and Tsai, H. L. (2017). 3D printing of large, complex metallic glass structures. *Materials and Design*, *117*, 213–222.

Shivam, P. (2016). Recent developments on biodegradable polymers and their future trends. *International Research. Journal of Science and Engineering*, *4*(1), 17–26.

Singh, S., Singh, G., Prakash, C., Ramakrishna, S., Lamberti, L., and Pruncu, C. I. (2020). 3D printed biodegradable composites: An insight into mechanical properties of PLA/chitosan scaffold. *Polymer Testing*, *89*, 106722.

Sivashankari, P. R., and Prabaharan, M. (2017). Chitosan/carbon based nanomaterials as scaffolds for tissue engineering. In *Biopolymer Based Composites*. Woodhead Publishing 381–397.

Sonia, T. A., and Sharma, C. P. (2012). An overview of natural polymers for oral insulin delivery. *Drug Discovery Today*, *17*(13–14), 784–792.

Stoltz, J. F., de Isla, N., Li, Y. P., Bensoussan, D., Zhang, L., Huselstein, C., and He, Y. (2015). Stem cells and regenerative medicine: Myth or reality of the 21th century. *Stem Cells International*, *2015*.

Subbiah, T., Bhat, G. S., Tock, R. W., Parameswaran, S., and Ramkumar, S. S. (2005). Electrospinning of nanofibers. *Journal of Applied Polymer Science*, *96*(2), 557–569.

Sun, J., and Tan, H. (2013). Alginate based biomaterials for regenerative medicine applications. *Materials*, *6*(4), 1285–1309.

Sutton, L., Moein, H., Rafiee, A., Madden, J. D., and Menon, C. (2016). Design of an assistive wrist orthosis using conductive nylon actuators. In *2016 6th IEEE International Conference on Biomedical Robotics and Biomechatronics (BioRob)*. IEEE, 1074–1079.

Swain, S. K., Pattanayak, A. J., and Sahoo, A. P. (2018). Functional biopolymer composites. In *Functional Biopolymers*. Springer, 159–182.

Theagarajan, R., Moses, J. A., and Anandharamakrishnan, C. (2020). 3D extrusion printability of rice starch and optimization of process variables. *Food and Bioprocess Technology*, *13*(6), 1048–1062.

Tiwari, N., Kumar, D., Priyadarshani, A., Jain, G. K., Mittal, G., Kesharwani, P., and Aggarwal, G. (2023). Recent progress in polymeric biomaterials and their potential applications in skin regeneration and wound care management. *Journal of Drug Delivery Science and Technology*, *27*, 104319.

Tonelli, F. M., Santos, A. K., Gomes, K. N., Lorencon, E., Guatimosim, S., Ladeira, L. O., and Resende, R. R. (2012). Carbon nanotube interaction with extracellular matrix proteins producing scaffolds for tissue engineering. *International Journal of Nanomedicine*, *7*, 4511.

Udayakumar, G. P., Muthusamy, S., Selvaganesh, B., Sivarajasekar, N., Rambabu, K., Banat, F., and Show, P. L. (2021). Biopolymers and composites: Properties, characterization and their applications in food, medical and pharmaceutical industries. *Journal of Environmental Chemical Engineering*, *9*(4), 105322.

Ulery, B. D., Nair, L. S., and Laurencin, C. T. (2011). Biomedical applications of biodegradable polymers. *Journal of Polymer Science Part B: Polymer Physics*, *49*(12), 832–864.

Vaithilingam, J., Kilsby, S., Goodridge, R. D., Christie, S. D., Edmondson, S., and Hague, R. J. (2015). Functionalisation of Ti6Al4V components fabricated using selective laser melting with a bioactive compound. *Materials Science and Engineering C*, *46*, 52–61.

Varma, K., and Gopi, S. (2021). Biopolymers and their role in medicinal and pharmaceutical applications. In *Biopolymers and Their Industrial Applications*. Elsevier, 175–191.

Vasita, R., and Katti, D. S. (2006). Nanofibers and their applications in tissue engineering. *International Journal of Nanomedicine*, *1*(1), 15.

Velu, R., Calais, T., Jayakumar, A., and Raspall, F. (2019). A comprehensive review on bio-nanomaterials for medical implants and feasibility studies on fabrication of such implants by additive manufacturing technique. *Materials*, *13*(1), 92.

Wade, R. J., and Burdick, J. A. (2014). Advances in nanofibrous scaffolds for biomedical applications: From electrospinning to self-assembly. *Nano Today*, *9*(6), 722–742.

Wang, L., Shi, J., Liu, L., Secret, E., and Chen, Y. (2011). Fabrication of polymer fiber scaffolds by centrifugal spinning for cell culture studies. *Microelectronic Engineering*, *88*(8), 1718–1721.

Wang, X. Q., Wang, F. P., Chen, W., Huang, J., Bazaka, K., and Ostrikov, K. K. (2016). Non-equilibrium plasma prevention of *Schistosoma japonicum* transmission. *Scientific Reports*, *6*(1), 1–9.

Wang, X. Q., Wu, D., Li, W., and Yang, L. (2022). Emerging biomaterials for reproductive medicine. *Engineered Regeneration*, *2*, 230–245.

Warner, E. L., Norton, I. T., and Mills, T. B. (2019). Comparing the viscoelastic properties of gelatin and different concentrations of kappa carrageenan mixtures for additive manufacturing applications. *Journal of Food Engineering*, *246*, 58–66.

Wróblewska-Krepsztul, J., Rydzkowski, T., Michalska-Pożoga, I., and Thakur, V. K. (2019). Biopolymers for biomedical and pharmaceutical applications: Recent advances and overview of alginate electrospinning. *Nanomaterials*, *9*(3), 404.

Wu, C. S. (2016). Modulation, functionality, and cytocompatibility of three-dimensional printing materials made from chitosan-based polysaccharide composites. *Materials Science and Engineering C*, *69*, 27–36.

Wu, C. S., Wang, Y., Streubel, P. N., and Duan, B. (2017). Living nanofiber yarn based woven biotextiles for tendon tissue engineering using cell tri culture and mechanical stimulation. *Acta Biomaterialia*, *62*, 102–115.

Xia, H., Chen, Q., Fang, Y., Liu, D., Zhong, D., Wu, H., and Sun, X. (2014). Directed neurite growth of rat dorsal root ganglion neurons and increased colocalization with Schwann cells on aligned poly (methyl methacrylate) electrospun nanofibers. *Brain Research*, *1565*, 18–27.

Xiang, N., Yuen Jr, J. S., Stout, A. J., Rubio, N. R., Chen, Y., and Kaplan, D. L. (2022). 3D porous scaffolds from wheat glutenin for cultured meat applications. *Biomaterials*, *285*, 121543.

Xu, F., Weng, B., Materon, L. A., Kuang, A., Trujillo, J. A., and Lozano, K. (2016). Fabrication of cellulose fine fiber based membranes embedded with silver nanoparticles *via* Force spinning. *Journal of Polymer Engineering*, *36*(3), 269–278.

Yadav, P., Yadav, H., Shah, V. G., Shah, G., and Dhaka, G. (2015). Biomedical biopolymers, their origin and evolution in biomedical sciences: A systematic review. *Journal of Clinical and Diagnostic Research, JCDR*, *9*(9), ZE21.

Yang, G., Li, X., He, Y., Ma, J., Ni, G., and Zhou, S. (2018). From nano to micro to macro: Electrospun hierarchically structured polymeric fibers for biomedical applications. *Progress in Polymer Science*, *81*, 80–113.

Yang, G., Xiao, Z., Ren, X., Long, H., Qian, H., Ma, K., and Guo, Y. (2016). Enzymatically crosslinked gelatin hydrogel promotes the proliferation of adipose tissue derived stromal cells. *PeerJ*, *4*, e2497.

Yang, Y., Wang, G., Liang, H., Gao, C., Peng, S., Shen, L., and Shuai, C. (2019). Additive manufacturing of bone scaffolds. *International Journal of Bioprinting*, *5*(1).

Yin, Z., Chen, X., Song, H. X., Hu, J. J., Tang, Q. M., Zhu, T., and Ouyang, H. W. (2015). Electrospun scaffolds for multiple tissues regeneration *in vivo* through topography dependent induction of lineage specific differentiation. *Biomaterials*, *44*, 173–185.

Zarekhalili, Z., Bahrami, S. H., Ranjbar-Mohammadi, M., and Milan, P. B. (2017). Fabrication and characterization of PVA/Gum tragacanth/PCL hybrid nanofibrous scaffolds for skin substitutes. *International Journal of Biological Macromolecules*, *94*, 679–690.

Zargar, V., Asghari, M., and Dashti, A. (2015). A review on chitin and chitosan polymers: Structure, chemistry, solubility, derivatives, and applications. *Chemical and Biochemical Engineering reviews*, *2*(3), 204–226.

Zhang, H., Zheng, X., Ahmed, W., Yao, Y., Bai, J., Chen, Y., and Gao, C. (2018). Design and applications of cell selective surfaces and interfaces. *Biomacromolecules*, *19*(6), 1746–1763.

Zhang, Z., Hu, J., and Ma, P. X. (2012). Nanofiber based delivery of bioactive agents and stem cells to bone sites. *Advanced Drug Delivery Reviews*, *64*(12), 1129–1141.

Zhao, D., Witte, F., Lu, F., Wang, J., Li, J., and Qin, L. (2017). Current status on clinical applications of magnesium based orthopaedic implants: A review from clinical translational perspective. *Biomaterials*, *112*, 287–302.

Zheng, L., Yu, Y., Tong, Z., Zou, Q., Han, S., and Jiang, H. (2019). The characteristics of starch gels molded by 3D printing. *Journal of Food Processing and Preservation*, *43*(7), e13993.

Zhou, H., Ge, J., Bai, Y., Liang, C., and Yang, L. (2019). Translation of bone wax and its substitutes: History, clinical status and future directions. *Journal of Orthopaedic Translation*, *17*, 64–72.

Zhu, Z., and Huangfu, D. (2013). Human pluripotent stem cells: An emerging model in developmental biology. *Development*, *140*(4), 705–717.

2 Applications of Biomaterials in Advanced Drug Delivery Systems

Nabajyoti Baildya, Subhankar Choudhury**, Poulami Jana***, Prosenjit Choudhury****, and Narendra Nath Ghosh*****,†*

*Department of Chemistry, Milki High School, Milki, Malda, West Bengal, India; **Department of Chemistry, Malda College, Malda, India; ***Department of Chemistry, Kaliachak College Sultanganj, Malda, West Bengal, India; ****Department of Physics, Dr. Meghnad Saha College, Itahar, India; *****Pakuahat A. N. M. High School, Malda, West Bengal, India

†Corresponding Author: ghosh.naren13@gmail.com

ABBREVIATIONS

AD	Alzheimer disease
AIDS	Acquired immune deficiency syndrome
ASD	Autism spectrum disorder
CD	Cyclodextrin
CMC	Critical micelle concentration
DNA	Deoxyribonucleic acid
DOPC	Dioleylphosphatidylcholine
DPPC	Dipalmitoylphosphatidylcholine
DPPG	Dipalmitoylphosphatidylglycerol
EGFR	Epidermal growth factor receptor
FDA	Food and Drug Administration
HBV	Hepatitis B virus
HIV	Human immunodeficiency virus
HPV	Human papillomavirus
MAA	Methacrylic acid
MRI	Magnetic resonance imaging
MS	Multiple sclerosis
NB	Neuroblastoma
NIPAAm	N-isopropylacrylamide
NP	Nanoparticle

DOI: 10.1201/9781032699882-2

NSAID	Non-steroidal anti-inflammatory drug
PAMAM	Polyamidoamine
PHLNP	Polymeric lipid hybrid nanoparticle
PLGA	Poly (D, L-lactic-co-glycolic acid)
RNA	Ribonucleic acid
SCID	Severe combined **immunodeficiency**
VLP	Virus-like particle
VNP	Virus-based nanoparticle

2.1 INTRODUCTION

The therapeutic efficacy and potential benefit of a drug largely depends on its delivery within the body system. A drug normally reaches the target sites repeatedly, ensuring remediation, but during this process, the concentration of the drug sometimes exceeds the tolerance level of the body, causing toxic side effects (Adeosun, Ilomuanya et al. 2020). Furthermore, the therapeutic activities of the drug mostly rely on the temperature, pH and water content of the body, and the alteration of these conditions can cause the drug to lose its activities (PS 2018). Hence, the biocompatibility and sustainable release of drugs are very crucial to reduce drug wastage and side effects. Therefore, overcoming the issues like poor solubility, high organ toxicity and poor selectivity and biodegradability lies in the proper understanding of the delivery process and the discovery of innovative drug nano-carrier. Biomaterials like lipids, proteins, vaccines, antibodies, peptides, medicines and enzymes, owing to their high biocompatibility as well as biodegradability issues, have enhanced delivery efficacy for a wide range of pharmaceutical compounds [6]. The progression in the field of organic and synthetic chemistry, genetic engineering, biotechnology and material science helps to improve the drug delivery process, particularly for polymer and lipid based materials [7]. These materials can be used in regenerative treatment and tissue engineering in bone (Tautzenberger, Kovtun et al. 2012), in the agriculture sector, such as in the overall development of plant health by the usage of silicon nanoparticles (Rastogi, Tripathi et al. 2017), and also in the biomedical sector.

In recent decades, nanotechnology has been widely applied for medical checkups and the treatment of different chronic illnesses *viz.* lower respiratory infections, tuberculosis, diarrhea, HIV, malaria, AIDS, cancer, infectious illnesses, diabetes, immedicable pain and autoimmune illnesses. In the therapeutic treatment of experimental autoimmune encephalomyelitis (EAE), it was found that the usual glucocorticoid treatment affecting the macrophages is less effective than glucocorticoid-loaded liposomes at lower doses (Rezaei, Safaei et al. 2019). The development of therapeutics for the treatment of hepatitis B virus (HBV) along with human papillomavirus (HPV) helps to improve the activity of several virus-based nanoparticles (VNPs) and virus-like particles (VLPs) in the human body [5]. Many critical diseases such as multiple sclerosis (MS), Alzheimer disease (AD), autism spectrum disorder (ASD) and other neurological disorders are improved due to the immense development of nanotechnology [6]. The usage of nanotechnology for the treatment of cancer by medical practitioners has been continuing for many years. For example, Abraxane and Doxil are two permitted treatments which help to enhance the activity of chemotherapy drugs. Abraxane nanoparticles are prepared from albumin protein bonded to a chemo-drug docetaxel and inhibit the proliferation of cancer cells. Abraxane was sanctioned by the FDA in 2005 to medicate breast and pancreatic cancers that have spread, as well as metastatic non-small-cell lung cancer. Polyethylene glycol-coated liposomes, known as Doxil, are an encapsulated form of a chemo-drug that is used primarily to medicate ovarian cancers, multiple myeloma and Kaposi's sarcoma.

Nowadays, it is very convenient to distinguish normal cells from cancer cells with the progression of nanotechnology, as it can identify small, unusual changes occurring in cells early. Thus, it can detect the cancer at its early stage, when just the cell division process has started abnormally. Hence, patients can be cured very easily. Tumors can be detected easily in imaging tests using nanotechnology (Jia, Han et al. 2022). To find cancer cells, nanoparticles coated with antibodies or other substances are employed that can easily attach to the cancer cells. Particles can also be coated with suitable elements that put out a signal when they get in touch with cancer cells. Appropriate materials attached to nanoparticles can emit signals when they get in touch with cancer cells. For instance, nanoparticles prepared from iron oxide attach to cancer cells and radiate a powerful indication that identifies the cancer on MRI examinations (Hosseini, Mohammadnejad et al. 2023). Medical practitioners can easily identify the location of cancer in the tissue or blood samples with the assistance of nanotechnology.

Currently, different drugs can be delivered with the advancement of synthetic routes for NPs to target sites like cells, tissues and organs (Jabbar, Ibrahim et al. 2022). Solid and colloidal forms of nanoparticles have nano-diameters of 10–200 nm (Dang and Guan 2020). They have three key interrelated physical characteristics: (1) they are extremely movable in the free state (e.g., without certain extra stimulus, the sedimentation rate of silica nanospheres with a 10 nm diameter is 0.01 mm/day in water under gravity); (2) they have large specific surface areas; and (3) they may show what are known as quantum effects. Therefore, nanoparticles have an enormous range of compositions, conditional on the use or variety of products (Kagdada, Bhojani et al. 2023). An important remedy in demanding research is paclitaxel (taxol). Nanoparticle-formulated paclitaxel can raise the cytotoxicity for cancer cells *in vitro* and simultaneously improve sustainable remedial effectiveness in an *in vivo* animal model (De Jong 2008). Paclitaxel enclosed in tocopherol TPGS-emulsified poly (D,L-lactic-co-glycolic acid) (PLGA) nanoparticles resulted in a prolonged level above the effective concentration *in vivo* (Feng, Zeng et al. 2007).

The chief objectives for the investigation of nano-bio-technologies in drug transportation comprise: (1) precise drug targeting, as nanoparticles can penetrate bio films and can enter cells, tissues and organs that lager size particles or drugs cannot penetrate and deliver (Barua 2014); (2) controlled and continued discharge of drugs during passage and at the site of localization; (3) increased drug therapeutic efficacy and a reduction in non-specific toxicity (Tiwari, Tiwari et al. 2012) and (4) precise discharge and drug degradation features that can be easily adjusted by improving the hydrophilicity and half-life of drug systemic transmission and decreasing immunogenicity (Shelley and Babu 2018). Nano-carriers provide diverse benefits over traditional drug delivery systems, such as the enhancement of plasma half-life, bio-distribution and delivery precision of a drug to the tumor microenvironment through endothelial layers. Nanoparticles assist in molecular directed cancer therapy and the identification of cancer lesions, as well as the ascertainment of molecular signatures of the tumor by non-invasive imaging (Kadian 2018).

2.2 DIFFERENT TYPES OF BIOMATERIALS USED AS DRUG NANO-CARRIERS

Biomaterials have been very popular systems over the last ten years due to their various biomedical applications. Liposomes, bio-responsive polymers like chitosan and dendrimers are categorized as nano-scale drug delivery vehicles that have been investigated over the years (You, Almeda et al. 2010; Abdelaziz, Gaber et al. 2018). Structurally, liposomes are concentric spheres of lipid bilayers separated by hydrophobic compartments made up of natural and synthetic phospholipids (Figure 2.1). Liposomes provide a safe platform for *in vivo* cancer therapy, as they can encapsulate many anticancer drug such as erlotinib and doxorubicin and thus improve cell type-specific delivery. The amphiphilic nanoparticle-encapsulated doxorubicin has been developed for the treatment of breast cancer and to reduce cardiotoxicity. Biomaterial-mediated drug transportation can be successfully used in the areas of prostate and breast cancer (Langasco, Cadeddu et al. 2017; Ruskowitz and DeForest 2018). Additionally, biomaterials have potential in combinational therapy, where the synchronized delivery of drugs to be combined with other therapies improves the therapeutic efficacy and lowers drug resistance.

2.2.1 Liposome-Mediated Drug Delivery Systems

Since their first report in the 1960s by Alec D Bangham, liposomes have been extensively applied as drug delivery tools. Liposomes are spherical in shape, with concentric lipid bilayers rendering discrete aqueous spaces. They are normally in the 50–450 nm size range (Etheridge, Campbell et al. 2013). Due to their favorable structure, they can be utilized for the delivery of both hydrophilic drugs by trapping them in the dissolved aqueous volume and hydrophobic drugs by encapsulating them in the phospholipid bilayer (Bangham and Horne 1964; Gordon, Schneider

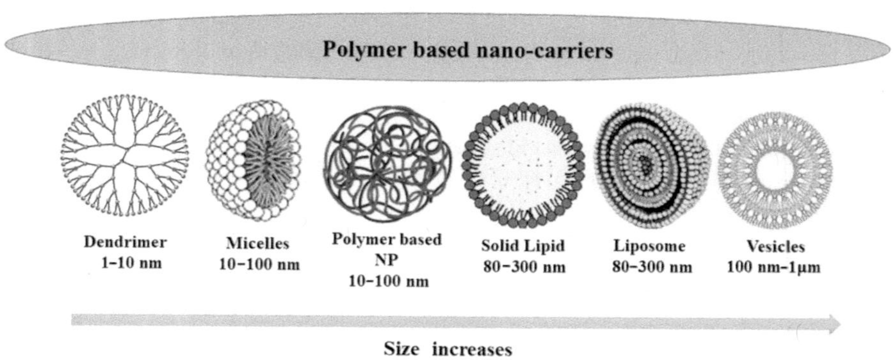

FIGURE 2.1 Different types of drug nano-carriers used in advanced drug delivery.

et al. 1975; Kinning and Thomas 1984). Liposome-based nano-carriers for the delivery of therapeutics like vaccines, antifungal medicines and anticancer therapies are used extensively in the pharmaceutical industry as agents for direct drug delivery. Among the most studied biomaterial-mediated nano-delivery systems, liposomes have an extensive variety of pharmaceutical industrial uses. Furthermore, because of their great biocompatibility, they are useful for the manufacturing of cosmetics like shampoos and other of skincare products. The cholesterol-modified lipid bilayer of liposomes can prevent lipid exchange and provide additional stabilization *in vivo* and also *in vitro* (Hissa, Oakes et al. 2017; Trucillo, Campardelli et al. 2017; Nakhaei, Margiana et al. 2021) (Figure 2.2). Table 2.1 summarizes the liposome-modified biomaterials for advanced drug delivery. Liposome NPs or cholesterol-functionalized liposome NPs have shown elevated levels of drug delivery efficiency without any toxic effects. Table 2.1 shows liposome and functionalized liposome nanoparticle-mediated selective and target-specific drug delivery.

Furthermore, liposome-mediated drugs like vinorelbine for solid tumors (Mayer and Janoff 2007), Cytarabine, daunorubicin for acute myeloid leukemia, siRNA for ovarian cancer (Aleku, Schulz et al. 2008; Li and Shen 2009) and Camptothecin for solid tumors (Huang, Hua et al. 2008) are in the investigational stage.

2.2.2 Bio-Responsive Polymer Materials as Nano-Carriers

Biodegradable and bio-absorbable polymers are attractive engineered materials for modern drug delivery. The polymer matrix provides a safe framework for transporting drugs and avoiding toxic effects to the body. Another advantage of polymers as drug nano-carriers is the ability to control their molecular weight by tuning the stoichiometry of the monomer units with different available polymerization strategies (Boyer, Bulmus et al. 2009; Matyjaszewski and Tsarevsky 2012). Different naturally occurring polymers like dextrin, cellulose, starch, arginine, proteins, peptides, DNA, RNA, chitosan, polysaccharides, poly (glycolic acid), poly (lactic acid) and hyaluronic acid have been successfully used for polymer-mediated drug delivery systems (Figure 2.3) (Kaur, Sood et al. 2023; Pulapura and Kohn 1992; Heller, Barr et al. 2002; Dechy-Cabaret, Martin-Vaca et al. 2004; Sung and Kim 2020). In this section, we broadly analyze the types of drugs delivered by polymer materials. Table 2.2 summarizes polymeric nanoparticles for their advanced selectivity and target-specific delivery of drugs.

2.2.2.1 Chitosan-Mediated Drug Delivery

Natural chitin-derived chitosan is one of the cationic polysaccharides that offer potential drug delivery vehicles. Chitosan, although it has less mechanical resistance and poor solubility, features enhanced biocompatibility and high target specificity, offering a high therapeutic index to the drugs associated with it (Garg, Chauhan et al. 2019; ur Rehman, Raza et al. 2023). Due to its cationic polymer matrix, chitosan has been used to harvest nano-composites with polyanions for smart drug transportation systems (Sung and Kim 2020). Chitosan is composed of a linear copolymer of glucosamine as well as N-acetyl glucosamine units through β-(1, 4) connections (Figure 2.3). Recent studies reported that chitosan NPs can be used for the delivery of siRNA through the mucosal surface barrier (Garg, Chauhan et al. 2019; Afrin, Geetha Bai et al. 2023).

TABLE 2.1
Liposome and Functionalized Liposome Nanoparticle-Mediated Advanced Drug Delivery

Sl. No.	Biomaterial	Drug Name	Disease Name	Activity	References
1	Liposome NPs	Topotecan	Antineoplastic agent used for the treatment of small-cell lung cancer, ovarian cancer and cervical cancer	Experts reported cytotoxic effects during the S-phase synthesis of DNA. Helps to release topoisomerase I twisting strain in DNA, which induces single-strand breaks in a reversible manner.	(Shaheen, Shakil Ahmed et al. 2006)
2	Conventional liposomes	Doxorubicin/ amphotericin	Used to treat blood, bladder and breast cancer	The therapeutic index of encapsulated doxorubicin has improved in encapsulated amphotericin liposomes, which have been applied for constant discharge of cytarabine.	(Papagiannaros, Hatziantoniou et al. 2006; Ellis, Bernsen et al. 2009)
3	Fusogenic liposomes (FLs)	Doxorubicin	Breast cancer	The transmission of doxorubicin and antibodies to the cytoplasm based on fusogenic liposomes is applied for the treatment of metastatic breast cancer.	(Tian, Nyberg et al. 2015)
4	Immunoliposomes	Doxorubicin and NGR (Asn-Gly-Arg) peptide targeting aminopeptidase	Neuroblastoma (NB) in SCID mice	Immunoliposomes can supply a great extent of 10B atoms into tumor cells to medicate neuroblastoma (NB) in SCID mice.	(Pastorino, Brignole et al. 2003)
5	Cholesterol-based liposomes	Cytarabine	Anticancer	Cholesterol + triolein + DOPC + DPPG shows improved level of drug delivery efficacy.	(Crommelin, van Hoogevest et al. 2020)
6	Cholesterol-based liposomes	Morphine sulfate	Pain control and management	Cholesterol + triolein + DOPC + DPPG shows improved level of drug delivery.	(Peravali, Brock et al. 2014)
7	Cholesterol-based liposomes	Minoxidil	Hair growth help for the treatment of male pattern baldness	α-DPPC + cholesterol enhances the drug-entrapment quantity due to the stability of cholesterol resides into the lipid bilayers.	(Lopez-Pinto, Gonzalez-Rodriguez et al. 2005)
8	Liposome NPs	Cytarabine	Lymphomatous meningitis	Improved level of delivery efficacy	(Wagner, Dullaart et al. 2006; Faraji and Wipf 2009)

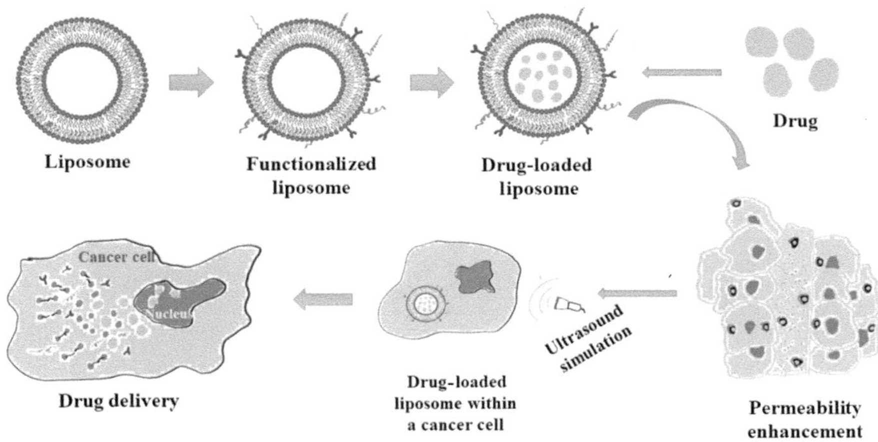

FIGURE 2.2 Mechanism of liposome-mediated anticancer drug delivery systems (Hossen, Hossain et al. 2019).

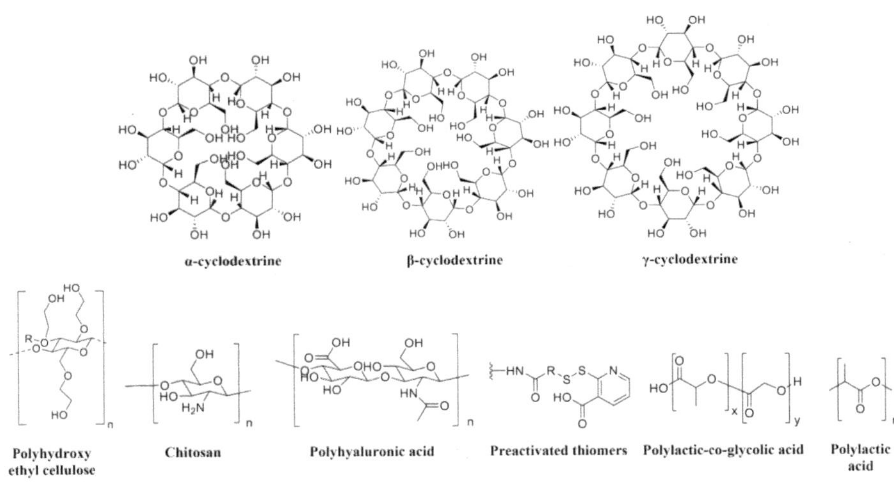

FIGURE 2.3 Polymer materials for enhanced drug delivery.

2.2.2.2 Cyclodextrin Derivative-Mediated Drug Delivery

Cyclodextrins are cyclic oligosaccharides comprising α-(1, 4) connected glucopyranose subunits and provide excellent nano-drug delivery opportunities. Depending upon available subunits, they are termed α, β and γ-cyclodextrins (CDs) comprising 6, 7 and 8 subunits, respectively, as shown in Figure 2.3. Due to their unique cavity size and high solubility, they form host–guest complexes very easily and deliver drugs to the target-specific sites (Manosroi, Apriyani et al. 2005; Karande and Mitragotri 2009; Rajamohan, Ashokkumar et al. 2023). α-CD and γ-CD showed

TABLE 2.2
Polymeric Lipid Hybrid Nanoparticles for Advanced Drug Delivery

Sl. No.	Biomaterial	Drug Name	Disease Name	Activity	References
1	Hydrophobically modified glycol chitosan NPs	Camptothecin	Colorectal and ovarian cancer	Exhibited noticeable anti-tumor properties as well as extraordinary tumor-targeting capabilities	(Nascimento, Singh et al. 2017)
2	Curcumin-loaded folate-modified chitosan NPs	Curcumin	Oxidative and inflammatory conditions, metabolic syndrome, arthritis, anxiety	Used as carriers for targeted therapy to deliver curcumin to cancerous cells	(Esfandiarpour-Boroujeni, Bagheri-Khoulenjani et al. 2017)
3	Poly D,L-lactic-co-glycolic acid (PLGA) NPs	Dexamethasone	Ulcerative colitis, arthritis, lupus, psoriasis, breathing disorders	Function by keeping down the passage of neutrophils and reducing lymphocyte colony proliferation	(Martín-Saldaña, Palao-Suay et al. 2017)
4	Poly(lactide)-tocopheryl polyethylene glycol succinate (PLA-TPGS) NPs	Erlotinib	Small-cell cancers (lung) or progressive metastatic pancreatic cancers	Prevents intracellular phosphorylation of tyrosine kinase with the epidermal growth factor receptor (EGFR)	(Zhou, Kennell et al. 2017)
5	poly D,L-lactic-co-glycolic acid (PLGA) NPs	Bevacizumab	Colorectal cancer, lung cancer, breast cancer, brain cancers	Electively binding circulating VEGF by blocking the binding of VEGF to its cell surface receptors. Thus, inhibition reduces microvascular growth against tumor blood vessels and thereby limits the blood supply to tumor tissues.	(Sousa, Dhaliwal et al. 2019)
6	PLGA-PEG NPs	Paclitaxel	Ovarian, breast, lung, pancreatic and cervical cancers; Kaposi's sarcoma	Paclitaxel targets microtubules. At high concentrations, Paclitaxel causes mitotic arrest at the G2/M phase, whereas at low concentrations, apoptosis is induced at the G0 and G1/S phases.	(Chan, Rhee et al. 2011)
7	PLGA-PEG NPs	Doxorubicin	Cancer of the blood, kidneys, nerves, bladder, breast, ovaries, stomach, lungs, thyroid, bones and soft tissues like muscles	Inhibition of macromolecular biosynthesis occurs from the interaction with DNA by intercalation, thereby inhibiting the progression of topoisomerase II, which is involved in transcription.	(Lv, Li et al. 2013)

enhanced selectivity for cyclosporin due to their aggregation effects (Jóhannsdóttir, Kristinsson et al. 2017). On the other hand, β-CD-maleic anhydride N-isopropyl acrylamide has accelerated the drug delivery of curcumin and doxorubicin hydrochloride for cancer cell targeting (Vickers 2017). Poly-β-CD can be used for the delivery of the antitubercular drug Ethionamide, as poly-β-CD has intrinsic antitubercular activity (Machelart, Salzano et al. 2019).

2.2.2.3 Dendrimers for Drug Delivery

Due to unique properties like lots of branching, globular geometry and high molecular weight, dendrimers are the one of the most promising, newest polymeric drug delivery vehicles (Choudhury, Gohil et al. 2018; Wang, Li et al. 2023). Generally, dendrimers deliver drugs via two different pathways. In the first approach, the drug is physically trapped in the dendrimer matrix by weak van der Waal forces of attraction, while in the second method, the drug is covalently bonded on dendrimers and delivered to the target sites (Chauhan 2018). A folic acid-modified 5.0G PAMAM dendrimer showed selectivity of borneol for targeting glioma diseases (Gauro, Nandave et al. 2021). A 4.0G PAMAM dendrimer showed elevated doxorubicin delivery with target specificity towards tumor cells for glioma treatment (Zhu, Liu et al. 2019).

2.2.2.4 Hydrogels as Drug Nano-Carriers

Hydrogels comprise lightly crosslinked copolymers of N-isopropylacrylamide and methacrylic acid with a specified composition and are suitable to detect minor alterations in blood pH and temperature for the transport of antithrombotic agents like streptokinase or heparin to blood clot sites (Peppas, Vakkalanka et al. 1996). Cholesterol-modified poly(ethylene glycol)–polylactide offers chondrocyte specificity due to its high mechanical strength, suitable pore size and potential adhesion properties, and this hydrogel assists as a valuable chondrocyte transporter (Wang, Feng et al. 2019). A recent study showed that hydrogel nano-sheets can be utilized for multistage drug transport for the active medication of corneal abrasion (Luo, Nguyen et al. 2022).

2.2.2.5 Solid Lipid Nanoparticles as Drug Nano-Carriers

Lipid nanoparticles exhibit important properties such as shape, size, aggregation behaviors and surface structure, making them potential players in the various fields of pharmaceutical science (Müller, Mäder et al. 2000; Mehnert and Mäder 2012; Lingayat, Zarekar et al. 2017). Magnetic nanoparticles are generally coated with organic compounds like fatty acids and polymers to develop biocompatibility and stability (Wu, Fu et al. 2004). In chemotherapy and gene transfer for cancer medication, they have emerged as highly efficient species. Inorganic and organic NPs have some merits and demerits. In order to overcome the demerits of organic and inorganic NPs, scientists have prepared hybrid NPs, which are more efficient in drug delivery, biocompatibility and biodegradability and reduce drug resistance due to the presence of multifunctional carriers (Huang, Xiao et al. 2019; Mottaghitalab, Farokhi et al. 2019). They can enclose both hydrophilic and hydrophobic drugs intended for providing a better remedial effect. Table 2.3 summarizes solid lipid and lipid hybrid nanoparticles for their advanced selectivity and target-specific delivery of drugs.

TABLE 2.3
Polymeric Lipid Hybrid Nanoparticles for Advanced Drug Delivery

Sl. No.	Sub-Sub Type	Drug Name	Disease Name	Activity	References
1	Polystyrene NPs	Polymyxin B	Eye infections, including acute bacterial conjunctivitis and blepharoconjunctivitis	The outer cell membrane of Gram-negative bacteria is disrupted, neutralizing lipopolysaccharides.	(Dubashynskaya and Skorik 2020)
2	Polymeric lipid hybrid nanoparticles (PHLNPs)	Laserphyrin	Pharynx chronic inflammatory disease	Due to photochemical and photophysical reactions between photo sensitizer and specific light, reactive oxygen species induce direct cytotoxicity.	(Bhattacharya 2021)
3	Solid lipid nanoparticles (SLNs)	Camptothecin	Leukemia	Camptothecin combines with topoisomerase I and DNA complex, causing a ternary complex that stabilizes, preventing DNA re-ligation.	(Li, Guo et al. 2014)
4	Solid lipid nanoparticles (SLNs)	Piroxicam	Pain, swelling and stiffness in osteoarthritis	Piroxicam is a potent inhibitor of prostaglandin (PG) synthesis *in vitro*.	(Mohammadi-Samani, Zojaji et al. 2018)

2.3 SYNTHESIS OF BIOMATERIALS

Two different techniques are available for the synthesis of nano-biomaterials. Techniques in which nano-sized materials are derived from their macro-range sources are known as "top-down", while "bottom-up" techniques involve building the NPs starting from single molecules. Generally, "bottom-up" methodologies are followed for the generation of a variety of nano-structured materials like micelles, liposomes, conjugated polymers, vesicles, dendrimers and capsules (Jana and Jana 2022). Polymers are supreme materials, and because of their unique chemical and mechanical characteristics, ease of synthesis and chemical tenability, they are excellent materials for biomedical applications.

2.3.1 Synthesis of Poly(D-Lactic Acid)

Poly(L-lactic acid) (PLLA) and poly(D-lactic acid) (PDLA) are hemi-crystalline and crystalline materials with a consistent chain, while poly(D,L-lactic acid) (PDLLA) exists in an amorphous form, and meso-PLA is attained by the polymerization of meso-lactide. The synthesis of poly(lactic acid) includes direct polymerization and ring-opening polymerization (ROP) (Xiao, Wang et al. 2012), as shown in Figure 2.4. Direct polymerization is less effective, while in the ROP process, D,L-lactide can be catalyzed by bis(trimethyl triazacyclohexane) praseodymium triflate [(Me3TAC)2 Pr(OTf)3](Köhn, Pan et al. 2003).

2.3.2 Synthesis of Liposomes, Vesicles and Micelles

Lipids and surfactant moieties can form supramolecular self-assemblies like liposome, vesicle and micelle NPs (Romero and Moya 2012). The driving force of self-assembly lies in the very low water solubility of the amphiphilic moieties. Normally, concentration, temperature, pH and ionic strength can be tuned to regulate the size and morphology of the micelles (Nelson, Rutledge et al. 1997). Surfactants like sodium dodecyl sulfate and cetyl trimethylammonium bromide form micelles with a hydrophobic chain with a length of 10–20 carbons. Often proteins and lipids can form aggregated micelles by the influence of heat to prepare soluble spherical aggregates

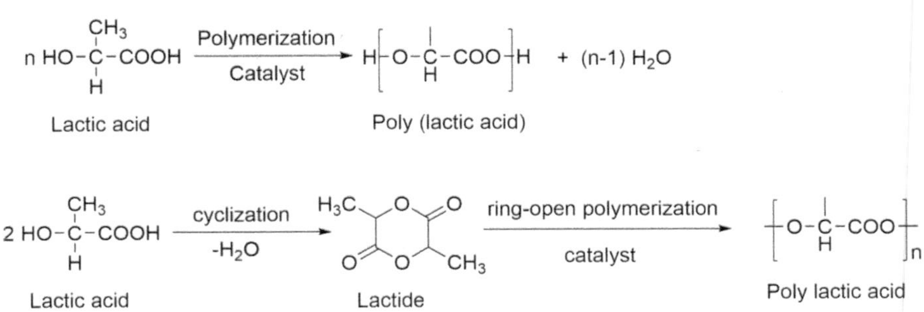

FIGURE 2.4 Poly(lactic acid) synthesis from a polymerization reaction.

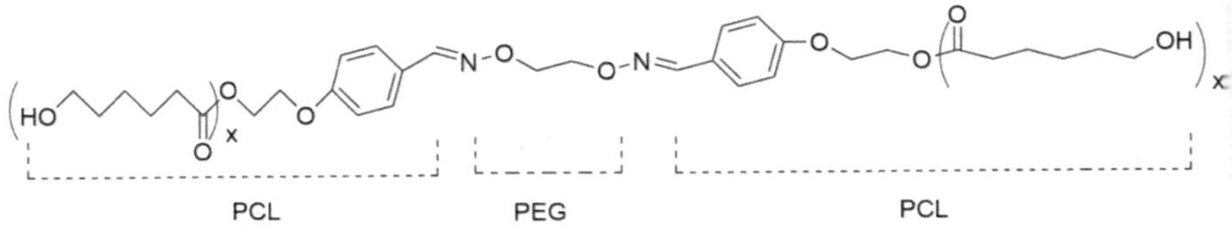

FIGURE 2.5 Structure of the polycaprolactone-oxime-poly(ethylene glycol)-oxime-polycaprolactone polymer.

in carbonate buffer at pH 8.25 (Brault, Kariapper et al. 2002; van Strien, Escalona-Rayo et al. 2023). Matthew B Francis et al. developed a new series of fusion proteins that can be transformed into stable self-assembled micelles of 27 nm in diameter, which can be applied as a drug nano-carrier (Klass, Smith et al. 2019).

Grazu et al. found larger, 146 nm-diameter micelles derived from folate-conjugated, amphiphilic, star-shaped block copolymers of folate-poly(ethylene glycol), poly(L-lactide) and methoxy poly (ethylene glycol) (Jesus and Grazu 2012). Jiao et al. produced amphiphilic block copolymers with the starting materials of methoxy poly (ethylene glycol) (MPEG) and poly(L-alanine) (PALA) coupled with folate to yield a drug nano-carrier that is efficient for tumor-specific paclitaxel drug delivery (Jiao et al. 2011). Recently, aggregation-induced emission (AIE) polymers composed of tetraphenylethene (TPE) and poly (aspartic acid)-block-poly (2-methacryloyloxyethyl phosphorylcholine) were synthesized using redox-sensitive disulfide bonds. These AIE polymer micelles offer *in vivo* imaging, which is tough to achieve using normal fluorescent agents. These micelles can be used for the encapsulation of doxorubicin (Dox) drug without creating many side effects (Hu, Zhuang et al. 2018). Thermosensitive micelles were prepared by Pourjavadi et al. from polylactide-functionalized chitosan. Here, the thermosensitivity of the chitosan polymer was presented by grafting these polymers with acrylamide polymers. Gold nanorods coupled with these micelles exhibited substantial drug discharge, preventing the progression of MCF7 cancer cells (Pourjavadi, Bagherifard et al. 2020). Liu et al. reported flower-like micelles that were built through oxime linkage between polycaprolactone (PCL) in addition to hydrophilic poly(ethylene glycol) (PEG) to produce polycaprolactone-oxime-poly(ethylene glycol)-oxime-polycaprolactone (Figure 2.5). The amphiphilic environment was efficient for drug delivery as well as the sustainable release of doxorubicin with higher-pH medium (Liu, Chen et al. 2014).

2.3.3 Synthesis of Cellulose Biomaterials

Commonly used cellulose materials include hydroxyethylcellulose (HEC), carboxymethylcellulose (CMC), hydroxypropyl methylcellulose (HPMC), cellulose acetate and hydroxypropylcellulose (HPC) (Helenius, Bäckdahl et al. 2006; Hasanin 2022). These cellulose materials are important for the applications of gel-based drug nanocarriers in drug delivery. Capitani et al. reported the synthesis of cellulose hydrogels utilizing CMC and HEC crosslinked with the help of divynilsulphone in a higher-pH

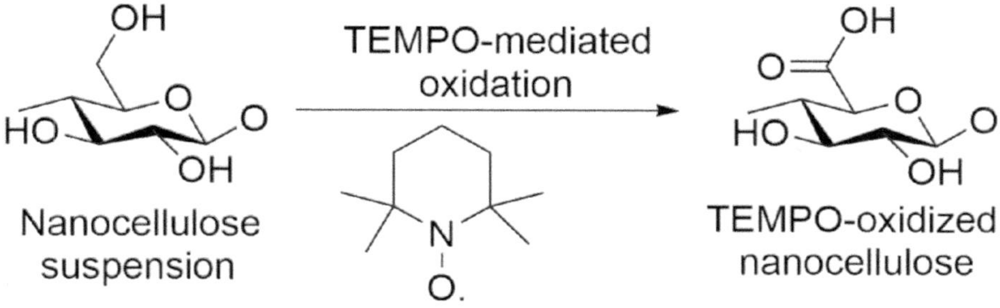

FIGURE 2.6 TEMPO (2,2,6,6-tetramethyl-piperidine-1-oxyl)-mediated oxidation and synthesis of nanocellulose.

region (Capitani, Del Nobile et al. 2000). Microporosity within these materials is achieved by dissolving the polymeric structure into acetone. Subramanian et al. synthesized cellulose nanocrystals (CNCs) by the hydrolysis of formic acid and TEMPO (2,2,6,6-tetramethyl-piperidine-1-oxyl)-facilitated oxidation (Figure 2.6). They also reported that these CNCs were added to different biopolymers like alginate (ALG), gelatin (GEL) and chitosan (CHI) to form different hydrogels. Using thermal gravity analysis, they showed that hydrogels strengthened with CNCs exhibited better thermal strength and miscibility without altering the main structure of the CNCs (Amebaw et al. 2022).

2.3.4 Synthesis of Chitosan Biomaterials

Chitosan NPs have been extensively studied over twenty years. Now a days it has been found that ionic gelation is one of the most powerful preparative techniques for the synthesis of chitosan nanoparticles. The fundamental technique here is established by ionic crosslinking that occurs in the existence of oppositely charged groups, *viz.* negatively charged moieties of the polyanion, that diffuse into positively charged protonated amino groups of chitosan, leading to the formation of nanoparticles (Yanat and Schroën 2021). A similar crosslinking technique is the reversed micelles method, which is based on covalent crosslinking, where the reverse micelle assemblies helped the synthesis of chitosan NPs (Singh, Mittal et al. 2021).

2.3.5 Synthesis of β-Cyclodextrin (CD) Nanoparticles

Feng Gao et al. reported β-cyclodextrin (CD) coupled with N-maleoyl chitosan (CD-g-NMCS) nanoparticles synthesized by ionic gelation from CD- and chitosan-bearing pendant cyclodextrin (CD-g-CS) nanoparticles. They showed that CD-g-NMCS nanoparticles were excellently stable compared to chitosan nanoparticles. Furthermore, they showed that water-insoluble drugs like ketoprofen (KTP) can be delivered with the help of these nano-carriers (Hou et al. 2017). On the other hand, due to its biocompatibility and nontoxic nature, the linear polysaccharide hyaluronic acid (HA) is extensively studied in the biomedical field. Numerous acid and hydroxyl groups existing in the structure of HA moiety make it a perfect material for structure modulation. HA-based hydrogels can be prepared from aqueous mixtures of HA and diverse concentrations of the acid derived from methylvinylether and maleic anhydride copolymer (Larrañeta, Henry et al. 2018). Hyaluronic acid-based hydrogels offer their excellent usage for encapsulating biomolecules, *viz.* small antioxidants and large proteins. The controlled release of these biomolecules can be achieved with the help of enzymatic degradation polymers (Lee, Lee et al. 2019).

2.4 MECHANISMS OF BIOMATERIAL-MEDIATED DRUG DELIVERY

Different nanoparticles applied in drug transportation are built up through "bottom-up" methods, attained by developing or accumulating building subunits. A notable fact is that a significant quantity of nanoparticles are created through the self-assembly of constructing subunits. Different types of noncovalent interactions operate in said processes and provide the strength of resulting nanostructures depending upon the features and structures of the building subunits (Lu, Wang et al. 2016). In the transportation procedure, the passive conveyance of drugs as "cargoes" by nano-vehicles is the most familiar procedure. The attachment of drugs to nano-carriers is accomplished via either chemical conjugation or physical encapsulation. Self-delivery is the other sub-route, which constructs nanostructures with drug molecules. The construction of precise nanostructures with distinctive properties, particularly through the self-assembly method, has been an exceedingly lively area in drug delivery research and assists in the controlled release of the drugs from the nano-carrier (Figure 2.7). Different types of noncovalent interactions, depending upon the structure and characteristics of building blocks, play important parts in the self-assembly procedures and provide the strength of resulting nanostructures. The passive delivery strategy of drugs by nano-carriers as "cargoes" is one of the most popular in the delivery process (Sen et al. 2024; Roy et al. 2022). The physical encapsulation and chemical conjugation are the main binding forces to tie up drugs with nano-carriers (Mondal et al. 2022).

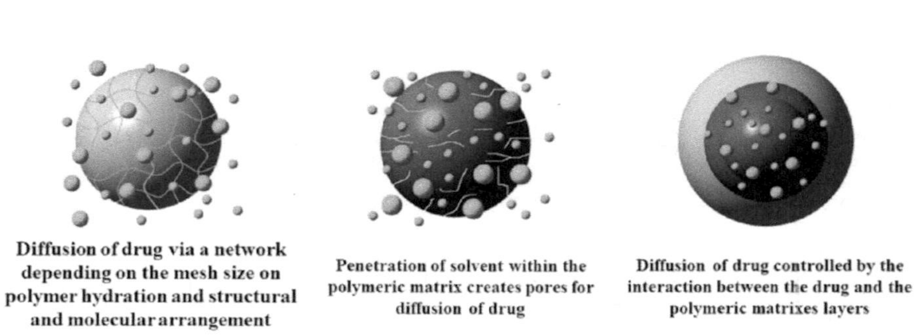

FIGURE 2.7 Sustainable discharge of a drug from a polymer network structure.

2.5 TYPES OF BONDING IN THE SELF-ASSEMBLY OF NANO-CARRIERS

Different nanostructures that are used in the drug transportation procedure are mostly made by self-assembly, a spontaneous route where precise geometries or orientations are built from building subunits (Ghosh et al. 2022). Several significant binding forces operate in the self-assembly process and mainly include noncovalent interactions (Mondal et al. 2022), like, hydrophobic, π–π staking, van der Waals interactions, hydrogen bonding, steric solvation, hydration forces and coordination bonding (Baildya et al. 2023). Various investigations indicate that with respect to covalent interaction, noncovalent interactions are much feebler; they exist mostly in the self-aggregated structure and provides opportunities for drug binding. Nevertheless, noncovalent interactions have the power to impact the complete structures of self-assembled nanostructures, separately or cooperatively.

2.5.1 Hydrophobic Effect

The hydrophobic effect is one of the most significant noncovalent interactions in the self-assembly procedure and is less directional than other noncovalent interactions (Pham, Chokamonsirikun et al. 2021). An extensive variety of constituents for self-assembly are amphiphilic molecules, comprising various synthetic structural subunits and biopolymers like proteins and lipids. The self-assembly of amphiphilic molecules can be promptly accomplished via microphase segregation compelled by thermodynamics due to the simultaneous presence of hydrophilic and hydrophobic parts. In aqueous media, the hydrophobic portions of the constituents will tend to associate with each other to reveal a minimum surface area towards water, whereas the hydrophilic parts try to enhance their relations with water. For example, in amphiphilic diblock copolymers, the nonpolar portion will gather to form a core when the concentration is greater than the critical micelle concentration (CMC), and the polar part expands in water and thus makes a shell around the nonpolar core (Vervald, Laptinskiy et al. 2019).

2.5.2 Electrostatic Interactions

Electrostatic interactions are attractive forces that operate between opposite charges and repulsive forces between like charges of atoms, ions and molecules; they play vital roles in self-assembly procedures. The strength provided through these interactions is about 50–300 kJ/mol, which is the highest among all noncovalent interactions (Faul and Antonietti 2003; Toksoz, Acar et al. 2010). Electrostatic interaction is the main binding force for stable nanoparticles formed from the interaction of cationic polymers with anionic proteins or genes in aqueous solutions (Cha, Kim et al. 2009; Bajpayee and Grodzinsky 2017). Cationic conjugated polymers that are water-soluble can attach to DNA through both ionic and hydrophobic interactions in the transportation of DNA. Sometimes, upon reduction of the hydrophobic effect, electrostatic interaction becomes one of the controlling factors to regulate the attachment between the hydrophilic conjugated polymer and DNA.

2.5.3 Hydrogen Bonds

Hydrogen bonds provide directional noncovalent interactions of two types: one is intermolecular and forms between different molecules, and the other is intramolecular and forms within a single molecule. They can occur in various types of molecules, like inorganic, organic and biomolecules like DNA and peptides (Kuo 2022). For example, hydrogen bonding is the main binding force that occurs between carbonyls and amide groups in the spine of β-sheets during the self-assembly of peptides and develops the strength of the self-assembled nano-carriers (Eckes, Mu et al. 2014). Hydrogen bonds in proper position can control the delivery of drugs to the target sites (Kim, Park et al. 2008; Kim, Lee et al. 2009).

2.5.4 π–π Stacking

π–π stacking plays a crucial role in building self-assembled nanostructures containing a π–conjugate system and provides their stability (Mao, Zhang et al. 2023; Sharma et al. 2023). It is much weaker (0–50 kJ/mol) and less directional than other noncovalent interactions. In case of the self-assembly process of diphenylalanine (FF), the π–π stacking of phenyl groups and hydrogen bonding are the main binding forces to form the stable self-assembled diphenylalanine (FF) nanostructures (Dinesh, Squillaci et al. 2015; Zhuang, Wang et al. 2019). Nevertheless, methotrexate could not build a polymeric structure because of the lack of hydrogen bonds.

The efficacy of drug delivery, including drug transportation and release at a suitable site, depends on many external parameters such temperature, pH of the medium and the nature of the solvent medium. Knowledge about the nature of the drug, nano-carrier and the binding force operating between them is very much essential to control the drug delivery process properly (Mondal et al 2022). In summary, a complete understanding of different noncovalent interactions is very important to manage these self-assembled nanostructures for successful drug delivery.

2.6 FUTURE PROSPECTS AND LIMITATIONS

In spite of the versatility and enormous potential of drug nano-carriers, there are some disadvantages regarding their toxicity, size, shape, synthesis, physical instability, aggregation, electromagnetic properties, solubility, surface chemistry and biodegradability aspects that can lead to problems in proper administration and storage (Khalaf, Alinejad et al. 2023; Taheri-Ledari, Tarinsun et al. 2023). The shape of most of nano-carriers is spherical, although different shapes can be provided during their synthesis. They can interact with living cells continuously, which could affect humans and animals adversely (San Anselmo Jarauta, Serrano Ostáriz et al. 2023; Cho, Wang et al. 2008). A novel approach, particle replication in no wetting templates (PRINT), has been under investigation to counter this problem. The PRINT method involves the production of uniform polymeric nanoparticles, which provide stability of size and shape and also allow customization such that the encapsulated-drug delivery process could be tailored as well (Saadli, Braunmiller et al. 2023). The application of biocompatible coatings on nanoparticles is a significant endeavor to minimize the toxicological effects (Bazi Alahri, Jibril Ibrahim et al. 2023). The future success of nanoparticle based drug delivery requires active collaborations among chemists, clinicians and bioengineers.

2.7 CONCLUSION

In this chapter, we have analyzed different prospects of drug nano-carriers used in advanced drug delivery systems. Innovative drug delivery systems not only diminish the side effects of drugs but also increase the carrier efficiency to deliver drugs to the target sites. Furthermore, changes in drug carrier morphology and hybrid nanostructure are beneficial to overcome limitations like poor target specificity, organ toxicity, solubility, biocompatibility and biodegradability issues. In this regard, advanced synthesis of polymeric, self-assembled, hydrogel nano-biomaterials should be emphasized for the controlled delivery and sustainable discharge of drugs to the target site while simultaneously minimizing their toxic and harmful effects to the body. Advances in biomaterial synthesis and applications will invite very safe and effective next-generation drug delivery strategies.

REFERENCES

Abdelaziz, H. M., M. Gaber, M. M. Abd-Elwakil, M. T. Mabrouk, M. M. Elgohary, N. M. Kamel, D. M. Kabary, M. S. Freag, M. W. Samaha and S. M. Mortada (2018). "Inhalable particulate drug delivery systems for lung cancer therapy: Nanoparticles, microparticles, nanocomposites and nanoaggregates." *Journal of Controlled Release* **269**: 374–392.

Adeosun, S. O., M. O. Ilomuanya, O. P. Gbenebor, M. O. Dada and C. C. Odili (2020). "Biomaterials for drug delivery: Sources, classification, synthesis, processing, and applications." *Advanced Functional Materials*: 141–167.

Afrin, H., R. Geetha Bai, R. Kumar, S. S. Ahmad, S. K. Agarwal and M. Nurunnabi (2023). "Oral delivery of RNAi for cancer therapy." *Cancer and Metastasis Reviews*: 1–26.

Aleku, M., P. Schulz, O. Keil, A. Santel, U. Schaeper, B. Dieckhoff, O. Janke, J. Endruschat, B. Durieux and N. Röder (2008). "Atu027, a liposomal small interfering RNA formulation targeting protein kinase N3, inhibits cancer progression." *Cancer Research* **68**(23): 9788–9798.

Amebaw, E., N. Sultan, E. Masrie, T. Argu, A. Ahmed and A. P. Rajan (2022). "Hydrogel synthesis from cellulose derivatives obtained from Yushania alpina bamboo for wound dressing applications." *Seybold Report* **11** (17): 2818.

Bajpayee, A. G. and A. J. Grodzinsky (2017). "Cartilage-targeting drug delivery: Can electrostatic interactions help?" *Nature Reviews Rheumatology* **13**(3): 183–193.

Baildya, N., S. Mazumdar, N. K. Mridha, A. P. Chattopadhyay, A. A. Khan, T. Dutta, M. Mandal, S. K. Chowdhury, R. Reza, and N. N. Ghosh (2023). "Comparative study of the efficiency of silicon carbide, boron nitride and carbon nanotube to deliver cancerous drug, azacitidine: A DFT study." *Computers in Biology and Medicine* **154**: 106593.

Bangham, A. D. and R. Horne (1964). "Negative staining of phospholipids and their structural modification by surface-active agents as observed in the electron microscope." *Journal of Molecular Biology* **8**(5): 660–668.

Barua, M. (2014). "Challenges associated with penetration of nanoparticles across cell and tissue barriers: A review of current status and future prospects." *Nano Today* **9**: 223–243.

Bazi Alahri, M., A. Jibril Ibrahim, M. Barani, H. Arkaban, S. M. Shadman, S. Salarpour, P. Zarrintaj, J. Jaberi and A. Turki Jalil (2023). "Management of brain cancer and neurodegenerative disorders with polymer-based nanoparticles as a biocompatible platform." *Molecules* **28**(2): 841.

Bhattacharya, S. (2021). "Methotrexate-loaded polymeric lipid hybrid nanoparticles (PLHNPs): A reliable drug delivery system for the treatment of glioblastoma." *Journal of Experimental Nanoscience* **16**(1): 344–367.

Boyer, C., V. Bulmus, T. P. Davis, V. Ladmiral, J. Liu and S. Perrier (2009). "Bioapplications of RAFT polymerization." *Chemical Reviews* **109**(11): 5402–5436.

Brault, P.-A., M. S. Kariapper, C. V. Pham, R. A. Flowers, W. T. Gunning, P. Shah and M. O. Funk (2002). "Protein micelles from lipoxygenase 3." *Biomacromolecules* **3**(4): 649–654.

Capitani, D., M. A. Del Nobile, G. Mensitieri, A. Sannino and A. L. Segre (2000). "13C solid-state NMR determination of cross-linking degree in superabsorbing cellulose-based networks." *Macromolecules* **33**(2): 430–437.

Cha, E.-J., J. E. Kim and C.-H. Ahn (2009). "Stabilized polymeric micelles by electrostatic interactions for drug delivery system." *European Journal of Pharmaceutical Sciences* **38**(4): 341–346.

Chan, J. M., J.-W. Rhee, C. L. Drum, R. T. Bronson, G. Golomb, R. Langer and O. C. Farokhzad (2011). "In vivo prevention of arterial restenosis with paclitaxel-encapsulated targeted lipid–polymeric nanoparticles." *Proceedings of the National Academy of Sciences* **108**(48): 19347–19352.

Chauhan, A. S. (2018). "Dendrimers for drug delivery." *Molecules* **23**(4): 938.

Cho, K., X. Wang, S. Nie, Z. Chen and D. M. Shin (2008). "Therapeutic nanoparticles for drug delivery in cancer." *Clinical Cancer Research* **14**(5): 1310–1316.

Choudhury, R. R., J. M. Gohil, S. Mohanty and S. K. Nayak (2018). "Antifouling, fouling release and antimicrobial materials for surface modification of reverse osmosis and nanofiltration membranes." *Journal of Materials Chemistry A* **6**(2): 313–333.

Crommelin, D. J., P. van Hoogevest and G. Storm (2020). "The role of liposomes in clinical nanomedicine development. What now? Now what?" *Journal of Controlled Release* **318**: 256–263.

Dang, Y. and J. Guan (2020). "Nanoparticle-based drug delivery systems for cancer therapy." *Smart Materials in Medicine* **1**: 10–19.

Dechy-Cabaret, O., B. Martin-Vaca and D. Bourissou (2004). "Controlled ring-opening polymerization of lactide and glycolide." *Chemical Reviews* **104**(12): 6147–6176.

De Jong, W. H. (2008). "Paul JA borm-drug delivery and nanoparticles: Application and hazards." *International Journal of Nanomedicine* **3**(2): 133–149.

Dinesh, B., M. A. Squillaci, C. Ménard-Moyon, P. Samorì and A. Bianco (2015). "Self-assembly of diphenylalanine backbone homologues and their combination with functionalized carbon nanotubes." *Nanoscale* **7**(38): 15873–15879.

Dubashynskaya, N. V. and Y. A. Skorik (2020). "Polymyxin delivery systems: Recent advances and challenges." *Pharmaceuticals* **13**(5): 83.

Eckes, K. M., X. Mu, M. A. Ruehle, P. Ren and L. J. Suggs (2014). "β Sheets not required: Combined experimental and computational studies of self-assembly and gelation of the ester-containing analogue of an Fmoc-dipeptide hydrogelator." *Langmuir* **30**(18): 5287–5296.

Ellis, M., R. Bernsen, H. Ali-Zadeh, J. Kristensen, U. Hedström, L. Poughias, M. Bresnik, A. Al-Essa and D. A. Stevens (2009). "A safety and feasibility study comparing an intermittent high dose with a daily standard dose of liposomal amphotericin B for persistent neutropenic fever." *Journal of Medical Microbiology* **58**(11): 1474–1485.

Esfandiarpour-Boroujeni, S., S. Bagheri-Khoulenjani, H. Mirzadeh and S. Amanpour (2017). "Fabrication and study of curcumin loaded nanoparticles based on folate-chitosan for breast cancer therapy application." *Carbohydrate Polymers* **168**: 14–21.

Etheridge, M. L., S. A. Campbell, A. G. Erdman, C. L. Haynes, S. M. Wolf and J. McCullough (2013). "The big picture on nanomedicine: The state of investigational and approved nanomedicine products." *Nanomedicine: Nanotechnology, Biology and Medicine* **9**(1): 1–14.

Faraji, A. H. and P. Wipf (2009). "Nanoparticles in cellular drug delivery." *Bioorganic & Medicinal Chemistry* **17**(8): 2950–2962.

Faul, C. F. and M. Antonietti (2003). "Ionic self-assembly: Facile synthesis of supramolecular materials." *Advanced Materials* **15**(9): 673–683.

Feng, S.-S., W. Zeng, Y. Teng Lim, L. Zhao, K. Yin Win, R. Oakley, S. Hin Teoh, R. C. Hang Lee and S. Pan (2007). "Vitamin E TPGS-emulsified poly (lactic-co-glycolic acid) nanoparticles for cardiovascular restenosis treatment." *Nanomedicine (Lond)* **2**(3): 333–344.

Fenton, O. S., K. N. Olafson, P. S. Pillai, M. J. Mitchell and R. Langer (2018). "Advances in biomaterials for drug delivery." *Advanced Materials* ***30***(29), 1705328.

Garg, U., S. Chauhan, U. Nagaich and N. Jain (2019). "Current advances in chitosan nanoparticles based drug delivery and targeting." *Advanced Pharmaceutical Bulletin* **9**(2): 195.

Gauro, R., M. Nandave, V. K. Jain and K. Jain (2021). "Advances in dendrimer-mediated targeted drug delivery to the brain." *Journal of Nanoparticle Research* **23**(3): 1–20.

Ghosh, A., S. K. Dubey, M. Patra, J. Mandal, N. N. Ghosh, P. Das, A. Bhowmick, K. Sarkar, S. Mukherjee, R. Saha and S. Bhattacharjee (2022). "Solvent- and substrate-induced chiroptical inversion in amphiphilic, biocompatible glycoconjugate supramolecules: Shape-persistent gelation, self-healing, and antibacterial activity." *Chemistry–A European Journal* **28**(63): e202201621.

Gordon, A., D. Schneider, J. Wilson, O. Bodansky, E. H. Cooper, J. Brachet and G. Brewer (1975). "Vol. 1. Plenum Press; London and New York, 1974. viii+ 316 pp. $28.90. Reviewed in: Nature, 12.6. 75,255, 566." *FEBS Letters*.

Hasanin, M. S. (2022). "Cellulose-based biomaterials: Chemistry and biomedical applications." *Starch-Stärke* **74**(7–8): 2200060.

Helenius, G., H. Bäckdahl, A. Bodin, U. Nannmark, P. Gatenholm and B. Risberg (2006). "In vivo biocompatibility of bacterial cellulose." *Journal of Biomedical Materials Research Part A: An Official Journal of the Society for Biomaterials, the Japanese Society for Biomaterials, and the Australian Society for Biomaterials and the Korean Society for Biomaterials* **76**(2): 431–438.

Heller, J., J. Barr, S. Y. Ng, K. S. Abdellauoi and R. Gurny (2002). "Poly (ortho esters): Synthesis, characterization, properties and uses." *Advanced Drug Delivery Reviews* **54**(7): 1015–1039.

Hissa, B., P. W. Oakes, B. Pontes, R.-S. Juan and M. L. Gardel (2017). "Cholesterol depletion impairs contractile machinery in neonatal rat cardiomyocytes." *Scientific Reports* **7**(1): 1–15.

Hosseini, S. M., J. Mohammadnejad, R. Najafi-Taher, Z. B. Zadeh, M. Tanhaei and S. Ramakrishna (2023). "Multifunctional carbon-based nanoparticles: Theranostic applications in cancer therapy and diagnosis." *ACS Applied Bio Materials* **6**(4): 1323–1338.

Hossen, S., M. K. Hossain, M. Basher, M. Mia, M. Rahman and M. J. Uddin (2019). "Smart nanocarrier-based drug delivery systems for cancer therapy and toxicity studies: A review." *Journal of Advanced Research* **15**: 1–18.

Hou, X., W. Zhang, M. He, Y. Lu, K. Lou and F. Gao (2017). "Preparation and characterization of β-cyclodextrin grafted N-maleoyl chitosan nanoparticles for drug delivery." *Asian Journal of Pharmaceutical Sciences* **12**(6): 558–568.

Hu, J., W. Zhuang, B. Ma, X. Su, T. Yu, G. Li, Y. Hu and Y. Wang (2018). "Redox-responsive biomimetic polymeric micelle for simultaneous anticancer drug delivery and aggregation-induced emission active imaging." *Bioconjugate Chemistry* **29**(6): 1897–1910.

Huang, W., Y. Xiao and X. Shi (2019). "Construction of electrospun organic/inorganic hybrid nanofibers for drug delivery and tissue engineering applications." *Advanced Fiber Materials* **1**(1): 32–45.

Huang, Z. R., S. C. Hua, Y. L. Yang and J. Y. Fang (2008). "Development and evaluation of lipid nanoparticles for camptothecin delivery: A comparison of solid lipid nanoparticles, nanostructured lipid carriers, and lipid emulsion." *Acta Pharmacologica Sinica* **29**(9): 1094–1102.

Jabbar, A. M., R. M. Ibrahim and A. A. Hussein (2022). "Antitumor activity of hesperidin extracted from citrus limon." *HIV Nursing* **22**(2): 327–330.

Jana, S. and S. Jana (2022). *Functional Biomaterials: Drug Delivery and Biomedical Applications*, Springer Nature.

Jesus, M. and V. Grazu (2012). *Nanobiotechnology: Inorganic Nanoparticles vs Organic Nanoparticles*, Elsevier.

Jia, W., Y. Han, X. Mao, W. Xu and Y. Zhang (2022). "Nanotechnology strategies for hepatocellular carcinoma diagnosis and treatment." *RSC Advances* **12**(48): 31068–31082.

Jiao, Z., X. Wang and Z. Chen (2011). "Folate-conjugated methoxy poly (ethylene glycol)/poly (L-Alanine) amphiphilic block copolymeric micelles for targeted delivery of paclitaxel." *Drug Delivery* **18**(7): 478–484.

Jóhannsdóttir, S., J. K. Kristinsson, Z. Fülöp, G. Ásgrímsdóttir, E. Stefánsson and T. Loftsson (2017). "Formulations and toxicologic in vivo studies of aqueous cyclosporin A eye drops with cyclodextrin nanoparticles." *International Journal of Pharmaceutics* **529**(1–2): 486–490.

Kadian, R. (2018). "Nanoparticles: A promising drug delivery approach." *Asian Journal of Pharmaceutical and Clinical Research* **11**(1): 30–35.

Kagdada, H. L., A. K. Bhojani and D. K. Singh (2023). "An overview of nanomaterials: History, fundamentals, and applications." *Nanomaterials*: 1–26.

Karande, P. and S. Mitragotri (2009). "Enhancement of transdermal drug delivery via synergistic action of chemicals." *Biochimica et Biophysica Acta (BBA)-Biomembranes* **1788**(11): 2362–2373.

Kaur, M., A. Sood and R. Gupta (2023). "Biobased materials in drug delivery." In *Advanced Applications of Biobased Materials*, Elsevier: 409–445.

Khalaf, M. M., S. S. Alinejad, O. Sajad and B. K. A. Rasool (2023). "Gastro-retentive drug delivery technologies and their applications with cardiovascular medications." *Journal of Population Therapeutics and Clinical Pharmacology* **30**(5): 1–19.

Kim, B.-S., H.-I. Lee, Y. Min, Z. Poon and P. T. Hammond (2009). "Hydrogen-bonded multilayer of pH-responsive polymeric micelles with tannic acid for surface drug delivery." *Chemical Communications* **28**: 4194–4196.

Kim, B.-S., S. W. Park and P. T. Hammond (2008). "Hydrogen-bonding layer-by-layer-assembled biodegradable polymeric micelles as drug delivery vehicles from surfaces." *ACS Nano* **2**(2): 386–392.

Kinning, D. J. and E. L. Thomas (1984). "Hard-sphere interactions between spherical domains in diblock copolymers." *Macromolecules* **17**(9): 1712–1718.

Klass, S. H., M. J. Smith, T. A. Fiala, J. P. Lee, A. O. Omole, B.-G. Han, K. H. Downing, S. Kumar and M. B. Francis (2019). "Self-assembling micelles based on an intrinsically disordered protein domain." *Journal of the American Chemical Society* **141**(10): 4291–4299.

Köhn, R. D., Z. Pan, J. Sun and C. Liang (2003). "Ring-opening polymerization of D, L-lactide with bis (trimethyl triazacyclohexane) praseodymium triflate." *Catalysis Communications* **4**(1): 33–37.

Kuo, S. W. (2022). "Hydrogen bonding mediated self-assembled structures from block copolymer mixtures to mesoporous materials." *Polymer International* **71**(4): 393–410.

Langasco, R., B. Cadeddu, M. Formato, A. J. Lepedda, M. Cossu, P. Giunchedi, R. Pronzato, G. Rassu, R. Manconi and E. Gavini (2017). "Natural collagenic skeleton of marine sponges in pharmaceutics: Innovative biomaterial for topical drug delivery." *Materials Science and Engineering: C* **70**: 710–720.

Larrañeta, E., M. Henry, N. J. Irwin, J. Trotter, A. A. Perminova and R. F. Donnelly (2018). "Synthesis and characterization of hyaluronic acid hydrogels crosslinked using a solvent-free process for potential biomedical applications." *Carbohydrate Polymers* **181**: 1194–1205.

Lee, S., Y. Lee, E.-M. Kim, K. W. Nam and I. Choi (2019). "Aqueous-phase synthesis of hyaluronic acid-based hydrogel nanoparticles for molecular storage and enzymatic release." *ACS Applied Polymer Materials* **2**(2): 342–350.

Li, J., X. Guo, Z. Liu, C. I. Okeke, N. Li, H. Zhao, M. O. Aggrey, W. Pan and T. Wu (2014). "Preparation and evaluation of charged solid lipid nanoparticles of tetrandrine for ocular drug delivery system: Pharmacokinetics, cytotoxicity and cellular uptake studies." *Drug Development and Industrial Pharmacy* **40**(7): 980–987.

Li, L. and Y. Shen (2009). "Overcoming obstacles to develop effective and safe siRNA therapeutics." *Expert Opinion on Biological Therapy* **9**(5): 609–619.

Lingayat, V. J., N. S. Zarekar and R. S. Shendge (2017). "Solid lipid nanoparticles: A review." *Nanoscience and Nanotechnology Research* **4**(2): 67–72.

Liu, B., H. Chen, X. Li, C. Zhao, Y. Liu, L. Zhu, H. Deng, J. Li, G. Li and F. Guo (2014). "pH-responsive flower-like micelles constructed via oxime linkage for anticancer drug delivery." *RSC Advances* **4**(90): 48943–48951.

Lopez-Pinto, J., M. Gonzalez-Rodriguez and A. Rabasco (2005). "Effect of cholesterol and ethanol on dermal delivery from DPPC liposomes." *International Journal of Pharmaceutics* **298**(1): 1–12.

Lu, H., J. Wang, T. Wang, J. Zhong, Y. Bao and H. Hao (2016). "Recent progress on nanostructures for drug delivery applications." *Journal of Nanomaterials* **2016**.

Luo, L.-J., D. D. Nguyen, C.-C. Huang and J.-Y. Lai (2022). "Therapeutic hydrogel sheets programmed with multistage drug delivery for effective treatment of corneal abrasion." *Chemical Engineering Journal* **429**: 132409.

Lv, S., M. Li, Z. Tang, W. Song, H. Sun, H. Liu and X. Chen (2013). "Doxorubicin-loaded amphiphilic polypeptide-based nanoparticles as an efficient drug delivery system for cancer therapy." *Acta Biomaterialia* **9**(12): 9330–9342.

Machelart, A., G. Salzano, X. Li, A. Demars, A.-S. Debrie, M. Menendez-Miranda, E. Pancani, S. Jouny, E. Hoffmann and N. Deboosere (2019). "Intrinsic antibacterial activity of nanoparticles made of β-cyclodextrins potentiates their effect as drug nanocarriers against tuberculosis." *ACS Nano* **13**(4): 3992–4007.

Manosroi, J., M. G. Apriyani, K. Foe and A. Manosroi (2005). "Enhancement of the release of azelaic acid through the synthetic membranes by inclusion complex formation with hydroxypropyl-β-cyclodextrin." *International Journal of Pharmaceutics* **293**(1–2): 235–240.

Mao, Y., Y. Zhang, Y. Yu, N. Zhu, X. Zhou, G. Li, Q. Yi and Y. Wu (2023). "Self-assembled supramolecular immunomagnetic nanoparticles through π–π stacking strategy for circulating tumor cells enrichment." *Regenerative Biomaterials*: rbad016.

Martín-Saldaña, S., R. Palao-Suay, M. R. Aguilar, R. Ramírez-Camacho and J. San Román (2017). "Polymeric nanoparticles loaded with dexamethasone or α-tocopheryl succinate to prevent cisplatin-induced ototoxicity." *Acta Biomaterialia* **53**: 199–210.

Matyjaszewski, K. and N. Tsarevsky (2012). "Atom transfer radical polymerization (ATRP): Current status and future perspectives." *Macromolecules* **45**: 4015–4039.

Mayer, L. D. and A. S. Janoff (2007). "Optimizing combination chemotherapy by controlling drug ratios." *Molecular Interventions* **7**(4): 216.

Mehnert, W. and K. Mäder (2012). "Solid lipid nanoparticles: Production, characterization and applications." *Advanced Drug Delivery Reviews* **64**: 83–101.

Mohammadi-Samani, S., S. Zojaji and E. Entezar-Almahdi (2018). "Piroxicam loaded solid lipid nanoparticles for topical delivery: Preparation, characterization and in vitro permeation assessment." *Journal of Drug Delivery Science and Technology* **47**: 427–433.

Mondal, M., S. Basak, D. Roy, M. S. Haydar, S. Choudhury, B. Ghosh, N. N. Ghosh, A. Dutta, P. Mandal, K. Roy, and A. Kumar (2022). "Probing the molecular assembly of a metabolizer drug with β-cyclodextrin and its binding with CT-DNA in augmenting antibacterial activity and photostability by physicochemical and computational methodologies. *ACS Omega* **7**(30): 26211–26225.

Mondal, M., S. Basak, S. Ali, D. Roy, S. Saha, B. Ghosh, N. N. Ghosh, K. Lepcha, K. Roy, and M. N. Roy (2022). Exploring inclusion complex of an anti-cancer drug (6-MP) with β-cyclodextrin and its binding with CT-DNA for innovative applications in antibacterial activity and photostability optimized by computational study. *RSC Advances* **12**(48): 30936–30951.

Mondal, M., S. Basak, D. Roy, S. Saha, B. Ghosh, S. Ali, N. N. Ghosh, A. Dutta, A. Kumar and M. N. Roy (2022). "Cyclic oligosaccharides as controlled release complexes with food additives (TZ) for reducing hazardous effects." *Journal of Molecular Liquids* **348**: 118429.

Mottaghitalab, F., M. Farokhi, Y. Fatahi, F. Atyabi and R. Dinarvand (2019). "New insights into designing hybrid nanoparticles for lung cancer: Diagnosis and treatment." *Journal of Controlled Release* **295**: 250–267.

Müller, R. H., K. Mäder and S. Gohla (2000). "Solid lipid nanoparticles (SLN) for controlled drug delivery–a review of the state of the art." *European Journal of Pharmaceutics and Biopharmaceutics* **50**(1): 161–177.

Nakhaei, P., R. Margiana, D. O. Bokov, W. K. Abdelbasset, M. A. Jadidi Kouhbanani, R. S. Varma, F. Marofi, M. Jarahian and N. Beheshtkhoo (2021). "Liposomes: Structure, biomedical applications, and stability parameters with emphasis on cholesterol." *Frontiers in Bioengineering and Biotechnology*: 748.

Nascimento, A. V., A. Singh, H. Bousbaa, D. Ferreira, B. Sarmento and M. M. Amiji (2017). "Overcoming cisplatin resistance in non-small cell lung cancer with Mad2 silencing siRNA delivered systemically using EGFR-targeted chitosan nanoparticles." *Acta Biomaterialia* **47**: 71–80.

Nelson, P. H., G. C. Rutledge and T. A. Hatton (1997). "On the size and shape of self-assembled micelles." *The Journal of Chemical Physics* **107**(24): 10777–10781.

Papagiannaros, A., S. Hatziantoniou, K. Dimas, G. T. Papaioannou and C. Demetzos (2006). "A liposomal formulation of doxorubicin, composed of hexadecylphosphocholine (HePC): Physicochemical characterization and cytotoxic activity against human cancer cell lines." *Biomedicine & Pharmacotherapy* **60**(1): 36–42.

Pastorino, F., C. Brignole, D. Marimpietri, M. Cilli, C. Gambini, D. Ribatti, R. Longhi, T. M. Allen, A. Corti and M. Ponzoni (2003). "Vascular damage and anti-angiogenic effects of tumor vessel-targeted liposomal chemotherapy." *Cancer Research* **63**(21): 7400–7409.

Peppas, N. A., S. Vakkalanka, C. S. Brazel, A. S. Luttrell and N. K. Mongia (1996). "Controlled release systems using swellable random and block copolymers and terpolymers." In *Advanced Biomaterials in Biomedical Engineering and Drug Delivery Systems*, Springer: 3–7.

Peravali, R., R. Brock, E. Bright, P. Mills, D. Petty and J. Alberts (2014). "Enhancing the enhanced recovery program in colorectal surgery-use of extended-release epidural morphine (DepoDur®)." *Annals of Coloproctology* **30**(4): 186.

Pham, D. T., A. Chokamonsirikun, V. Phattaravorakarn and W. Tiyaboonchai (2021). "Polymeric micelles for pulmonary drug delivery: A comprehensive review." *Journal of Materials Science* **56**: 2016–2036.

Pourjavadi, A., M. Bagherifard and M. Doroudian (2020). "Synthesis of micelles based on chitosan functionalized with gold nanorods as a light sensitive drug delivery vehicle." *International Journal of Biological Macromolecules* **149**: 809–818.

Pulapur.

Rajamohan, R., S. Ashokkumar, S. Ramasundaram and Y. R. Lee (2023). "Development of non-toxic and water-soluble nanofibers from oseltamivir in the presence of cyclodextrins for drug release." *Journal of Molecular Liquids* **371**: 121141.

Rastogi, A., Tripathi, D. K., Yadav, S., Chauhan, D., K. Živčák, M., Ghorbanpour, M., El-Sheery, N.,I., and Brestic, M (2019). "Application of silicon nanoparticles in agriculture". *3 Biotech*. Mar; **9**: 1–1.

Rezaei, R., M. Safaei, H. R. Mozaffari, H. Moradpoor, S. Karami, A. Golshah, B. Salimi and H. Karami (2019). "The role of nanomaterials in the treatment of diseases and their effects on the immune system." *Open Access Macedonian Journal of Medical Sciences* 7(11): 1884.

Roy, A., R. Das, D. Roy, S. Saha, N. N. Ghosh, S. Bhattacharyya, and M. N. Roy. (2022). Encapsulated hydroxychloroquine and chloroquine into cyclic oligosaccharides are the potential therapeutics for COVID-19: Insights from first-principles calculations. *Journal of Molecular Structure* **1247**: 131371.

Romero, G. and S. E. Moya (2012). "Synthesis of organic nanoparticles." *Frontiers of Nanoscience* **4**: 115–141.

Ruskowitz, E. R. and C. A. DeForest (2018). "Photoresponsive biomaterials for targeted drug delivery and 4D cell culture." *Nature Reviews Materials* **3**(2): 1–17.

Saadli, M., D. L. Braunmiller, A. Mourran and J. J. Crassous (2023). "Thermally and magnetically programmable hydrogel microactuators." *Small*: 2207035.

San Anselmo Jarauta, M., J. L. Serrano Ostáriz and S. Hernández Ainsa (2023). "Novel dendritic multifunctional nanocarriers and their application in biomedicine." Universidad de Zaragoza, 2021.

Sharma, A., Bomzan, P., Roy, D., Chhetri, A., Choudhury, S., Ghosh, N.N., Ali, S., Bk, P., Ghosh, S., Dutta, A. and Kumar, A., 2023. Molecular Assembly of Rhodanine with Torus-Shaped Cyclodextrins and Their Innovative Applications by Physicochemical Contrivance Simultaneously Optimized by Computational Study. ChemistrySelect, 8(11), p.e202300417.

Sen, S., N. Baildya, M. Alphonse-Mendoza, B. Singh, S. Chakraborty, N. Nath Ghosh, and G. Biswas. "Experimental and theoretical study on supramolecular encapsulation of molnupiravir by Cucurbit [7] uril: A potential formulating agent for COVID-19." *Journal of Molecular Liquids* (2023): 123877.

Shaheen, S. M., F. Shakil Ahmed, M. N. Hossen, M. Ahmed, M. S. Amran and M. Ul-Islam (2006). "Liposome as a carrier for advanced drug delivery." *Pakistan Journal of Biological Sciences* **9**(6): 1181–1191.

Shelley, H. and R. J. Babu (2018). "Role of cyclodextrins in nanoparticle-based drug delivery systems." *Journal of Pharmaceutical Sciences* **107**(7): 1741–1753.

Singh, A., A. Mittal and S. Benjakul (2021). "Chitosan nanoparticles: Preparation, food applications and health benefits." *Science Asia* **47**: 1–10.

Sousa, F., H. K. Dhaliwal, F. Gattacceca, B. Sarmento and M. M. Amiji (2019). "Enhanced anti-angiogenic effects of bevacizumab in glioblastoma treatment upon intranasal administration in polymeric nanoparticles." *Journal of Controlled Release* **309**: 37–47.

Sung, Y. K. and S. W. Kim (2020). "Recent advances in polymeric drug delivery systems." *Biomaterials Research* **24**(1): 1–12.

Taheri-Ledari, R., N. Tarinsun, F. Sadat Qazi, L. Heidari, M. Saeidirad, F. Ganjali, F. Ansari, F. Hassanzadeh-Afruzi and A. Maleki (2023). "Vancomycin-loaded Fe3O4/MOF-199 core/shell cargo encapsulated by guanidylated– β-cyclodextrine: An effective antimicrobial nanotherapeutic." *Inorganic Chemistry* **62**(6): 2530–2547.

Tautzenberger, A., A. Kovtun and A. Ignatius (2012). "Nanoparticles and their potential for application in bone." *International Journal of Nanomedicine* **7**: 4545.

Tian, X., S. Nyberg, P. S. Sharp, J. Madsen, N. Daneshpour, S. P. Armes, J. Berwick, M. Azzouz, P. Shaw and N. J. Abbott (2015). "LRP-1-mediated intracellular antibody delivery to the Central Nervous System." *Scientific Reports* **5**(1): 1–14.

Tiwari, G., R. Tiwari, B. Sriwastawa, L. Bhati, S. Pandey, P. Pandey and S. K. Bannerjee (2012). "Drug delivery systems: An updated review." *International Journal of Pharmaceutical Investigation* **2**(1): 2.

Toksoz, S., H. Acar and M. O. Guler (2010). "Self-assembled one-dimensional soft nanostructures." *Soft Matter* **6**(23): 5839–5849.

Trucillo, P., R. Campardelli and E. Reverchon (2017). "Supercritical CO2 assisted liposomes formation: Optimization of the lipidic layer for an efficient hydrophilic drug loading." *Journal of Co2 Utilization* **18**: 181–188.

ur Rehman, M. S., Z. A. Raza, Z. A. Rehan, M. J. Bakhtiyar, F. Sharif and M. Yousaf (2023). "Citric acid crosslinked biocompatible silk fibroin-mediated porous chitosan films for sustained drug release application." *Materials Today Communications*: 105373.

van Strien, J., O. Escalona-Rayo, W. Jiskoot, B. Slütter and A. Kros (2023). "Elastin-like polypeptide-based micelles as a promising platform in nanomedicine." *Journal of Controlled Release* **353**: 713–726.

Vervald, A. M., K. A. Laptinskiy, S. A. Burikov, T. V. Laptinskaya, O. A. Shenderova, I. I. Vlasov and T. A. Dolenko (2019). "Nanodiamonds and surfactants in water: Hydrophilic and hydrophobic interactions." *Journal of Colloid and Interface Science* **547**: 206–216.

Vickers, N. J. (2017). "Animal communication: When I'm calling you, will you answer too?" *Current Biology* **27**(14): R713–R715.

Wagner, V., A. Dullaart, A.-K. Bock and A. Zweck (2006). "The emerging nanomedicine landscape." *Nature Biotechnology* **24**(10): 1211–1217.

Wang, C., N. Feng, F. Chang, J. Wang, B. Yuan, Y. Cheng, H. Liu, J. Yu, J. Zou and J. Ding (2019). "Injectable cholesterol-enhanced stereocomplex polylactide thermogel loading chondrocytes for optimized cartilage regeneration." *Advanced Healthcare Materials* **8**(14): 1900312.

Wang, J., B. Li, U. B. Kompella and H. Yang (2023). "Dendrimer and dendrimer gel-derived drug delivery systems: Breaking bottlenecks of topical administration of glaucoma medications." *MedComm–Biomaterials and Applications* **2**(1): e30.

Wu, N., L. Fu, M. Su, M. Aslam, K. C. Wong and V. P. Dravid (2004). "Interaction of fatty acid monolayers with cobalt nanoparticles." *Nano Letters* **4**(2): 383–386.

Xiao, L., B. Wang, G. Yang and M. Gauthier (2012). "Poly (lactic acid)-based biomaterials: Synthesis, modification and applications." *Biomedical Science, Engineering and Technology* **11**: 247–282.

Yanat, M. and K. Schroën (2021). "Preparation methods and applications of chitosan nanoparticles; with an outlook toward reinforcement of biodegradable packaging." *Reactive and Functional Polymers* **161**: 104849.

You, J.-O., D. Almeda, G. J. Ye and D. T. Auguste (2010). "Bioresponsive matrices in drug delivery." *Journal of Biological Engineering* **4**(1): 1–13.

Zhou, Z., C. Kennell, M. Jafari, J.-Y. Lee, S. J. Ruiz-Torres, S. E. Waltz and J.-H. Lee (2017). "Sequential delivery of erlotinib and doxorubicin for enhanced triple negative Breast cancer treatment using polymeric nanoparticle." *International Journal of Pharmaceutics* **530**(1–2): 300–307.

Zhu, Y., C. Liu and Z. Pang (2019). "Dendrimer-based drug delivery systems for brain targeting." *Biomolecules* **9**(12): 790.

Zhuang, W.-R., Y. Wang, P.-F. Cui, L. Xing, J. Lee, D. Kim, H.-L. Jiang and Y.-K. Oh (2019). "Applications of π-π stacking interactions in the design of drug-delivery systems." *Journal of Controlled Release* **294**: 311–326.

3 Biomaterials in Ophthalmology

Advancements, Applications, and Challenges

Harshit Sajal, Yuvaraj Sivamani**, Ramyakrishna A Rangaswamy*, Apoorva M Venkatesh*, and Sumitha Elayaperumal*,†*

*Department of Biotechnology and Bioinformatics JSS Academy of Higher Education and Research, Mysore, Karnataka, India; **Department of Pharmaceutical Chemistry, Cauvery College of Pharmacy, Mysore, India

†Corresponding Author: esmirthit@gmail.com

ABBREVIATIONS

ADH	Adipic dihydrazide
BG	Bioactive glass
BGC	Bioactive glass–ceramics
CAB	Cellulose acetate butyrate
CAD	Computer-aided design
CAM	Computer-aided manufacturing
CF	Perfluoropropane
CT	Computerized tomography
DED	Dry eye disease
DES	Dry eye syndrome
EDC	ethyl-(dimethyl aminopropyl) carbodiimide
GAG	Glycosaminoglycan
HA	Hyaluronic acid
HA'	Hydroxyapatite
HIV	Human immunodeficiency virus
IOL	Intraocular lens
IOP	Intraocular pressure
KCS	Keratoconjunctivitis sicca
NMDA	N-methyl-d-aspartate
NSAID	Non-steroidal anti-inflammatory drug
OOKP	Osteo-odonto-keratoprosthetic

DOI: 10.1201/9781032699882-3

OS	Silicone oil
PDA	Polydopamine
PEG	Polyethylene glycol
PFCL	Perfluorocarbon fluids
PMMA	Polymethyl methacrylate
PTFE	Polytetrafluoroethylene
PTMC	Poly(trimethylene carbonate)
PVA	Polyvinyl alcohol
PVD	Posterior vitreous detachment
RGC	Retinal ganglion cell
ROS	Reactive oxygen species
RPE	Retinal pigment epithelium
SELP	Silk-elastin-like protein polymer
SF	Silk fibroin
SF	Sulfur hexafluoride
SFA	Semi-fluorinated alkane
STD	Dysfunctional tear syndrome
STMP	Sodium trimetaphosphate

3.1 INTRODUCTION

The term "biomaterial" was first used by the European Society for Biomaterials in 1987. Biomaterials refer to non-biological constituents employed in medical devices to treat living systems. Biomaterials interact with a biological system for therapeutic or diagnostic reasons in medicine, and they have been developing over time (Williams 2009). Biomaterials can substitute or enhance an organ or function and can be manufactured from a variety of materials. These materials are used to make devices that replace a body part or function in a safe, reliable, economical, and physiologically acceptable way. Biomaterials have had an enormous impact on medical applications in recent years. The global market for biomaterials reached USD 35.5 billion in the year 2020 and is expected to increase to USD 7.5 billion by 2025 (www.marketsandmarkets.com 2022). The market for biomaterials in emerging economies is expected to grow significantly due to the surge in patient cases, increased use of implantable technologies, increased awareness of cardiovascular disease, increased disposable income, improved healthcare infrastructure, and relaxed regulatory guidelines.

The effects of an aging society on the healthcare system have become a major concern. Adequate vision care is critical to the elderly's independence. Aging affects all tissues and aspects of the eye to some extent. The most prevalent vision issues linked to aging include presbyopia, cataracts, dry eyes, and glaucoma (Chirila and Harkin 2016). Unlike our other organs, the eye is a very complex organ that is easy to perceive and offers a comparatively easy approach for surgery. It was also the first organ to have an external substance inserted into it to serve as what is now known as a biomaterial. The variety of ophthalmic biomaterials has expanded significantly with the development of synthetic hydrogels and polymers that, without dissolving in an aqueous medium, can interact with and hold water. Specifically, the application of ophthalmic biomaterials, and biomaterials in general, is increasing (Amato 2015). These materials incorporate knowledge, concepts, and ideas from a variety of disciplines, including engineering, biology, chemistry, physics, medicine, and materials science.

The oldest and best-known ophthalmic biomaterials are contact lenses, which are currently made of silicone hydrogels and hydrogels. Cataract procedures involve the removal of the clouded eye lens, which can be replaced with intraocular lenses. They typically contain silicone copolymers or derivative acrylics (Winterton et al. 2007; Powell et al. 2010). Artificial tears, used primarily to treat dry eyes, are another type of biomaterial that is widely marketed. They improve lubrication, reduce friction, stabilize the tear film, lessen symptoms of irritability, and guard against dehydration. They are applied as ointments, gels, or eye drops. Presbyopia is treated with inlays, which function in several different ways (Pearson and Hopkins 2007; Moarefi et al. 2017). Several authors have suggested possible areas for ophthalmic applications of biomaterials (Ankita et al. 2022; Nguyen et al. 2019; Khan et al. 2013). Both soft contact lenses and artificial tears are acceptable for the anterior segment. The lens can incorporate inlays and intraocular lenses. The application of biomaterials to the posterior segment primarily involves vitreous substitutes.

Silk fibroin (SF), extracted from silkworm silk, is a natural unique protein. This biopolymer possesses excellent mechanical attributes, including biodegradability, biocompatibility, and bioresorbability. This has attracted researchers for medical applications including tissue engineering and other biologically related applications. Tissue engineering might benefit from the use of silk fibroin. Another important biomaterial is collagen, an important class of structural proteins that are expressed in various tissues and have unique and variable characteristics. Collagen gels, films, and shields have been extensively used in infected corneal tissue, corneal tissue engineering, and drugs and antibiotic delivery. Table 3.1 presents the primary categories of ophthalmic applications that utilize biomaterials.

TABLE 3.1
Ophthalmic Applications of Biomaterials (Based on Ferraz 2022)

Clinical Application	Material
Contact lenses	PMMA
	HEMA hydrogel
	Silicone hydrogel
	PVA
Intraocular lenses	PMMA
	Hydrophobic acrylate polymers
	Hydrophilic acrylate polymers
	Siloxanes
	Collamer
Inlays	Hydrophilic hydrogels
Vitreous substitutes	Gas (air, sulfur hexafluoride and perfluoropropane
	Liquid (physiological solution, perfluorocarbon fluids [PFCL], semi-fluorinated alkanes [SFAs])
	Natural and semi-synthetic polymers (hyaluronic acid, chitosan, silicone oil)
	Hydrogels

(PMMA: polymethyl methacrylate; HEMA: hydroxyethyl methacrylate; PVA: polyvinyl alcohol)

TABLE 3.2
Summary of Common Colloidal Biodegradable Nanoparticles in Ophthalmology (Source: Tsai et al. 2018)

Carriers	Administration Methods	Diseases	Argument
Liposomes	Topical administration Subconjunctival injection Intravitreal injection	Dry eye syndrome Fungal keratitis Age-related macular degeneration Glaucoma Autoimmune uveoretinitis	Phospholipid bilayer structure with high biocompatibility Could carry both hydrophilic and lipophilic drugs High transfection efficiency Popular and well-researched vehicle
Chitosan nanoparticles	Topical administration Corneal stroma injection Subretinal injection	Bacterial endophthalmitis Inherited corneal diseases RPE-associated genetic diseases	Low production costs Mucoadhesive property that could prolong drug retention time on the ocular surface Ability of breaking through tight junction gaps to overcome the ocular barriers
PLGA nanoparticles	Topical administration Intravitreal injection	Corneal inflammatory disorders Uveitis Retinal inflammatory disorders	Well-researched material Superior hydrophilicity Biodegradable and good biocompatibility Could protect the drug from degrading quickly Controlled drug release
Gelatin nanoparticles	Topical administration Intravitreal injection	Anterior ocular bacterial disease Dry eye syndrome Corneal neovascularization	Low production costs Component of corneal stroma Polyampholyte Good biocompatibility and biodegradable Easy surface modification Easy and efficient encapsulation of drug molecules or genes

Polydopamine nanoparticles have proven to be strong candidates for drug delivery and cancer treatment. Due to its superior biocompatibility, biodegradability, and photothermal transfer ability, polydopamine (PDA) has been extensively used in biomedical applications. It contains a lot of phenolic groups; PDA can scavenge ROS and is used to treat inflammation and injury caused by ROS. A brief overview of typical biodegradable colloidal nanoparticles used in the field of ophthalmology is provided in Table 3.2. Ceramics have been well recognized for their advantages in biomedical applications due to their extraordinary diversity of physico-chemical, mechanical, and biological characteristics. Ocular keratoprosthesis, orbital implants for patients with anophthalmia, and oculoplastic surgery for orbital floor repair are three ophthalmic surgical specialties where bioceramics have been tested and used (artificial corneas). Alumina, polyethylene, and hydroxyapatite are currently the most popular biomaterials used in ocular surgery. The performance of ocular implants can be enhanced by bioactive glasses (BGs), bioactive glass–ceramics (BGC), and polyethylene. The ability of bioactive glasses to adhere to both bone and muscle tissue—a primary characteristic of implants used in reconstructive surgery—revealed their extreme promise for the treatment of defects and fractures of the orbital floor.

3.2 ANATOMY OF THE EYE

The anatomy of the eye is depicted in Figure 3.1. The eye is the visual organ that is located in the bony cavity known as the orbit. The orbit was observed to be significantly larger than the soft tissue eyeball. The connective tissue, i.e., Tenon's capsule and fat, occupy the space between the eyeball and orbit. This capsule renders a smooth socket, aiding free moments. It is encircled by the choroid and sclera and connected to the brain via optic pathways, two protective and nutritional membranes. The hollow, circular eye is surrounded by an attachment fabricated

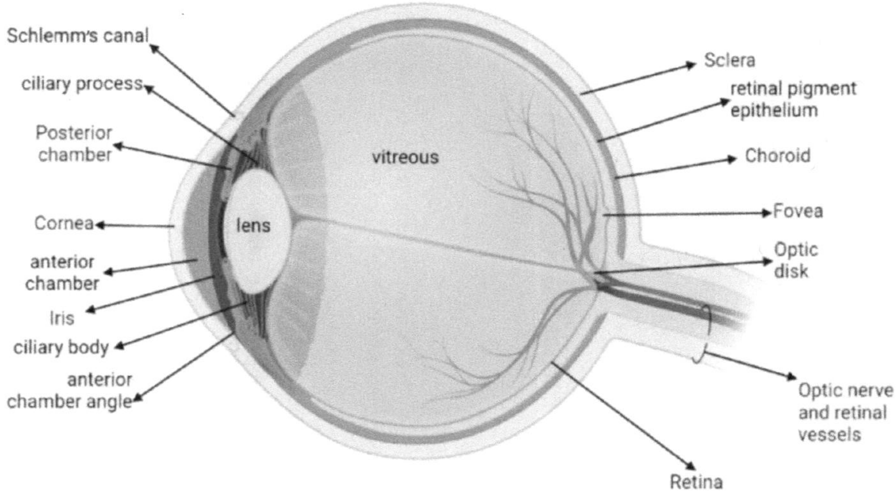

FIGURE 3.1 Anatomy of the eye.

from motor membrane or protective membrane. It has been well established that the physiology and anatomy of the eye are incredibly intricate (Friedman and Kaiser 2007; Basak 2019). The structure and organization of the eye is illustrated in Figure 3.1.

The eyeball is roughly spherical and approximately 2.5 cm in diameter. It has three layers: a fibrous outer layer, a vascular middle layer, and a light-sensitive inner layer. The cornea and sclera (the white portion), which are continuous, make up the outer fibrous coat (the transparent part). The retina is supported by a vascular membrane called the choroid, which is found at the back of the eye. The retina, a light-sensitive membrane that lines the inside of the eye, converts the intensity of light into electrical signals. Light enters the pigmented cells of the retina and stimulates the photoreceptor cells, the rods and cones, after first passing through the cornea, anterior and posterior chambers, aqueous humor, lens, and vitreous body. Rods provide movement and shape to the eye in dim light. Cones are color and shape receptors and exhibit bright light sensitivity. These cells are stimulated by light, which produces nerve impulses that travel from the eye to the brain via the optic nerve.

The anterior and posterior chambers of the eye are filled with the aqueous humor and vitreous humor, which nourish the avascular cornea and lens, respectively. An intraocular pressure of 24 mmHg is maintained by the sustained release and drainage of fluid. Suspensory ligaments exert tension on the transparent lens, which is sandwiched between the anterior chamber and the vitreous humor. Other macromolecules like crystalline proteins and glycosaminoglycans are also present in the collagenous tissue that makes up the eye's lens, vitreous body, cornea, and sclera. Several eye tissues contain type I collagen, but the degree of posttranslational modification varies among the various eye tissues. About 80% of the eye is made up of a gel-like substance called the vitreous body. The vitreous body contains small-diameter type II collagen fibrils that are encased in a hyaluronic acid matrix and are primarily made up of water (Bhat 2002).

Tear fluid continuously bathes the eye. A stable, continuous layer is developed across the cornea as a result of the regular production of tears by the lacrimal system for the feeding of the cornea, antibacterial defense, and clearance of cellular debris and foreign matter, among other objectives. This results in a high-quality optical surface. The apparatus has a functional drainage system to get rid of the extra lachrymal fluid and cell debris. It is made up of the canaliculi, pieta lachrymal, nasolacrimal duct, and lacrimal sac. During the blinking relaxation phase, tears are pulled into the canaliculi and subsequently released along through the inferior and superior puncta, which is further shut. Thus, efficient tear drainage depends just on the blink function. Tear production can be significantly increased by a variety of chemical, physical, thermal, and emotional factors (Holland et al. 2013).

The transplant of the cornea is arguably the most frequent clinical allotransplant. Within an hour after death, the eye needs to be taken out of the body, though a five-hour gap is permitted. The entire eye is typically preserved when a graft is needed and placed in 3–5°C sterile liquid paraffin. Since they are still avascular, the corneal transplant and the neighboring corneal tissue effectively continue to be separated from the host's cells.

3.3 THE USE OF BIOMATERIALS IN OPHTHALMOLOGY

Ophthalmology is one of the branches of medicine focusing on the health of the eye and includes eye anatomy, physiology, and diseases affecting the eye. As the population ages, eye problems become more prevalent, and biomaterials are increasingly being used to restore vision and enhance patients' quality of life. Proper care is crucial, as the eye is responsible for vision (Chirila and Harkin 2016). Aging tissues and all aspects of the eye can lead to common vision issues like dry eyes, cataracts, glaucoma, and age-related vision issues (Friedman and Kaiser 2007).

Ophthalmic biomaterials have a relatively recent history. Onofrio Abbate implanted an external substance resembling a biomaterial in 1862. It was an artificial cornea made of a glass disc encased in two rings. Although it was tested on animal corneas, it was impossible to leave the device in place for longer than a week. Later, Dimmer tried to create an artificial cornea out of celluloid (a material consisting of stabilizers, nitrocellulose, and camphor), inserting it in four patients, but the device was rejected within a short period. It took 50 years before polyvinyl alcohol (PVA) gel, an implantable ophthalmic biomaterial, was created using a synthetic polymer. Polymethyl methacrylate (PMMA) was used to construct the very first artificial cornea (Santos et al. 2011) A few years later, the original vitreous humor was replaced with a man-made polymer known as poly (1-vinyl-2-pyrrolidone). The invention of synthetic hydrogels is largely accountable for the development of biomaterials to treat ocular lesions.

New generations of biomaterials are being developed with the primary goal of filling in gaps or flaws present in earlier generations while also enhancing comfort, effectiveness, and safety. Innovations were developed to raise production standards, increase output, or boost productivity to cut costs. Cost-cutting pressures from the market are present to boost competition and improve accessibility. The use of ophthalmic biomaterials has increased significantly over the past few years. They are currently very sophisticated technologies. Ophthalmic biomaterials need to be able to provide tissues oxygen, alter the refractive index, protect surrounding tissue during surgery, harmonize with the tissue around them, and control the healing process, among other requirements.

3.4 HYDROGELS IN OPHTHALMOLOGY

Hydrogels were the first biomaterials developed for use in the human body. They are water-swollen polymeric materials with a distinct three-dimensional structure. Although several ophthalmic applications for hydrogels have already been approved, others are still being looked into. In situ gelling vehicles for ocular medication delivery, as well as soft contact lenses and foldable intraocular lenses, are all effectively marketed as hydrogels. Advancements are being made for the continuous discharge of nucleic acids, therapeutic proteins, anti-inflammatory drugs, and antibiotics (Findl and Leydolt 2007). Hydrogels may be made from a wide variety of organic, semi-synthetic, and synthetic polymers. Alginate, hyaluronic acid (HA), and collagen are a few examples of natural-origin polymers. Synthetic materials that form gels include polymers based on acrylate monomers, polyethylene glycol, polyvinyl alcohol, and siloxanes (Kirchhof et al. 2015).

3.4.1 Contact Lenses

It may be necessary to use an optical correction device to achieve good visual acuity. Contact lenses with convergent or divergent powers—measured in diopters—can be used for this. Myopia, hypermetropia, astigmatism, and presbyopia are the four most prevalent refractive disorders. In the 19th century, glass contact lenses made their debut. First-generation scleral glass lenses were invented in the 1880s by Adolf Fick (Amato 2015). The creation of contact lenses was reported in the 1888s. Polymethyl methacrylate (PMMA), which is thought to be biologically inert, light, simple to manufacture, and break-resistant, was first introduced by Rohm and Haas in 1936. The invention of hard lenses, which caused the widespread use of contact lenses, is thought to have resulted from a manufacturing error when producing PMMA scleral lenses (Efron et al. 2021).

In the 1960s, silicone elastomer lenses were developed as soft silicone contact lenses that have a hydrophobic surface, are highly permeable to gasses, and do not retain water. With the release of the soft lens in 1972, which was a huge success due to its comfort and superior biocompatibility, hydrophilic lenses came into existence. However, researchers needed to increase their gas permeability, so they chose to make them thinner and more aqueous in composition (Efron et al. 2021). The initial rigid gas-penetrable lenses were produced in 1974. Cellulose acetate butyrate (CAB) was one of the initial components, which was more likely to deform than PMMA but had a higher gas permeability. Norman Gaylord successfully added silicone to the basic PMMA structure to create a new series of silicone acrylate contact lenses. The first regular contact lenses were created in 1994 thanks to a method that significantly cut production costs. Strenuous research and development over more than a decade were required to create silicone hydrogel contact lenses that reduced hypoxia-related contact lens issues (Hom and Bruce 2006; Guillon et al. 2019).

About 88% of all lenses worn are soft contact lenses, making them the most common type. The stable polymer used to create hydrogel contact lenses can bind to or absorb water. The material becomes hydrated as a result of the liquid's ability to pass through polymer pores. The lens must be comfortable, ion-penetrable to maintain eye movement, sustainable, inert, non-toxic, biocompatible, simple to make, and able to create a steady and constant tear film to keep the basic metabolism rate of the cornea. These requirements are necessary due to the unique conditions of the eye (Guillon et al. 2019; Pillay et al. 2020).

3.4.2 Intraocular Lenses

The most common cause of blindness worldwide is cataracts, which is a clouding of the lens. It is brought on by natural aging-related changes in lens proteins, which can also be exacerbated by other factors like smoking or UV exposure. A polymer-based substitute for the biological lens is used for treatment. Phacoemulsification is the most common procedure; this requires making a minor corneal incision, breaking up the cloudy lens with a probe, and suctioning it out of the eye. In the preserved capsular bag, an artificial intraocular lens (IOL) is then inserted (Khandelwal et al. 2019; Chirila and Harkin 2016).

The initial IOL was made of rigid, non-collapsible, hydrophobic PMMA and required a significant incision. The first folding silicone lens was created by Thomas Mazzocco, for which a 3 mm incision may be used (Pillay et al. 2020). The ideal

IOL must be simple to implant without causing any difficulties for the surgeon and should offer the patient clear eyesight for a substantial length of time. For the IOL to be accessible, the production line must be relatively straightforward, and the material and design must permit a minimal amount of postoperative inflammation.

To block UV light, all IOLs currently on the market contain a chromophore. Due to the increased oxidative stress caused by blue light, it is dangerous and can harm the retina. IOLs fall into one of two categories: an acrylic/methacrylate polymer made up of hydrophilic silicone/silicon elastomers and hydrophobic (flexible) silicone/hydrophilic gel (either rigid or flexible) or acrylic. Due to the size of the incision required for implantation, non-folding PMMA lenses from the class of acrylic polymers are exceedingly uncommon in Europe and the USA (Khandelwal et al. 2019; Leung et al. 2014).

3.4.3 Artificial Tears

A multifactorial disease of the ocular surface, dry eye is characterized by symptoms like hyperosmolarity of the tear film, instability, an abnormal ocular surface, inflammation, and sensorineural abnormalities. The disruption of lacrimal homeostasis is one of its defining characteristics. It is an ocular surface disorder that affects millions of people all over the world to varying degrees of severity, from minor irritation to pain or shifting vision. Some of the names for dry eyes are dry eye syndrome (DES), keratoconjunctivitis sicca (KCS), dry eye disease (DED), and dysfunctional tear syndrome (DTS). KCS is the common name for the condition that causes the ocular surface to become dry and inflamed. The phrase most commonly used is DES or DED. Environmental, aqueous tear deficiency-related, and evaporative factors are frequently used to categorize the causes of DED. DED, which frequently has a multifactorial origin, can be brought on by a problem with lipid secretion, mucins, water, or a rise in tear film evaporation. The prevalence of DED rises with age and is typically associated with other pathologies. It can also be brought on by the environment or as a side effect of medication. To enhance diagnosis and care, dry eye is categorized based on risk factors

TABLE 3.3
Main Components and Functions of Artificial Tears (Source: Ferraz 2022)

Component	Main Function
Viscosity-improving agents (carbomer 0, carboxymethyl cellulose [CMC], hyaluronic acid [HA], hydroxypropylmethylcellulose [HPMC], polyvinylpyrrolidone [PVP])	Increase the time of permanence in the eye due to their mucoadhesive properties
Osmoprotectors	Maintain normal cellular metabolism, even under extreme osmotic stress
Trehalose	Bioprotection and osmoprotection
Quercetin, epigallocatechin gallate, n-propyl gallate, and gallic acid	Protect the corneal epithelium from oxidative damage
Benzalkonium chloride (BAC), sodium perborate, sodium chlorite, polyquaternium-1	Preservatives

and disease pathogenesis characteristics (Yao et al. 2011; Holland et al. 2013). The main components of artificial tears and their primary functions are listed in Table 3.3.

3.4.4 Drug Delivery Systems

The wide range of uses for hydrogels in ocular drug administration is illustrated by the fact that they are helpful in the effective delivery of medications to the eye. Drugs are frequently administered topically by using eye drops to deliver the medication to the eye, but these are ineffective and can have negative systemic effects. Only about 5% of the drug incorporated can reach intraocular tissue, and 95% is lost through tear drainage. Eye drops are rapidly eliminated from the eyes and have poor ophthalmic bioavailability because of the drugs' insufficient absorption. Furthermore, to achieve therapeutic efficacy for a sufficiently long duration, their short-term retention frequently calls for a frequent dosing schedule. These difficulties have compelled researchers to create drug delivery methods that deliver medications with a longer ocular residence time. Hydrogels can also be used to stop ocular discharge due to their elastic properties, which will make patients' eyes feel better and less gritty. Because they are easy to administer as a liquid and maintain their properties as a gel for a long time after administration, in situ-forming hydrogels are especially desirable serving as vehicles for eye medicine delivery. For instance, the in situ gelling system of alginate with high guluronic acid content is used in the delivery of pilocarpine to the eye. Without this system, pilocarpine nitrate solution only lasts for 3 hours. This system has extended the duration of pilocarpine's pressure-lowering effect to 10 hours (Wu et al. 2019; Lin et al. 2004).

3.4.5 Vitreous Substitutes

The "vitreous body", often known as the "vitreous" or "vitreous humor", is present in the posterolateral portion of the eye between the retina and the lens. It takes up more than two-thirds of the eye's volume. It is an opaque gel that contains several elements of various densities and biological compositions and is very inhomogeneous. Proteins (mainly collagen) and glycosaminoglycans (GAGs; consisting of hyaluronic acid, chondroitin sulfate, and heparan) as well as ascorbic acid, metabolites (lactic acid and glucose), enzymes, and ascorbic acid make up the vitreous. Hyalocytes, macrophages, fibrocytes/fibroblasts, amino acids, fatty acids, ascorbic acid, prostaglandin, proteins, and water are additional constituents that makes up the vitreous. Fibers give the vitreous its viscoelastic properties, and hyaluronic acid gives it its shock-absorbing qualities. The vitreous serves four primary purposes: structurally, it supports the growth, volume, and elasticity of the eye; optically, it maintains transparency and enhanced accommodation; biochemically, it acts as a barrier; and nutritionally, it serves as a source of nutrients and supports metabolism. Age causes the vitreous body to gradually liquefy from its completely gelatinous state at birth. This vitreous liquefaction, which corresponds to the vitreous cortex disassociation of the retina, is a contributing element to posterior vitreous detachment (PVD) (Donati et al. 2014; Kleinberg et al. 2011).

The following requirements must be fulfilled by a perfect vitreous substitute: it must (i) always be safe for use with ocular tissues and biocompatible with them; (ii) be transparent and clear, with a density and refractive index close to that of genuine glass; (iii) act as a buffering agent; (iv) enable the movement of proteins, solutes, and metabolites; and (v) be non-absorbable. Because it does not yet exist, the ideal vitreous replacement is still a work in progress.

The many vitreous substitutes that are currently accessible enable the replacement of the vitreous' mechanical function but are toxic over time. The following general categories can be used to classify them: liquid (physiological solution, perfluorocarbon fluids [PFCL], semi-fluorinated alkanes [SFA], natural and semi-synthetic polymers like hyaluronic acid and chitosan); silicone oil and experimental substitutes; and gas (air, sulfur hexafluoride [SF6], and perfluoropropane [C3F8]). Despite having considerable clinical limitations, silicone oil (SO) is the sole material now utilized for long-term vitreous replacement.

Identifying experimental replacements entails looking for a material with the same molecular makeup as the vitreous and similar chemical and physiological characteristics. The majority of these replacements are constructed from artificial polymers, particularly hydrogels, which are further classified as normal hydrogels and smart hydrogels. A relatively new category of stimulus-sensitive hydrogels is known as smart hydrogels. Since smart hydrogels have excellent transparency and outstanding biocompatibility, they seem to be strong contenders for long-term vitreous replacements. They have the same general characteristics as regular hydrogels and can react to many different signals, such as light, PH, temperature, electric fields, pressure, and chemicals. Drug diffusion, better gelation, and gel expansion are the results of these interactions. Information on their toxicity or inflammatory effects is still lacking, though. Since some complications are still not fully understood, these materials remain in the experimental stage. Since smart hydrogels have excellent transparency and outstanding biocompatibility, they seem to be strong contenders for long-term vitreous replacements (Barros et al. 2020).

Cross-linked hydrogels are a common component of recent research on vitreous substitutes; these materials exhibit improved retention times in the eye and can serve as tamponade agents. It has been reported that established hydrogel-based vitreous substitutes have undergone new developments. According to research, PVA hydrogels with rheological characteristics similar to those of the natural vitreous body may be made by cross-linking using non-toxic trisodium trimetaphosphate (STMP). After injection, these qualities remained intact, and in vitro cytotoxicity showed promising results (Leone et al. 2010). This promising material still needs to undergo in vivo studies to demonstrate its compatibility over an extended period. Swindle-Reilly copolymerized acrylamide with bis-acryloylcystamine (Davis et al. 2017). In vivo animal tests showed acceptable biocompatibility, and the goal was to achieve mechanical qualities that were similar to those of genuine vitreous humor. The need for further testing remains. Two interacting PEG derivatives were used by Tao et al. (2013) to study alternative cross-linking methods, which they tested on rabbit models. The obtained hydrogel possessed mechanical and optical characteristics that were highly similar to those of the normal vitreous body, showed no adverse effects, and was stable during the nine-month in vivo rabbit trial (Ferraz 2022; Gao et al. 2015).

Hyaluronic acid (HA) is the most promising of the natural polymers studied for vitreous replacement. Using a variety of cross-linkers, such as adipic dihydrazide (ADH), photopolymerization of glycidyl methacrylate groups, and

1-ethyl-3-(3-dimethyl aminopropyl) carbodiimide (EDC), two distinct HA hydrogels were evaluated by Schramm et al. for their potential as a vitreous replacement (Schramm et al. 2012). The ADH/EDC cross-linked hydrogels tested on in vitro cell cultures marginally damaged the cells, but photopolymerized HA gels had no toxic effects. The photopolymerized gels showed sufficient biocompatibility throughout a six-week in vivo test. Similar ADH cross-linked HA hydrogels, according to another study, exhibited no negative impacts either in vitro or in vivo (Ferraz 2022).

3.5 SILK FIBROIN IN OPHTHALMOLOGY

The natural protein silk fibroin (SF), which has superior mechanical qualities as well as being biodegradable, biocompatible, and bioresorbable, has drawn a lot of interest for use in medical applications. Silk fibers are derived from a variety of sources, including spiders, silkworms, scorpions, mites, and flies. A good source to produce biomedical devices is silkworm silk. Good cytocompatibility, configurable biodegradability, acceptable mechanical qualities, and limited inflammatory responses are all characteristics of devices with silk fibroin made by silkworms (Nguyen et al. 2019). Fibroin proteins have a secondary structure that gives them the mechanical qualities of silk threads, making them ideal biomaterials in tissue engineering as well as other biomedical applications. Silk cloth has been prized by humans for millennia due to its glossy texture and superior physical attributes. It has been genuinely transformative to be capable of removing the silk thread from the cocoon and utilizing the washed thread to weave clothing. The use of sterile silk sutures, particularly for delicate procedures like eye surgery, changed the medical landscape when silk fiber was repurposed for medical purposes (Sun et al. 2021).

3.5.1 Silk Structure

Fibroin and sericin, the two main proteins present *Bombyx mori* silk, are the building blocks of silk fibers. Fibroin microfibrils that have been strung together to form filaments make up silk fibers. Two fibroin threads, each produced by a different salivary gland in the worm, are spun into silk by workers. To form a structural unit, both filaments are wrapped in the adhesive and hydrophilic protein sericin. Domesticated *B. mori* silkworms construct their cocoons primarily out of two proteins: silk fibroin and sericin. Unlike silk fibroin, sericin is a single hydrophilic protein that ranges in molecular weight from 20 to 400 kDa. Several components make up silk fibroin, including the heavy chain, light chain, and glycoprotein P25. The C-terminus of silk fibroin contains a single disulfide bond that covalently connects the light chain, which does not contain a repeating amino acid sequence, to the heavy chain. Glycoprotein P25 connects with the heavy–light chain complex via hydrophobic interactions rather than being covalently attached to the heavy chain and is approximately the same size as the light chain (27 kDa) (Kunz et al. 2016).

The primary structure of the H chain is composed of 11 non-repeated hydrophilic sections and 12 repetitive hydrophobic domains. Silk I, II, and III, three distinct SF polymorphs, have been discovered. Arthropod gland silk contains a coiled form of silk I. Aqueous dispersions that have been regenerated in vitro exhibit the same conformation. During the spinning process, silk I is converted into silk II, which has the same structure and mechanical properties. Silk II is produced by laboratories and used as biomaterials for bone fracture fixation devices, scaffolds for tissue engineering, biosensors, and nanoparticles for drug delivery. After spinning silk, an antiparallel-sheet crystal structure called silk III is created. To create this polymorph, silk I is subjected to a variety of mechanical, physical, and chemical processes in the lab, including agitation, heating, methanol exposure, and water tempering. The repeated regions that make up the heavy chain of SF can be rearranged, allowing for the creation of heavy chain structure as well as intra- and intermolecular interactions including hydrogen bonds and van der Waals interactions (Zafar et al. 2015).

3.5.2 Silk for Ocular Tissue Engineering

The leading cause of blindness, corneal disease, affects about 27.9 million people worldwide. The only effective treatment for restoring visual acuity at this time is corneal transplantation, but most developing nations have lengthy waiting lists for this procedure due to the Eye Bank's limited supply of donor corneas and growing demand for them. Since there are not many human corneas available, corneal tissue engineering has made some important strides, especially the development of corneal cells using silk films as substrates for ocular surface repair in any of the cornea's five layers (from outermost to innermost: the epithelial layer, the Bowman's layer, the Descemet's membrane, the stroma, and the endothelium) (Tran et al. 2018).

3.5.3 Corneal Epithelium

The surgical membrane of preference for the reconstruction of the corneal epithelium is now the human amniotic membrane because of its capacity to reduce angiogenesis, tissue scarring, and inflammation. However, there are some disadvantages to using this membrane. First off, the amniotic membrane is mechanically weak, especially in comparison to other synthetic membranes like silk fibroin, which makes handling it challenging. Second, the semi-transparent nature of the amniotic membrane can have a negative impact on light transmission, a crucial feature of the corneal surface. Finally, because human donors provide the human amniotic membrane, there is a chance that diseases (like HIV, hepatitis, etc.) could be transmitted. Liu and colleagues demonstrated in preclinical studies that by employing human amniotic membranes as the reference material, the usage of silk fibroin can prevent these possible problems (Tan et al. 2012).

By solution casting *B. mori* silk fibroin and water annealing to create beta-sheets, Liu et al. created silk fibroin membranes for epithelial cell sheet synthesis (Liu et al. 2012). This silk fibroin film was approximately 40 mm thick, 14 mm wide, and very translucent. Even after handling, it was still able to keep its form. On the other hand, when handled with forceps in a similar preparation, the human amniotic membrane was semi-transparent and prone to folding. After 72 hours of cultivation, cells on the amniotic membrane differentiated more quickly and, compared to cells sown on the silk fibroin membrane, produced a density that was three times greater. The number of cells per inch of amniotic membrane after 144 hours, however, was equivalent to that on the silk fibroin membrane. The amount of keratin 3 and P63a expressed by corneal epithelial cells was constant across all culture substrates.

The effectiveness of silk fibroin and human amniotic membranes for generating human limbal epithelial stem cells was directly compared by Biazar and colleagues in an in vitro investigation (Biazar et al. 2015). Three distinct seeding techniques were examined in the study. Human limbal stem cells were planted onto orientated nanofibrous silk mats, randomized nanofibrous silk mats, and human amniotic membranes to test if they would maintain their limbal stem cell properties. When cultivated on silk film substrates, corneal limbal epithelial stem cells were able to preserve their non-differentiated stem cell stage and also develop into healthy corneal epithelium in a rabbit model of limbal stem cell deficit. Less clear corneas and increased neovascularization are typical in patients lacking limbal stem cells.

3.5.4 Corneal Stroma

About 90% of the cornea's thickness is made up of the stroma, which is primarily made of cells, collagen, and proteoglycans. It is a complicated layer with intricate microstructures that communicate with nerve cells and the epithelium layer. Diseases like corneal ulcers have been related to impaired corneal innervation, which includes altered corneal epithelium, nerves, endothelium, and keratocytes together with reduced corneal sensitivity (Biazar et al. 2015).

The most recent study by Wang et al. (2017) examined the creation of a silk corneal scaffold with stroma, epithelium, and innervation. The authors used chicken dorsal root ganglion, which can interact with human cells and resemble corneal innervation, human corneal stromal stem cells, and human corneal epithelial cells. On a template made of polydimethylsiloxane (either patterned or plain), silk fibroin spiked with polyethylene glycol (PEG) was solution cast to create the films, which were then dried and water annealed. To produce porous silk sheets that might eventually allow for mass transportation, the samples were then leached from the PEG. The films either had patterns or had been stamped to become biofunctional (with keratinocyte growth factor, hepatic growth factor, nerve growth factor, and epithelial growth factor). Human corneal stromal stem cells and patterned silk sheets were separately seeded with human corneal cells. Seeds from chicken dorsal root ganglions were found in the silk sponge. By layering cell-seeded patterned and plain silk sheets, the 3D corneal tissue model was developed. A porous silk sponge was then used to enclose the model and provide innervation. These liquid or air-liquid interface-grown three-dimensional co-cultures were studied in comparison to single cultures.

3.5.5 Corneal Descemet Membrane

When treating eye conditions affecting the corneal endothelium, surgical techniques like Descemet stripping, automated endothelial keratoplasty, and Descemet membrane endothelial keratoplasty are frequently used. In these procedures, the Descemet membrane and endothelium from the donor graft are transplanted into the patient. Silk fibroin-based tissue engineering may eventually eliminate the need for donor grafts. It has been demonstrated by Vazquez and colleagues, who also created an artificial endothelial graft, that silk fibroin substrates may be used to cultivate corneal endothelial cells that perform similarly to the Descemet membrane (Vázquez et al. 2017). After casting the silk sheet from a 5% w/v silk fibroin solution, scientists were left with a thin, 10 mm thick film. By using water annealing, the completed silk fibroin film was produced.

To effectively create endothelial grafts, human and rabbit corneal endothelium cells were cultivated on silk fibroin. The thickness and cell density of endothelial grafts composed of rabbit silk fibroin were equivalent to those of the contralateral cornea and integrated well into the corneal tissue. Furthermore, there were no indications of immunological rejection in the endothelium grafts. Conversely, the corneas of the rabbits in the control group, who simply had the Descemet membrane removed, did not throughout the 6-week follow-up phase and had edema. The rabbits that did not receive cultivated corneal endothelium cells as a component of a silk fibroin transplant showed the same results (Vázquez et al. 2017).

3.5.6 Retinal Bruch's Membrane

Transplanting monolayers of retinal pigment epithelial cells is one method for treating retinal degeneration brought on by conditions like age-related macular degeneration. In this field, exciting developments are taking place. For instance, using porous polyester membranes covered with fibronectin, phase I clinical studies have demonstrated the effective transplant of retinal pigment epithelium made using human embryonic stem cells (da Cruz et al. 2018). Transwells® for cell culture were used to make these non-biodegradable membranes. However, the transplanted retinal pigment epithelial cell sheet's propensity for folding and the membrane's durability are two downsides of this kind of treatment. The Bruch's membrane may be replaced after transplantation if retinal pigment epithelial cells are used as a material for in vitro proliferation of silk fibroin (Biazar et al. 2015).

A thin, mechanically sturdy support must be biocompatible because it will be placed next to neurological tissue in the restructuring of the retina. Before cell seeding, to create silk fibroin beta-sheet, Shadforth and associates used water annealing at room temperature (Shadforth et al. 2017). Within 12 weeks, the 3 mm thick silk fibroin film's cells demonstrated cobblestone morphology and pigmentation, characteristics present in adult retinal pigment epithelial cells. During this time, the retinal pigment cells multiplied and gradually built up surface microvillous structures with high density. Although the in vivo implantation of a synthetic Bruch's membrane was not evaluated in this work, the published findings indicate that such a treatment strategy for retinal degenerative disorders may be possible.

3.5.7 Ocular Drug Delivery

The most common route for drug delivery in intraocular infections, direct ingestion, has many issues with drug bioavailability. This has unintended consequences. The use of nanoparticles has benefits including enhanced local penetration of large, poorly water-soluble molecules like glucocorticoids and immune-related medications, as well as cyclosporine for diseases that threaten vision. Many drugs are unable to effectively pass through some sort of barrier that partially isolates the eye from the rest of the body, leading to minimal dose absorption. These barriers include the corneal epithelium, which has numerous tight junctions and desmosomes; the windowless iris vessels; the mucosal aqueous layer of the tear film, which protects the ciliary body; the unpigmented layer of the tear film; the corneal epithelium; and the front surface of the eye. Along with the retinal blood vessel endothelium, the inner and outer hemorrhagic retina is made from the retinal pigment epithelium (RPE) and safeguards the blood–water barrier by preventing molecules from the blood from entering the eye's interior, creating a physical barrier that blocks blood molecules from reaching the retina's vitreous-cavity border (Agrahari et al. 2016).

There are multiple ways to administer drugs to the eye, including eye drops, therapeutic contact lenses, therapeutic intraocular lenses, periocular injections (such as subconjunctival or sub-tenon injections), drug-eluting implants, intravitreal injections, and intracameral injections, which are illustrated in Figure 3.2. Both autoimmune uveitis, a serious intraocular inflammatory condition, and glaucoma, a common eye disease requiring management of intraocular pressure, have seen promising advancements in treatment using nanoparticle-mediated drug delivery. The drug has more time to come into contact with its target tissue as a result. Nanocarriers enable the transmucosal delivery of the non-steroidal anti-inflammatory drug indomethacin

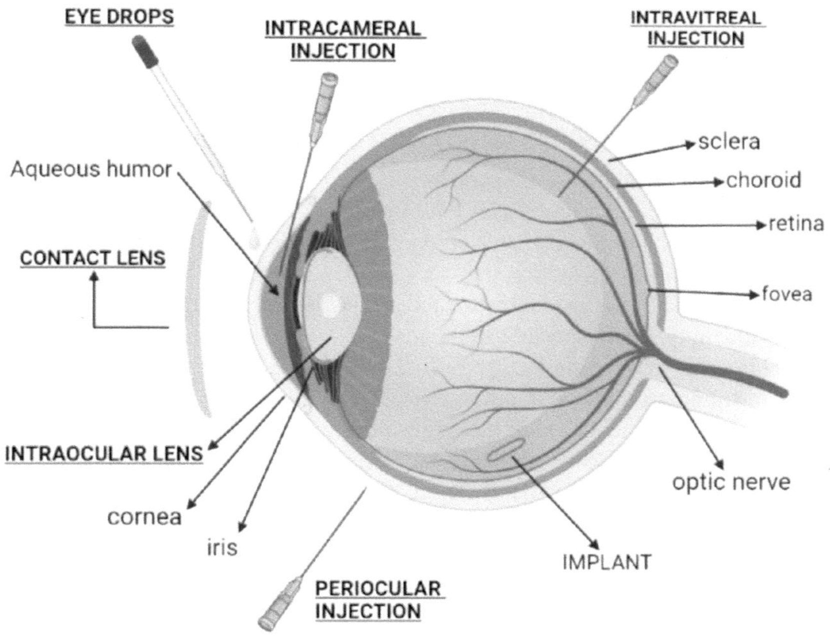

FIGURE 3.2 Various routes of ocular drug administration include eye drops, therapeutic contact lenses, therapeutic intraocular lenses, periocular injections (such as subconjunctival or sub-tenon injections), drug-eluting implants, and intravitreal and intracameral injections.

to internal ocular structures. To treat severe retinal conditions, the application of nanoparticles to deliver unstable molecules like nucleic acids shows promise (Zhou et al. 2013). Silk-elastin-like protein polymers (SELPs) were created by combining the properties of silk and elastin in hydrogels. Gelation time and polymer concentration can be used to control the water content of SELP hydrogels. SELP hydrogels have been used to release small molecules like cytochrome c, vitamin B, and theophylline. DNA release control has also been accomplished using SELP hydrogels. DNA size, shape, and concentration were used to determine the DNA release rates from SELP hydrogels (Huang et al. 2015).

3.6 COLLAGEN AS A BIOMATERIAL IN OPHTHALMOLOGY

Collagens are a significant class of structural proteins that are expressed in various tissues and have unique and variable characteristics. Although collagens do not impart transparency to the skin, they do so to the cornea and crystalline lens of the eye. There are different types of collagens that all have the same triple-helix structure but have different chain compositions, giving them different properties. The varying tissue morphology is also influenced by the different ways that collagen fibers are organized. Collagen has been investigated and used as a biomaterial as a result of its significant capacity to form various tissues. Collagen type I (Col-I) and collagen type IV are the two primary collagens found in the tissues of the cornea and lens. For clear vision, both collagens offer structure and transparency. This review investigates the use of these two types of collagens as novel biomaterials in the bioengineering of special tissue that may be used to treat a range of eye conditions that result in blindness.

3.6.1 Structure of Collagen

Astbury (1938) was the first to propose a collagen structure in 1938 that mixed trans and cis peptide units, and the model Pauling and Corey proposed in 1951 featured the same characteristics having three coaxial helices. However, neither of these models matched the X-ray diffraction pattern of collagen fibers. The first group to propose that collagen has a triple helical structure was Ramachandran's team in Madras, India (Bhattacharjee and Bansal 2005).

To create the three-stranded, rope-like collagen molecule, three polypeptide chains are wound around one another. Every chain has a unique twist that faces the other way. High glycine and amino acid residue content is the main factor influencing how a helix forms. Covalent bonds and hydrogen bonding between neighboring CO and NH groups hold the strands together in a substantial part. The primary collagen molecule has a rod-like shape, a molecular mass of about 300 kDa, and measurements of roughly 3000 Å in length and 15 Å in diameter. Glycine, proline, and hydroxyproline are the three fundamental amino acids that make up the triple-helix structure. The specific repeating pattern in the collagen triple helix is Gly-X-Y, where X can be any amino acid except cysteine and Y is usually proline or hydroxyproline. Collagen performs specific functions as a result of particular amino acids. Hydrogen bonds maintain the integrity of the helix structure by tying together peptide bonds (Khan and Khan 2013).

Individual triple helices, sometimes referred to as tropocollagen molecules, are shaped into highly elastic, tensile-strengthening fibrils that may be further assembled and cross-linked to efficiently sustain stress. Many connective tissue illnesses are caused by anomalies in the collagen chemical composition or its arrangement into mature fibers, including Ehlers–Danlos syndrome, osteogenesis imperfecta, some types of osteoporosis, and arthritis.

3.6.2 Collagen Films

Collagen films are primarily used as barrier membranes in biomaterials. Films made of biodegradable materials and resembling ophthalmological shields are produced by air-drying a casted collagen preparation, ranging in thickness from 0.01 to 0.5 mm. Hydrogen bonds, covalent bonds, or just plain entrapment can all be used to load the drugs into collagen membranes. They are tough enough to tolerate manipulation even after being hydroxylated, sterilized, and rendered flexible (easily bent). Collagen films, sheets, or discs are used in the treatment of tissue infections, particularly those of infected corneal tissue. Additionally, they serves as a medication delivery system for medicines like tetracycline (Minabe et al. 1989).

3.6.3 Collagen Shields

The collagen corneal shield is a multipurpose ophthalmic lens made of collagen, a natural protein. Collagen-based drug delivery systems are frequently used because the formulation offers the potential for self-administration and is easy to apply to the ocular surface. The shield's mechanical properties prevent corneal epithelial damage during blinking while the eye is healing. For collagen shields to deliver drugs, the medication must first be loaded into the shield before it can release be released. Drugs are trapped in the collagen matrix's interstices and act as a reservoir in the matrix of collagen. A layer of biocompatible collagen solution is left behind when the barrier crumbles and shreds through it, which appears to lubricate the eye's surface, reduce lid rubbing onto the cornea, increase the duration of the drug's interaction with the cornea, and accelerate epithelial healing. What improves the medicine's impact is a large dosage release of the substance from the lenses (Khan and Khan 2013).

3.6.4 Collagen Gels

Due to their flowability, collagen gels raise the prospect of a simple-to-inject, biocompatible drug delivery matrix. Injectable systems are the main application for collagen gels. These injectable collagen gels can be found most commonly in two different forms: collagen fibers suspended for injection, and viscous solutions that are not fibrillar in an aqueous medium. Patented ophthalmic formulations start as liquids but change to gels once they are applied to the eye. When applied, the gel will adhere to the eye's cul-de-sac far longer than liquid versions and allow for prolonged administration of antibiotics or non-steroidal anti-inflammatory drugs (NSAIDs).

3.7 POLYDOPAMINE NANOPARTICLES IN OPHTHALMOLOGY

A natural bioadhesive and bioactive polymer with high chemical versatility, polydopamine (PDA) is an intriguing candidate for numerous biomedical applications. Due to its superior biocompatibility, biodegradability, and photothermal transfer ability, polydopamine (PDA) has been extensively exploited in biomedical applications. Because it contains a lot of phenolic groups, PDA can scavenge ROS and has been used to treat inflammation and injury caused by ROS (Cheng et al. 2019). PDA therapy significantly reduced ROS production and proinflammatory cytokines in models of lung inflammation and peritonitis that were created acutely. PDA has been suggested by Bao and colleagues to reduce periodontal inflammation. PDA has also been investigated as a drug carrier due to its excellent drug-loading capacity through stacking interaction and hydrogen bond (Lou et al. 2021).

Many anticancer medications, including doxorubicin, oxaliplatin, prostate-specific membrane antigen inhibitor, and many more, were shown to be encapsulated and administered by PDA. MiR-21-5p, a negatively charged microRNA, was administered via cationic PDA nanoparticles (PDA-polyethyleneimine) to treat glaucoma by increasing the permeability of the outflow route and thereby lowering intraocular pressure (IOP). Therefore, it was proposed that PDA nanoparticles could serve as therapeutic nanoplatforms to halt retina ganglion cells (RGCs) egeneration based on scavenging ROS and delivering therapeutic agents (Lou et al. 2021).

Brimonidine, a selective alpha-2 adrenoceptor agonist, is employed in medicine to reduce IOP. Through regulating the activity of the postsynaptic excitatory N-methyl-d-aspartate (NMDA) receptor, brimonidine also has neuroprotective effects on retinal ganglion cells (RGCs). Brimonidine is frequently administered as topical eye drops (brimonidine tartrate, Alphagan®), but this form of medication has a low drug bioavailability (1–7%) and quick clearance. Along with other negative effects, it also raises the risk of periocular allergic reactions (12.7.%) (e.g., itching, shallow breathing, and puffy eye). Therefore, brimonidine can be delivered directly into the vitreous chamber utilizing nanoencapsulation, which has the potential to increase bioavailability and prevent unwanted side effects (Cantor 2006; Jordan and Bawazeer 2001).

3.8 BIOCERAMICS IN OPHTHALMOLOGY

Due to their extraordinary diversity of physical, chemical, mechanical, and biological characteristics, ceramics have been widely praised for their benefits in biomedical applications. By expertly adjusting the composition, porosity, and surface texture of ceramics, these characteristics can be precisely tailored, increasing their adaptability and suitability for particular healthcare applications. Bioceramics have historically been used for the repair of hard tissues, such as bone and teeth, due to their suitable strength for load-bearing applications, wear resistance (especially alumina, zirconia, and composites thereof), and, in some cases, bone-bonding ability (bioactive glasses and calcium orthophosphates). Even though their use in this field has been supported by science since the late 1700s, bioceramics have also been used in other medical fields, such as ophthalmic surgery. However, the potential and importance of ceramic ocular implants still seem to be underappreciated, and there is currently a dearth of thorough, critical analysis in the pertinent literature. Ocular keratoprosthesis, orbital implants for patients with anophthalmia, and oculoplastic surgery to repair the orbital floor are three ophthalmic surgical specialties where bioceramics have been tested and used (artificial cornea). Alumina, polyethylene, and hydroxyapatite are currently the most popular biomaterials used in ocular surgery (Petrović 2021).

The Boston keratoprosthesis (B-KPro) is currently the most commonly used artificial cornea or keratoprosthesis. This treatment alternative is utilized for corneal disorders that are not responsive to standard penetrating keratoplasty (PKP) or corneal transplantation. The three components that constitute the B-KPro include a front plate with an optical stem, a back plate, and a titanium locking c-ring. A schematic of the miniaturized B-KPro was developed to implant into mouse eye by Salvador-Culla and Kolovou (2016).

3.8.1 Hydroxyapatite

The main component of mammalian hard tissues is hydroxyapatite (HA'), a naturally occurring biological nanomaterial. It can be found in enamel as high-aspect-ratio rods with a diameter of 20–40 nm or in dentin and bone as 5–20 nm thick platelets. The implant serves as a bone graft during orbital floor repair, providing structural support where the bone defect is (fracture). To stabilize the orbital implant in ophthalmic patients and to guarantee proper ocular prosthesis motility, porous bioceramics encourage fibrovascular in-growth. The main application of bioceramics in the field of keratoprosthesis is to make a skirt that connects the central optical portion of the prosthesis with the host tissue.

Porous HA': At the end of the 19th century, porous orbital implants were developed as a solution to the problems associated with glass orbital implants, also known as "glass eyes", such as their fragility and potential for implosion. After cancellous bone spheres were thermally processed, all that was left was the CaP (calcium and phosphate) mineral framework, which was primarily made up of ultramicroscopic HA' crystals and trace amounts of calcium carbonate and calcium citrate. This is how the first orbital implant was made. Prior to World War II, Spaeth referred to the Guist's sphere, an implant made of calcined bovine bone, as "the most satisfactory of all orbital implants", and the use of Schmidt's bone-derived HA porous spheres was documented up until 1930 (Baino 2014).

Coralline HA': A coralline porous HA' sphere (Bio-Eye) was first used as an orbital implant after primary enucleation in the middle of the 1980s in the field of ophthalmic surgery. Coralline HA's porous, networked structure allows for host fibrovascular in-growth, which may lower the danger of infection, migration, and extrusion while preventing bacterial colonization of the implant surface. A few months after surgery, it may also be possible to drill a hole in the frontal region of the Bio-Eye to insert a peg. This peg can then be paired with the posterior surface of the ocular prosthesis to give the artificial eye a realistic range of motion. For the time being, surgeons still favor non-porous polymeric implants for children (like solid silicone and PMMA spheres). However, there is one unavoidable disadvantage to coralline HA' orbital implants: since HA' is delicate, it is impossible to simply suture the extraocular muscles to the implant (Elmazar et al. 2003; Nam et al. 2006).

Synthetic HA': Advanced manufacturing techniques were used to produce 3D porous implants for repairing the orbital floor using powders of artificial HA' that had been chemically created on the spot or purchased from a supplier. The computer-aided design/computer-aided manufacturing (CAD/CAM) technique was used to create the custom HA' scaffolds using computerized tomography (CT) data as a high-accuracy virtual 3D template. Simon et al. reported on a 3D periodic scaffold made of microporous HA' rods that were put together to create porous structures that were size-matched to trabecular bone (Simon et al. 2007). The potential value of the created construction materials for craniofacial and orbital bone reconstruction was also emphasized. Theoretically, autologous grafts and polymeric materials throughout orbital floor surgery can be replaced by quickly created synthetic HA' scaffolds. However, there are still brittleness problems, including intraoperative implantation difficulties and postoperative loss of structural and mechanical integrity, much like with coralline HA'. In the middle of the 1990s, synthetic HA' orbital implants (FCI3) were used for the first time in ophthalmic surgery. It has recently been suggested that synthetic HA' is a promising substance for anchoring the porous skirt of an experimental keratoprosthesis (Petrović 2021; Jordan and Bawazeer 2001).

HA' coating: HA' has also been tested as a coating material for porous orbital implants and solid polymeric or carbon substrates for keratoprosthetics. The polymeric sponge replication method was used to create a synthetic HA'-coated porous alumina (Al_2O_3) orbital implant to address the shortcomings of the Bio-Eye. The 20 μm thick HA' coating layer was intended to provide enhanced biocompatibility and long-term consistency in the eye while acting as a load-bearing structure on top of the porous alumina skeleton. HA-coated porous carbon matrices were used as artificial dental laminate replacements in the osteo-odonto-keratoprosthetic (OOKP) design for artificial corneas. The keratocytes' adhesion to the carbon mesh was significantly increased by the HA' coating created by sonoelectrochemical deposition, but the adherent keratocytes did not produce an excessive number of cytokines. Additionally, cytokine IL-8 was significantly adsorbed by the porous matrices themselves, which helped to reduce inflammation (Wang et al. 2011).

3.8.2 Bioactive Glass–Ceramics and Bioactive Glasses

Numerous other biomaterials have recently undergone extensive research for use in ocular surgery, including bioactive glass–ceramics (BGCs) and bioactive glasses (BGs). These biomaterials' extraordinary adaptability, which largely stems from the flexibility of their composition, enables a variety of applications in the field of ophthalmology. BGs and BGCs may have a unique capacity to promote in vivo cell activity and tissue regeneration, according to a recent theory. The performance of ocular implants can be enhanced by BGs and BGCs. The ability of bioactive glasses to adhere to both bone and muscle tissue—the primary characteristic of implants used in reconstructive surgery—makes them very promising for the treatment of orbital floor fractures and the repair of defects (Kinnunen et al. 2000; Peltola et al. 2008).

S53P4 glass plates appear to be a promising and dependable option for orbital floor reconstruction due to their biocompatibility, bioactivity (ability to stimulate new bone growth), and gradual biodegradability (ensuring adequate structural strength while the bone regenerates). Additionally, if the size and shape of the glass implant are properly chosen, excellent aesthetic and functional results can be achieved. In addition to their use in the bone-regenerating substance of orbital oculoplastic, silicate BG formulations have also been proposed for the creation of explorative porous orbital implants. A special mention should be made of the use of BGs and BGCs for synthetic corneas. In the past three decades, a few BG compositions have indeed been tested for such fabrication of the prosthetic skirt to improve the integration of the device with the host tissue. Typically, glass was used to fabricate the optical part of the keratoprosthesis (the transparent core) (Chirila 2001; Baino 2014).

3.8.3 Alumina and Polyethylene

In addition to its well-known uses in orthopedics for the fabrication of femur heads as well as acetabular cups for artificial hip joints and condylar elements and tibial plates for artificial knees, alumina is used in the production of porous orbital implants and keratoprosthesis in the field of ophthalmology. In the late 1990s, it was suggested that porous alumina be used to make orbital implants for ophthalmic surgery; in 2000, the Food and Drug Administration (FDA) approved this kind of technology, which is now marketed as a "bioceramic implant" (Rahaman et al. 2007; Morel et al. 1998).

HA is utilized in the production of HA/PE composite implants. Under the brand name HAPEXTM, they have been used successfully for the past 20 years in otolaryngology (middle ear bone prosthesis) and orbital floor repair. Low-modulus, tough, and bioinert PE is combined with stiff, osteoconductive, but brittle HA to produce a biomedical composite with desired traits for bone replacement (Meijer et al. 2002; Zhang et al. 2007)

Several recent studies have focused on the development and testing of a nanosized HA/polyvinyl alcohol (PVA) composite hydrogel as an artificial cornea fringe to improve the firm fixation of the keratoprosthesis to surrounding host tissues. This composite, according to Xu et al. was highly biocompatible with corneal fibroblasts in a test tube, had a network of interconnected pores, and could hold more water compared to non HA/PVA material (Xu et al. 2008). Co-precipitation and compression molding were used to produce sheets of b-TCP/poly(trimethylene carbonate) (PTMC) composite material with a thickness of about 1.0 mm, and it was suggested that these sheets be used as materials for orbital floor repair. In the 1970s, interest in Protoplast I, an inert composite material that was commercially available and made of polytetrafluoroethylene (PTFE) (Teflon) and vitreous carbon fibers, increased in the fields of maxillofacial, oculoplastic, and corneal surgery. This composite looked like black felt, had pores that ranged in size from 100 to 500 ml and was wettable (Baino 2014).

3.9 FUTURE PROSPECTS AND LIMITATIONS

Biomaterials have the potential to significantly improve the diagnosis, treatment, and management of various ophthalmic conditions. In ophthalmology, biomaterials are used to repair, replace, or regenerate damaged or diseased ocular tissues. Some of the future prospects and limitations of biomaterials in ophthalmology are discussed below.

Future Prospects:

I. **Improved Diagnostics:** Biomaterials can be used to develop new diagnostic tools for ophthalmic diseases. For example, biomaterials can be used to develop biosensors that can detect specific biomarkers in tears or other ocular fluids, which can aid in the diagnosis of various ocular diseases.
II. **Advanced Therapeutics:** Biomaterials can be used to develop advanced therapeutics for the treatment of various ocular diseases. For example, sustained-release drug delivery systems can be developed using biomaterials that can deliver drugs directly to the affected site in a controlled manner.
III. **Tissue Regeneration:** Biomaterials can be used to promote tissue regeneration in the eye. For example, biomaterials can be used to develop scaffolds that can support the growth and differentiation of stem cells for the regeneration of damaged or diseased ocular tissues.
IV. **Implantable Devices:** Biomaterials can be used to develop implantable devices for the treatment of various ocular conditions. For example, intraocular lenses made of biomaterials can be used to replace damaged lenses in cataract surgery.

Biomaterials have significant potential in ophthalmology, and ongoing research and development are likely to result in the development of more effective and safe biomaterials for the treatment of ocular diseases. However, several limitations need to be addressed to enable their widespread use in clinical settings.

Limitations:

I. **Biocompatibility:** One of the major limitations of biomaterials in ophthalmology is biocompatibility. The biomaterials used in ophthalmology should be biocompatible and should not elicit any adverse immune response or toxic reactions.
II. **Long-Term Stability:** Biomaterials used in ophthalmology should be stable over a long period. However, the ocular environment is complex and dynamic, which can affect the long-term stability of biomaterials.
III. **Cost:** The development of biomaterials for ophthalmic applications can be costly, which can limit their widespread use.
IV. **Regulatory Approval:** Biomaterials used in ophthalmology should meet regulatory requirements for safety and efficacy. The regulatory approval process can be lengthy and costly, which can limit the availability of biomaterial-based treatments.

3.10 CONCLUSION

Biomaterials have revolutionized the field of ophthalmology by providing innovative solutions for the repair, replacement, and regeneration of ocular tissues. Biomaterials have a broad range of applications in ophthalmology, including drug delivery, tissue engineering, diagnostic tools, and implantable devices. The use of biomaterials in ophthalmology has significantly improved the diagnosis, treatment, and management of ocular diseases, enhancing patient outcomes and quality of life. Despite the tremendous progress in this area, several challenges, including biocompatibility, long-term stability, regulatory approval, and cost, still need to be addressed to enable their widespread use. With ongoing research and development, it is expected that more effective and safe biomaterials will be developed for the treatment of ocular diseases, leading to improved ophthalmic care in the future. Overall, biomaterials have a significant impact on the field of ophthalmology, offering exciting opportunities for the development of innovative therapies for ocular diseases.

REFERENCES

Agrahari, Vibhuti, Abhirup Mandal, Vivek Agrahari, Hoang M. Trinh, Mary Joseph, Animikh Ray, Hicheme Hadji, Ranjana Mitra, Dhananjay Pal, and Ashim K. Mitra. "A Comprehensive Insight on Ocular Pharmacokinetics." *Drug Delivery and Translational Research* 6, no. 6 (December 1, 2016): 735–754. https://doi.org/10.1007/S13346-016-0339-2.

Amato, S.F. *Regulatory Affairs for Biomaterials and Medical Devices*. Regulatory Affairs for Biomaterials and Medical Devices, 2015: 79–92. www.sciencedirect.com/science/article/pii/B9780857095428500061.

Ankita Sachdev, I.V., Sourya Acharya, Tejas Gadodia, Samarth Shukla, Harshita J, Chinmay Akre, Mansi Khare, and Shreyash Huse. "A Review on Techniques and Biomaterials Used in 3D Bioprinting." *Cureus* 14, no. 8 (August 27, 2022). https://doi.org/10.7759/CUREUS.28463.

Astbury, W.T. "X-ray adventures among the proteins." *Transactions of the Faraday Society* 34 (1938): 378–388.

Baino, Francesco, and Chiara Vitale-Brovarone. "Bioceramics in Ophthalmology." *Acta Biomaterialia* 10, no. 8 (2014): 3372–3397. https://doi.org/10.1016/J.ACTBIO.2014.05.017.

Barros, Joana Alberta Ribeiro, Luís Daniel Rodrigues de Melo, Rita Araújo Reis da Silva, Maria Pia Ferraz, Joana Cecília Valente de Rodrigues Azeredo, Victor Manuel de Carvalho Pinheiro, Bruno Jorge Antunes Colaço, Maria Helena Raposo Fernandes, Pedro de Sousa Gomes, and Fernando Jorge Monteiro. "Encapsulated Bacteriophages in Alginate-Nanohydroxyapatite Hydrogel as a Novel Delivery System to Prevent Orthopedic Implant-Associated Infections." *Nanomedicine: Nanotechnology, Biology, and Medicine* 24 (February 1, 2020). https://doi.org/10.1016/J.NANO.2019.102145.

Basak, Samar K. *Essentials of Ophthalmology*. Jaypee Brothers Medical Publishers, 2019.

Bhat, Sujata V. "Overview of Biomaterials." In *Biomaterials*. Springer, 2002: 1–11.

Bhattacharjee, Arnab, and Manju Bansal. "Collagen Structure: The Madras Triple Helix and the Current Scenario." *IUBMB Life* 57, no. 3 (March 2005): 161–172. https://doi.org/10.1080/15216540500090710.

Biazar, Esmaeil, Alireza Baradaran-Rafii, Saeed Heidari-Keshel, and Sara Tavakolifard. "Oriented Nanofibrous Silk as a Natural Scaffold for Ocular Epithelial Regeneration." *Journal of Biomaterials Science, Polymer Edition* 26, no. 16 (November 2, 2015): 1139–1151. https://doi.org/10.1080/09205063.2015.1078930.

"Biomaterials Market Worth $47.5 Billion by 2025." Accessed November 29, 2022. www.marketsandmarkets.com/PressReleases/global-biomaterials.asp.

Cantor, Louis B. "Brimonidine in the Treatment of Glaucoma and Ocular Hypertension." *Therapeutics and Clinical Risk Management* 2, no. 4 (2006): 337. https://doi.org/10.2147/TCRM.2006.2.4.337.

Cheng, Wei, Xiaowei Zeng, Hongzhong Chen, Zimu Li, Wenfeng Zeng, Lin Mei, and Yanli Zhao. "Versatile Polydopamine Platforms: Synthesis and Promising Applications for Surface Modification and Advanced Nanomedicine." *ACS Nano* 13, no. 8 (August 27, 2019): 8537–8565. https://doi.org/10.1021/acsnano.9b04436.

Chirila, Traian V. "An Overview of the Development of Artificial Corneas with Porous Skirts and the Use of PHEMA for Such an Application." *Biomaterials* 22, no. 24 (December 15, 2001): 3311–3317. https://doi.org/10.1016/S0142-9612(01)00168-5.

Chirila, Traian V., and D. Harkin. *ScienceDirect. Biomaterials and Regenerative Medicine in Ophthalmology.* Woodhead Publishing, 2016.

da Cruz, L., K. Fynes, O. Georgiadis, J. Kerby, Y. H. Luo, A. Ahmado, A. Vernon, J. T. Daniels, B. Nommiste, S. M. Hasan, S. B. Gooljar, A. F. Carr, A. Vugler, C. M. Ramsden, M. Bictash, M. Fenster, J. Steer, T. Harbinson, A. Wilbrey, A. Tufail, . . . P. J. Coffey. "Phase 1 Clinical Study of an Embryonic Stem Cell-Derived Retinal Pigment Epithelium Patch in Age-Related Macular Degeneration." *Nature Biotechnology* 36, no. 4 (2018): 328–337. https://doi.org/10.1038/nbt.4114.

Davis, J. T., P. D. Hamilton, and N. Ravi. "Poly(acrylamide co-acrylic acid) for Use as an In Situ Gelling Vitreous Substitute." *Journal of Bioactive and Compatible Polymers* 32, no. 5 (2017): 528–541. doi:10.1177/0883911516688482.

Donati, Simone, Simona Maria Caprani, Giulia Airaghi, Riccardo Vinciguerra, Luigi Bartalena, Francesco Testa, Cesare Mariotti, Giovanni Porta, Francesca Simonelli, and Claudio Azzolini. "Vitreous Substitutes: The Present and the Future." *BioMed Research International* 2014 (2014). https://doi.org/10.1155/2014/351804.

Efron, Nathan, Lyndon W. Jones, Phillip B. Morgan, and Jason J. Nichols. "Bibliometric Analysis of the Literature Relating to Scleral Contact Lenses." *Contact Lens and Anterior Eye* 44, no. 4 (2021): 65.

Elmazar, H., I. Jackson, D. Degner, T. Miyawaki, K. Barakat, L. Andrus, and M. Bradford. "The Efficacy of Gore-Tex vs. Hydroxyapatite and Bone Graft in Reconstruction of Orbital Floor Defects." *Undefined* (2003). https://doi.org/10.1007/S00238-002-0448-7.

Ferraz, Maria Pia. "Biomaterials for Ophthalmic Applications." *Applied Sciences* 12, no. 12 (June 9, 2022): 5886. https://doi.org/10.3390/APP12125886.

Findl, Oliver, and Christina Leydolt. "Meta-Analysis of Accommodating Intraocular Lenses." *Journal of Cataract & Refractive Surgery* 33, no. 3 (2007): 522–527. https://doi.org/10.1016/j.jcrs.2006.11.020.

Friedman, Neil J., and Peter K. Kaiser. *Essentials of Ophthalmology.* Elsevier Health Sciences, 2007.

Gao, Qian Ying, Yue Fu, and Yan Nian Hui. "Vitreous Substitutes: Challenges and Directions." *International Journal of Ophthalmology* 8, no. 3 (June 18, 2015): 437–440. https://doi.org/10.3980/J.ISSN.2222-3959.2015.03.01.

Guillon, Michel, Trisha Patel, Kishan Patel, Ruchi Gupta, and Cecile A. Maissa. "Quantification of Contact Lens Wettability after Prolonged Visual Device Use under Low Humidity Conditions." *Contact Lens and Anterior Eye* 42, no. 4 (2019): 386–391.

Holland, Edward J., Mark J. Mannis, and W. Barry Lee. *Ocular Surface Disease: Cornea, Conjunctiva and Tear Film: Expert Consult-Online and Print.* Elsevier Health Sciences, 2013.

Hom, Milton M., and Adrian S. Bruce. *Manual of Contact Lens Prescribing and Fitting.* Elsevier Health Sciences, 2006.

Huang, Wenwen, Alexandra Rollett, and David L. Kaplan. "Silk-Elastin-like Protein Biomaterials for the Controlled Delivery of Therapeutics." *Expert Opinion on Drug Delivery* 12, no. 5 (May 2015): 779–791. https://doi.org/10.1517/17425247.2015.989830.

Jordan, David R., and Ahmed Bawazeer. "Experience with 120 Synthetic Hydroxyapatite Implants (FCI3)." *Ophthalmic Plastic and Reconstructive Surgery* 17, no. 3 (2001): 184–190. https://doi.org/10.1097/00002341-200105000-00007.

Khan, Ruby, and Mohd Haroon Khan. "Use of Collagen as a Biomaterial: An Update." *Journal of Indian Society of Periodontology* 17, no. 4 (July 2013): 539–542. https://doi.org/10.4103/0972-124X.118333.

Khandelwal, Sumitra S., Jason J. Jun, Selene Mak, Marika Suttorp Booth, and Paul G. Shekelle. "Effectiveness of Multifocal and Monofocal Intraocular Lenses for Cataract Surgery and Lens Replacement: A Systematic Review and Meta-Analysis." *Graefe's Archive for Clinical and Experimental Ophthalmology = Albrecht von Graefes Archiv Fur Klinische Und Experimentelle Ophthalmologie* 257, no. 5 (May 8, 2019): 863–875. https://doi.org/10.1007/S00417-018-04218-6.

Kinnunen, Ilpo, Kalle Aitasalo, Matti Pöllönen, and Matti Varpula. "Reconstruction of Orbital Floor Fractures Using Bioactive Glass." *Journal of Cranio-Maxillo-Facial Surgery: Official Publication of the European Association for Cranio-Maxillo-Facial Surgery* 28, no. 4 (2000): 229–234. https://doi.org/10.1054/JCMS.2000.0140.

Kirchhof, Susanne, Achim M. Goepferich, and Ferdinand P. Brandl. "Hydrogels in Ophthalmic Applications." *European Journal of Pharmaceutics and Biopharmaceutics* 95 (2015): 227–238.

Kleinberg, Teri T., Radouil T. Tzekov, Linda Stein, Nathan Ravi, and Shalesh Kaushal. "Vitreous Substitutes: A Comprehensive Review." *Survey of Ophthalmology* 56, no. 4 (July 2011): 300–323. https://doi.org/10.1016/J.SURVOPHTHAL.2010.09.001.

Kunz, Regina Inês, Rose Meire Costa Brancalhão, Lucinéia De Fátima Chasko Ribeiro, and Maria Raquel Marçal Natali. "Silkworm Sericin: Properties and Biomedical Applications." *BioMed Research International* 2016 (2016). https://doi.org/10.1155/2016/8175701.

Leone, G., M. Consumi, M. Aggravi, A. Donati, S. Lamponi, and A. Magnani. "PVA/STMP Based Hydrogels as Potential Substitutes of Human Vitreous." *Journal of Materials Science: Materials in Medicine* 21, no. 8 (2010): 2491–2500. https://doi.org/10.1007/s10856-010-4092-7.

Leung, Theresa G., Kristina Lindsley, and Irene C. Kuo. "Types of Intraocular Lenses for Cataract Surgery in Eyes with Uveitis." *The Cochrane Database of Systematic Reviews* 3, no. 3 (March 4, 2014). https://doi.org/10.1002/14651858.CD007284.PUB2.

Lin, Hong Ru, K. C. Sung, and Wen Jong Vong. "In Situ Gelling of Alginate/Pluronic Solutions for Ophthalmic Delivery of Pilocarpine." *Biomacromolecules* 5, no. 6 (November 2004): 2358–2365. https://doi.org/10.1021/BM0496965.

Liu, J., B. D. Lawrence, A. Liu, I. R. Schwab, L. A. Oliveira, and M. I. Rosenblatt. "Silk Fibroin as a Biomaterial Substrate for Corneal Epithelial Cell Sheet Generation." *Investigative Ophthalmology & Visual Science* 53, no. 7 (2012): 4130–4138. https://doi.org/10.1167/iovs.12-9876.

Lou, Xiaotong, Yuanyuan Hu, Hong Zhang, Jia Liu, and Yin Zhao. "Polydopamine Nanoparticles Attenuate Retina Ganglion Cell Degeneration and Restore Visual

Function after Optic Nerve Injury." *Journal of Nanobiotechnology* 19, no. 1 (2021) 436. https://doi.org/10.1186/s12951-021-01199-3.

Meijer, Astrid G. W., Hans M. Segenhout, Frans W. J. Albers, and Han J. L. van de Want. "Histopathology of Biocompatible Hydroxylapatite-Polyethylene Composite in Ossiculoplasty." *ORL* 64, no. 3 (2002): 173–179.

Minabe, Masato, Atsuo Uematsu, Kayo Nishijima, Eiko Tomomatsu, Toshiyuki Tamura, Toshio Hori, Toshio Umemoto, and Tsunetoshi Hino. "Application of a Local Drug Delivery System to Periodontal Therapy: I. Development of Collagen Preparations with Immobilized Tetracycline." *Journal of Periodontology* 60, no. 2 (February 1989): 113–117. https://doi.org/10.1902/JOP.1989.60.2.113.

Moarefi, M. Amir, Shamik Bafna, and William Wiley. "A Review of Presbyopia Treatment with Corneal Inlays." *Ophthalmology and Therapy* 6, no. 1 (June 1, 2017): 55–65. https://doi.org/10.1007/S40123-017-0085-7.

Morel, X., A. Rias, B. Briat, A. El Aouni, F. D'Hermies, J. P. Adenis, J. M. Legeais, and G. Renard. "Biocompatibility of a Porous Alumina Orbital Implant. Preliminary Results of an Animal Experiment." *Journal Francais D'ophtalmologie* 21, no. 3 (1998): 163–169.

Nam, Su Bong, Yong Chan Bae, Jae Sul Moon, and Young Seok Kang. "Analysis of the Postoperative Outcome in 405 Cases of Orbital Fracture Using 2 Synthetic Orbital Implants." *Annals of Plastic Surgery* 56, no. 3 (March 2006): 263–267. https://doi.org/10.1097/01.SAP.0000199173.73610.BC.

Nguyen, Thang Phan, Quang Vinh Nguyen, Van Huy Nguyen, Thu Ha Le, Vu Quynh Nga Huynh, Dai Viet N. Vo, Quang Thang Trinh, Soo Young Kim, and Quyet Van Le. "Silk Fibroin-Based Biomaterials for Biomedical Applications: A Review." *Polymers* 11, no. 12 (December 1, 2019). https://doi.org/10.3390/POLYM11121933.

Pauling, L., and R. B. Corey. "The Structure of Fibrous Proteins of the Collagen Gelatin Group." *Proceedings of the National Academy of Sciences* 37 (1951): 272–281.

Pearson, R. M. (Richard M.), and G. A. Hopkins. *Ophthalmic Drugs: Diagnostic and Therapeutic Uses*, 5th ed. Butterworth Heinemann, 2007.

Peltola, Matti, Ilpo Kinnunen, and Kalle Aitasalo. "Reconstruction of Orbital Wall Defects with Bioactive Glass Plates." *Journal of Oral and Maxillofacial Surgery: Official Journal of the American Association of Oral and Maxillofacial Surgeons* 66, no. 4 (April 2008): 639–646. https://doi.org/10.1016/J.JOMS.2007.11.019.

Petrović, Nenad. "Application of Bioceramics in Ophthalmology." In *Encyclopedia of Materials: Composites*, Elsevier. 2021: 326–334, ISBN 9780128197318, https://doi.org/10.1016/B978-0-12-819724-0.00047-1.

Pillay, Rayishnee, Rekha Hansraj, and Nishanee Rampersad. "Historical Development, Applications and Advances in Materials Used in Spectacle Lenses and Contact Lenses." *Clinical Optometry* 12 (2020): 157.

Powell, Charles H., John M. Lally, Lisa D. Hoong, and Stanley W. Huth. "Lipophilic versus Hydrodynamic Modes of Uptake and Release by Contact Lenses of Active Entities Used in Multipurpose Solutions." *Contact Lens & Anterior Eye: The Journal of the British Contact Lens Association* 33, no. 1 (February 2010): 9–18. https://doi.org/10.1016/J.CLAE.2009.10.006.

Rahaman, Mohamed N., Aihua Yao, B. Sonny Bal, Jonathan P. Garino, and Michael D. Ries. "Ceramics for Prosthetic Hip and Knee Joint Replacement." *Journal of the American Ceramic Society* 90, no. 7 (July 1, 2007): 1965–1988. https://doi.org/10.1111/J.1551-2916.2007.01725.X.

Salvador-Culla, B., and P. E. Kolovou. "Keratoprosthesis: A Review of Recent Advances in the Field." *Journal of Functional Biomaterials* 7, no. 2 (2016): 13. https://doi.org/10.3390/jfb7020013.

Santos, Lívia, Maria Pia Ferraz, Yuki Shirosaki, Maria Ascensao Lopes, Maria Helena Fernandes, Akiyoshi Osaka, and José Domingos Santos. "Degradation Studies and Biological Behavior on an Artificial Cornea Material." *Investigative Ophthalmology & Visual Science* 52, no. 7 (2011): 4274–4281.

Schramm, Charlotte, Martin S. Spitzer, Sigrid Henke-Fahle, Gabriele Steinmetz, Kai Januschowski, Peter Heiduschka, Jürgen Geis-Gerstorfer, Tilo Biedermann, Karl U. Bartz-Schmidt, and Peter Szurman. "The Cross-Linked Biopolymer Hyaluronic Acid as an Artificial Vitreous Substitute." *Investigative Ophthalmology & Visual Science* 53, no. 2 (2012): 613–621.

Shadforth, Audra M.A., Shuko Suzuki, Christina Theodoropoulos, Neil A. Richardson, Traian V. Chirila, and Damien G. Harkin. "A Bruch's Membrane Substitute Fabricated from Silk Fibroin Supports the Function of Retinal Pigment Epithelial Cells in Vitro." *Journal of Tissue Engineering and Regenerative Medicine* 11, no. 6 (June 1, 2017): 1915–1924. https://doi.org/10.1002/TERM.2089.

Simon, Joshua L., Sarah Michna, Jennifer A. Lewis, E. Dianne Rekow, Van P. Thompson, James E. Smay, Andrew Yampolsky, J. Russell Parsons, and John L. Ricci. "In Vivo Bone Response to 3D Periodic Hydroxyapatite Scaffolds Assembled by Direct Ink Writing." *Journal of Biomedical Materials Research. Part A* 83, no. 3 (November 1, 2007): 747–758. https://doi.org/10.1002/JBM.A.31329.

Sun, Weizhen, David Alexander Gregory, Mhd Anas Tomeh, and Xiubo Zhao. "Silk Fibroin as a Functional Biomaterial for Tissue Engineering." *International Journal of Molecular Sciences* 22, no. 3 (February 1, 2021): 1–28. https://doi.org/10.3390/IJMS22031499.

Tan, Donald T.H., John K.G. Dart, Edward J. Holland, and Shigeru Kinoshita. "Corneal Transplantation." *Lancet (London, England)* 379, no. 9827 (2012): 1749–1761. https://doi.org/10.1016/S0140-6736(12)60437-1.

Tao, Y., X. Tong, Y. Zhang, J. Lai, Y. Huang, Y. R. Jiang, and B. H. Guo. "Evaluation of an In Situ Chemically Crosslinked Hydrogel as a Long-Term Vitreous Substitute Material." *Acta biomaterialia* 9, no. 2 (2013): 5022–5030. https://doi.org/10.1016/j.actbio.2012.09.026.

Tran, S. H., C. G. Wilson, and F. P. Seib. "A Review of the Emerging Role of Silk for the Treatment of the Eye." *Pharmaceutical Research* 35, no. 12 (2018): 248. https://doi.org/10.1007/s11095-018-2534-y.

Tsai, C. H., P. Y. Wang, I. C. Lin, H. Huang, G. S. Liu, and C. L. Tseng. "Ocular Drug Delivery: Role of Degradable Polymeric Nanocarriers for Ophthalmic Application." *International Journal of Molecular Sciences* 19, no. 9 (2018): 2830. https://doi.org/10.3390/ijms19092830.

Vázquez, Natalia, Carlos A. Rodríguez-Barrientos, Salvador D. Aznar-Cervantes, Manuel Chacón, José L. Cenis, Ana C. Riestra, Ronald M. Sánchez-Avila, et al. "Silk Fibroin Films for Corneal Endothelial Regeneration: Transplant in a Rabbit Descemet Membrane Endothelial Keratoplasty." *Investigative Ophthalmology & Visual Science* 58, no. 9 (July 1, 2017): 3357–3365. https://doi.org/10.1167/IOVS.17-21797.

Wang, Liqiang, Kyung Jae Jeong, Homer H Chiang, David Zurakowski, Irmgard Behlau, James Chodosh, Claes H. Dohlman, Robert Langer, and Daniel S. Kohane. "Hydroxyapatite for Keratoprosthesis Biointegration." *Investigative Ophthalmology & Visual Science* 52, no. 10 (September 2011): 7392–7399. https://doi.org/10.1167/iovs.11-7601.

Wang, S., C. E. Ghezzi, R. Gomes, R. E. Pollard, J. L. Funderburgh, and D. L. Kaplan. "In Vitro 3D Corneal Tissue Model with Epithelium, Stroma, and Innervation." *Biomaterials* 112 (2017): 1–9. https://doi.org/10.1016/j.biomaterials.2016.09.030.

Williams, David F. "On the Nature of Biomaterials." *Biomaterials* 30, no. 30 (October 1, 2009): 5897–5909. https://doi.org/10.1016/J.BIOMATERIALS.2009.07.027.

Winterton, Lynn C., John M. Lally, Karen B. Sentell, and L. Lawrence Chapoy. "The Elution of Poly (Vinyl Alcohol) from a Contact Lens: The Realization of a Time Release Moisturizing Agent/Artificial Tear." *Journal of Biomedical Materials Research. Part B, Applied Biomaterials* 80, no. 2 (February 2007): 424–432. https://doi.org/10.1002/JBM.B.30613.

Wu, Yumei, Yuanyuan Liu, Xinyue Li, Dereje Kebebe, Bing Zhang, Jing Ren, Jun Lu, Jiawei Li, Shouying Du, and Zhidong Liu. "Research Progress of In-Situ Gelling Ophthalmic Drug Delivery System." *Asian Journal of Pharmaceutical Sciences* 14, no. 1 (January 1, 2019): 1–15. https://doi.org/10.1016/J.AJPS.2018.04.008.

Xu, Fenglan, Yubao Li, Yingpin Deng, and Jie Xiong. "Porous Nano-Hydroxyapatite/Poly(Vinyl Alcohol) Composite Hydrogel as Artificial Cornea Fringe: Characterization and Evaluation in Vitro." *Journal of Biomaterials Science. Polymer Edition* 19, no. 4 (April 1, 2008): 431–439. https://doi.org/10.1163/156856208783719473.

Yao, William, Richard S. Davidson, Vikram D. Durairaj, and Christopher D. Gelston. "Dry Eye Syndrome: An Update in Office Management." *The American Journal of Medicine* 124, no. 11 (2011): 1016–1018. https://doi.org/10.1016/J.AMJMED.2011.01.030.

Zafar, Muhammad S., David J. Belton, Benjamin Hanby, David L. Kaplan, and Carole C. Perry. "Functional Material Features of Bombyx Mori Silk Light versus Heavy Chain Proteins." *Biomacromolecules* 16, no. 2 (February 2015): 606–614. https://doi.org/10.1021/bm501667j.

Zhang, Y., K. E. Tanner, N. Gurav, and L. Di Silvio. "In Vitro Osteoblastic Response to 30 Vol% Hydroxyapatite-Polyethylene Composite." *Journal of Biomedical Materials Research. Part A* 81, no. 2 (May 2007): 409–417. https://doi.org/10.1002/JBM.A.31078.

Zhou, Hong-Yan, Ji-Long Hao, Shuang Wang, Yu Zheng, and Wen-Song Zhang. "Nanoparticles in the Ocular Drug Delivery." *International Journal of Ophthalmology* 6, no. 3 (2013): 390–396. https://doi.org/10.3980/j.issn.2222-3959.2013.03.25.

4 Use of AI and Machine Learning for the Analysis of Cellular Images in Breast Cancer

Reena Thakur, Pradnya Borkar**, Parul Bhanarkar*, and Prashant Panse****

*Jhulelal Institute of Technology, Nagpur, India;
**Symbiosis Institute of Technology, Symbiosis International (Deemed University), Pune, India;
***Department of IT, Medi-Caps University, Indore, India

ABBREVIATIONS

ANN	Artificial neural network
CNN	Convolutional neural network
DT	Decision tree
EFuNN	Evolving fuzzy neural network
GAN	Generative adversarial network
GMM	Gaussian mixture model
IPI	International prediction index
ML	Machine learning
RBF	Radial basis function
RF	Random forest
SNP	Single nucleotide polymorphism
SVM	Support vector machine

4.1 INTRODUCTION

Cancer develops when a cluster of cells in one area of the body multiplies uncontrollably. The most common type of cancer in women is breast cancer. As breast cancer progresses over the years, its precursor stages change. Tumors arise when cells divide abnormally and quickly, leading to a mass or severely distorted structure. Women risk developing breast cancer more than men (Akay, 2009; Wolberg & Mangasarian, 1990). It is possible to exert some control over breast cancer by being aware of the numerous risk factors. In addition, if the numerous signs of this condition are recognized early, treatment is typically relatively simple (Ryu & Chandrasekaran, 2007). Invasive and

DOI: 10.1201/9781032699882-4

noninvasive breast cancers are the two main subtypes. The invasive kind of breast cancer is characterized by invading malignant cells into neighboring tissues and organs (Sahan et al., 2007). Noninvasive breast cancer occurs when malignant cells do not expand beyond the tumor's original site. There has been significant progress in analyzing, identifying, and classifying breast cancer (Ubeyli, 2007). There have been many successful and unsuccessful attempts to create fully automated categorization systems. Creating cutting-edge, improved methods can significantly aid radiologists' ability to diagnose an illness accurately. The author (Ubeyli, 2007) reviewed some seminal studies and papers that have contributed to our understanding of identifying and categorizing breast cancer.

To identify breast cancer, the Babu et al. developed a feed-forward neural network employing the back propagation algorithm (Babu et al., 2013). Using kernel functions, the Reddy and Reddy created a support vector machine approach for the classification of breast cancer (Reddy & Reddy, 2014). Rajaguru and Prabhakar utilized RBF and the gaussian mixture model (GMM) to investigate breast cancer categorization (Rajaguru & Prabhakar, 2017a) thoroughly. Many support vector machine (SVM) kernel functions were investigated and evaluated by Hussain et al. for application in the detection of breast cancer (Hussain et al., 2011). To identify breast cancer, the Abbass proposed the traditional artificial neural network (ANN) approach (Abbass, 2002). In order to categorize breast cancer, several authors have employed mammography to identify breast masses using neural networks that used form, textural characteristics, and edge sharpness (Andre & Rangayyan 2006; Rajaguru & Prabhakar, 2017). Radial basis functions (RBF) and support vector machine (SVM) classifiers were employed by researchers to perform breast cancer diagnosis based on the features provided by the genetic algorithm (Guo & Nandi, 2006; Iranpour & Almassi, 2007). In addition to using a self-organizing map for cluster analysis on a database of breast cancer cases, several authors developed an intelligent decision support system to help with breast cancer identification (Janghel et al., 2010; Markey et al., 2003). Using an ANN to extract characteristics, the (Abdolmaleki et al., 2001) employed dynamic magnetic resonance imaging to classify breast cancer. In this study, the authors categorized the likelihood of acquiring breast cancer using the Bayesian discriminant classifier (Abdolmaleki et al., 2001).

Unfortunately, there is currently no known cure for cancer. The sole treatment option for someone with cancer is to amputate the damaged limb or organ. Preventing a person from ever having cancer through early detection is ideal. Machine learning is a method that can "learn" and "retrieve" information from data and then utilize that "gained" knowledge to anticipate the desired results. Early cancer detection is only one area where machine learning algorithms have proven invaluable. Machine learning is divided into three subfields in computer science: supervised learning, unsupervised learning, and reinforcement learning. In supervised learning, labels are provided so a computer may make predictions about unlabeled input characteristics; in unsupervised learning, features are provided, but no labels or output classes are known in advance. During reinforcement learning, which is the method of allowing the models to learn independently, the machine executes a task and then rewards or punishes itself according to a predetermined set of rules, aiming to increase the reward's overall value. Predicting if a person has a benign or malignant cancer using a combination of machine learning algorithms would be fast and accurate.

4.2 PREDICTION OF BREAST CANCER USING MACHINE LEARNING

For a long time now, machine learning has been used extensively in the study of cancer. Since approximately two decades ago, decision trees (DTs) and artificial neural networks (ANNs) have been employed in the detection and diagnosis of cancer (Simes, 1985). Nowadays, machine learning is employed for a wide range of applications, including the detection and classification of cancer in X-ray and CRT images, as well as the classification of malignancies based on proteomic and genomic (microarray) testing (Maclin & Dempsey, 1991; Zhou et al., 2004; Wang et al., 2005; Petricoin & Liotta, 2005; Bocchi et al., 2004). Machine learning has been chiefly used in diagnosing and detecting cancer (McCarthy et al., 2004). Recently, scientists studying cancer have attempted to use machine learning to assess and predict cancer prognosis.

The goals of cancer diagnosis and detection differ from those of prognosis and course prediction. The three most crucial cancer prognosis and prediction components are survival, recurrence, and susceptibility (risk assessment). In the first case, a person is attempting to predict a tumor to foretell their likelihood of contracting a specific type of cancer before the illness manifests itself. In the latter situation, someone is attempting to predict the chance of cancer recurrence after the condition has appeared to be conquered. When a disease is identified, predictions about how it will turn out (life expectancy, survival, progression, tumor-drug sensitivity) are made. The accuracy of the diagnosis determines whether the prognostic prediction is correct in the latter two situations. Other factors need to be considered when creating a prognostic projection, and a prognosis for a condition can only be determined once a medical diagnosis has been made (Hagerty et al., 2005).

A multidisciplinary team of professionals frequently determines the prognosis for cancer based on the patient's age and general health, the location and kind of cancer, the disease stage, and the tumor's size and grade. The attending physician typically must carefully integrate histological (cell-based), clinical (patient-based), and demographic (population-based) data in order to arrive at a credible prognosis. A subfield of AI called "machine learning" uses statistical, probabilistic, and optimization algorithms to "learn" from data and then apply that understanding to categorize new data, find novel patterns, and forecast novel trends (Thomas et al., 2020).

4.2.1 Prediction of Cancer Risk or Susceptibility

One intriguing study created a method to forecast the occurrence of "spontaneous" breast cancer in the past using the single nucleotide polymorphism (SNP) profiles of steroid metabolizing enzymes (CYP450s) (Cruz & Wishart, 2006). This study's premise was that specific SNP combinations in genes that regulate steroid metabolism would raise the risk of breast cancer by enabling the buildup of environmental hormones or poisons in breast tissue. The researchers compared 63 breast cancer patients to 74 healthy controls using SNP data (98 SNPs from 45 distinct cancer-associated genes) The study's success may be primarily attributed to the authors' employing many strategies to reduce the sample-to-feature ratio and exploring numerous machine learning strategies to choose the optimal classifier. For instance the authors efficiently narrowed a starting sample of 98 SNPs down to just 2–3 SNPs that seemed to be the most important.

This improved the sample-per-feature ratio from roughly 3:2 (for three SNPs) to 45:1 (for two SNPs) to 68:1 (if all 98 SNPs had been utilized). Thus, the so-called "curse of dimensionality" was averted in the research. When the sample size was decreased, several machine learning (ML) techniques were used, including a sophisticated support vector machine (SVM), several decision tree models, and a naive Bayes model. The decision tree classifier exhibited maximum accuracy with only two SNPs, while the SVM and naive Bayes classifiers only needed a set of three SNPs each.

According to the SVM classifier, it was 69% accurate, whereas naive Bayes and decision tree classifiers were 67% and 68% accurate, respectively. The study's cross-validation and confirmation efforts are also noteworthy. The accuracy of each model's predictions was verified using at least three different methods. The training was evaluated and monitored using 20-fold cross-validation. By performing the cross-validation five times and averaging the results, the author used a bootstrap resampling approach to lessen the randomness caused by sample partitioning. In order to eliminate bias in feature selection (i.e., discover the most informative subset of SNPs), the feature selection procedure was performed 100 times inside each fold (five times for each of the 20 folds). The results were then contrasted with those of a random permutation test, which revealed a probability of accurately predicting the future of no more than 50%.

Although the authors made every effort to reduce the unpredictability caused by sample splitting, leave-one-out cross-validation might have been a more successful method. The authors disregarded this standard deviation as meaningless because all strategies outperformed chance by more than 25%. Standard deviations for all reported accuracies from the various cross-validations were below 4%. Although no external validation set was published, people found similar results in follow-up research with 200 more participants (Collins et al., 2016). In conclusion, the author's research proves that with the proper planning, cautious execution, careful data selection, and exhaustive validation of several machine learners, an accurate and robust cancer risk prediction tool may be created. This study also demonstrates how machine learning may help us understand the polygenic risk factors and underlying molecular mechanisms that might lead to sporadic or non-hereditary breast cancer.

4.2.2 Prediction of Cancer Survivability

Roughly 50% of the machine learning studies on cancer prediction used forecasts of 0%, 5%, 10%, 15%, 20%, 25%, and 30%. About 5% of studies used the fundamental Bayes Genetic Engineering Soft Logic Choice SVM ANN Tree Clustering Image 5 for malignancies of the throat, prostate, and other organs. A histogram displaying the distribution of cancer predictions was made using several machine learning techniques (Cruz & Wishart, 2006). However, many malignancies from different organs or tissues seem consistent with machine learning predictions. The two most common kinds of cancer are breast and prostate. Cancers categorized as "other" include brain, cervical, esophageal, thoracic, thyroid, ophthalmic, and head and neck cancers; leukemia; osteosarcoma; pleural mesothelioma; and trophoblastic tumor types (uterine) Verma et al., 2020).

Deaths from DLBCL were accurately predicted by this classifier 73.2% of the time. Several "evolving fuzzy neural network" (EFuNN) classifiers were created in addition to the Bayesian classifier to process the genomic data. The top EFuNN classifier involved the incomplete use of 17 genes from the microarray data. The precision of this ideal EFuNN was 78.5%. A consensus forecast was reached by combining the EFuNN and Bayesian classifiers into a hierarchical modular system. The hybrid classifier outperformed all the individual classifiers employed with an accuracy of 87.5%. The top machine learning classifier (77.6% through SVMs) outperformed this method by 10% (Krithiga & Geetha, 2020).

The efficacy of the EFuNN classifier was examined using leave-one-out cross-validation. In this case, there was also no external validation set to test the model's generalizability. The sample per feature ratio (SFR) was somewhat greater than three due to the small number of samples (56 patients) used (17 gene characteristics). As a result, the authors went to great lengths to explain how their classifier operates to defend their strategy. They covered the basics of EFuNN, the construction of the Bayesian classifier, and the combination of the two into a single prediction. The authors also performed independent verification of the microarray data from the clinical data. For a machine learning analysis, the depth of this presentation is impressive. This study demonstrates that the accuracy of cancer prognosis predictions can be considerably increased by the capacity to mix clinical and genetic data.

4.2.3 Prediction of Cancer Recurrence

In approximately half (43%) of the studies considered in the analysis of prediction of cancer recurrence, machine learning was used. Researchers followed breast cancer patients for a median of five years to determine whether their disease would return (Bosco, 2009). Seven other predictive factors were combined with the patient's age, tumor size, and the number of axillary metastases. The data set also included protein indicators like progesterone and estrogen receptor concentrations. This study aimed to develop an automated, quantitative prognostic method that would perform better than the current TNM staging approach. TNM is mainly based on the expert clinical judgment of a pathologist with training in the field.

Each of the 2441 patients with breast cancer contributed seven data points to the study, resulting in a dataset with over 17,000 data points generated using an ANN-based model. This meant that the sample-to-feature ratio never dropped below the recommended threshold of 5. The data was divided into three equal portions for optimization and validation: training data (one-third), monitoring data (one-third), and test data (one-third). The researchers also acquired a second batch of 310 breast cancer patient samples from a separate institution for external validation. This allowed them to test how well their model would work outside their own organization.

Data handling and processing are exceptional due to the large amount of data used, the thoroughness of validation, and the stringent quality control measures.

For instance, to maintain high standards, the referring physicians independently examined the data after it was entered manually into a relational database. The sample size of 2441 patients and 17,000 data points after partitioning still allowed for the assumption of a normally distributed population of breast cancer patients. However, the authors tested this assumption by comparing the patient data distributions over all four sets (training, test, monitoring, and external) and finding that these parameters were comparable. The authors created a reliable and accurate classifier because of the rigorous quality assurance testing the author performed.

Because the study aimed to develop a model that predicted relapses more accurately than the standard TNM staging system, comparing the ANN model to the TNM staging system was essential. Comparisons were made using receiver operator characteristic curves (ROC curves). In terms of area under the ROC curve, the ANN model (0.72) beat the TNM system (0.677). This research is a prime illustration of how machine learning may be effectively used in various contexts.

There was sufficient data acquired, and the amount and quality of the data for each sample were independently checked. In order to evaluate the generalizability of the machine learning model, blinding sets from both the original data set and an external source were supplied. In conclusion, the model's performance was directly contrasted with that of TNM staging, a standard prognostic approach. This study's limitations may stem from the researchers focusing solely on one specific machine learning (ANN) technique. Another machine learning approach may have surpassed their ANN model, given the nature and quantity of the data collected.

4.3 AI AND MACHINE LEARNING APPROACHES FOR CANCER CELL PREDICTION IN BREAST CANCER

AI and machine learning algorithms have been effectively used for predicting diseases and performing detailed analysis of the test data for further treatment of the disease. Breast cancer prediction is now implemented through machine learning algorithms, as the analysis, diagnosis, and prediction involve complex data sets. So far, ANNs and decision trees based on machine learning have shown superior results in predicting cancer cells.

The cell lines in breast cancer are helpful for breast cancer analysis and modeling, as the cell lines contain a vast number of details in order to study the tumors. The cell lines can quickly accumulate mutations during the study and analysis of the cell lines, as the recent study (Naji et al., 2021) mentions that the breast cancer mortality rate in 2021 in India was around 12.7 per 10,000 women with an average age of approximately 25 years. This increase has alarmed us about the increasing cases of breast cancer worldwide. Machine and AI technology can help in the initial diagnosis and detection of cancer cells with better accuracy. The techniques applied so far from the machine learning family include support vector machines, decision trees, logistic regression, and k-nearest neighbors. The accuracy and precision of these listed methods and hence the efficiency of the detection can be figured out through a confusion matrix (Naji et al., 2021).

4.3.1 AI in Breast Imaging

With the advent of new imaging technologies, there is a vast scope for improvement in the interpretive tasks of cancer imaging. The advancements in the AI model-based computer-aided detection system have majorly worked better in detecting cancer cells and thus caused a reduction in false positives. Specific computer vision methods have recently been useful for pattern recognition in breast imaging. The most used systems, like ImageChecker M1000, also use computer vision to solve their purpose. There is a drastic increase in the AI technologies for breast cancer screening, where technologies like digital breast tomosynthesis came into existence along with other technologies, including the Tomo detection and screen point medical transparency techniques (Cruz & Wishart, 2007).

Recently, breast cancer has been a major cause of increased deaths in women worldwide. Keeping this in mind, it is correct to mention and consider that modern methodologies, including AI concepts, will work in the direction of diagnosing malignant lesions as early as possible to decrease the risk of more damage.

4.3.1.1 Image Processing: AI-Based Methods for Breast Cancer Diagnosis

Certain image processing methods are being used for breast cancer diagnosis, including mammography, thermography, immune imaging, etc. It is essential to screen the deadly disease's early symptoms so that the affected can receive necessary treatment. Many imaging techniques are available for the early diagnosis of breast cancer, but mammography is the most crucial. Mammography is an effective method for detecting breast cancer; however, it has had less success in cases where the breasts are dense. Diagnostic sonography is also one of the methods of image processing utilized for early identification of malignancy. These technologies can be further improved to handle factors like noise in the image, perception ability of the radiologists, poor contrast, insufficient clarity, etc. Mammography uses X-rays at low levels for imaging. Ultrasound is a highly sensitive and quick method for cancer detection. Thermography is a noninvasive breast cancer early detection method that is applicable to muscle tissues. The steps involved in this diagnosis include the following:

1. Image acquisition or image data collection
2. Image preprocessing and cleaning
3. Image segmentation
4. Feature extraction concerning the detection problem
5. Image categorization or classification

Regarding detecting breast cancer, feature extraction is considered the most crucial step. Some important breast tissue features include mean, skewness, kurtosis, energy, sum variance, contrast, homogeneity, etc.

4.3.1.1.1 Support Vector Machines

A spectral technique used for image classification for the images of breast tissues is the support vector machine. SVM has been successfully applied in MR image classification as it has a better classification rate and likelihood ratio (Lo & Wang, 2012).

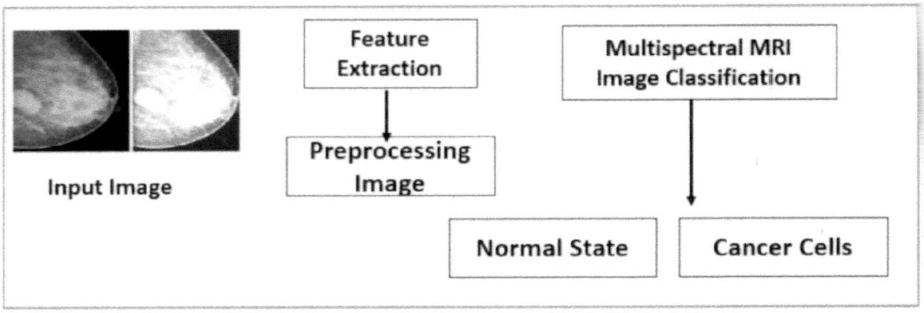

FIGURE 4.1 SVM-based multispectral MRI classification.

Multispectral MR image classification is successfully applied for the detection of breast cancer. The technique provides the capability of soft tissue characterization with the help of a hyperplane classifier. Figure 4.1 shows SVM-based multispectral MRI classification.

A Wisconsin diagnostic breast cancer dataset was analyzed with the SVM model for breast cancer prediction (Naji et al., 2021). The analysis covered primary classifiers, including KNN, decision tree, logistic regression, etc. Predictions were evaluated based on accuracy, precision, sensitivity, and F1 score. The SVM represents one of the best choices for efficient AI techniques for cancer cell detection.

4.3.1.1.2 Artificial Neural Networks

Many medical procedures have been implemented for years with the support of artificial neural networks (ANNs). The ANNs can handle a wide range of problems related to pattern recognition. ANN's are able to deal with different statistical classification methods like linear and non-linear regression techniques. ANN models can be trained to evaluate the threat of breast cancer based on mammographic and demographic image data. ANN has been successfully applied for the detection of problems in significant types of cancer. The mammography logistic regression model and the mammography ANN have resolved breast cancer-related issues. Building an ANN model requires less domain knowledge, and several user-friendly software interfaces are available. The ANNs are most suitable for modeling complex relationships that involve prior knowledge of the given data. ANN can model any arbitrary relationships between the variables.

4.3.1.1.3 Genetic Algorithms

Researchers have had several discussions over the years about the use of genetic algorithms to create techniques to diagnose breast cancer using the data provided. Neural networks have successfully implemented several image classification applications for breast cancer detection. Genetic algorithms combined with support vector machines can improve breast cancer detection efficiently. Genetic algorithms have the capability for better feature extraction and require less training time and comparatively less execution time. The genetic algorithms are categorized as evolutionary algorithms for solving complex problems like breast cancer prediction and analysis. A model based on genetic algorithms and SVM is shown in Figure 4.2.

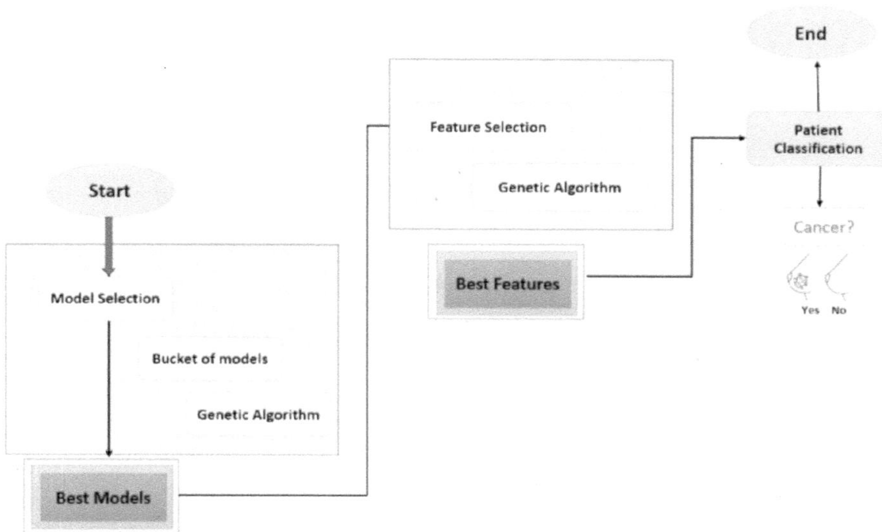

FIGURE 4.2 Genetic algorithm- and SVM-based breast cancer prediction.

4.3.1.2 Machine Learning-Based Techniques

4.3.1.2.1 Deep CNN for the Detection of Cell Abnormality (Krithiga & Geetha, 2020)

Detecting the early signs of starting breast cancer is better than starting the treatment process. A critical first step in the therapy of breast cancer is the diagnosis of the condition. Many computer-aided diagnosis systems have been created recently to find the anomalies in breast tissues. The detection of cancer cells has improved because of the use of CNN, which is based on deep learning. Deep learning, a branch of machine learning, has emerged as a solution to many challenges in medical research. The application of CNN helps to perform the feature extraction and classification tasks better for diagnosing breast cancer cells. The advantages of combining the features of deep learning with the CNN structure are high performance and the capability to deal with high dimensional data. Issues related to breast cancer imaging and diagnosis include image enhancement, bettering image segmentation, and classification as benign or malignant cells. The deep CNN-based model for breast cancer detection is given in Figure 4.3.

4.3.1.2.2 Machine Learning-Based Breast Cancer Detection Algorithms

Machine learning has been used in the diagnosis and treatment of breast cancer all over the world. Among the many technologies used in improving breast cancer detection and prediction are the support vector regression, random forest, support vector machine, k-nearest neighbor, naive Bayes, decision trees, back propagation neural networks, etc. (Qin et al., 2022). The primary stages of breast cancer detection are as shown in Figure 4.4.

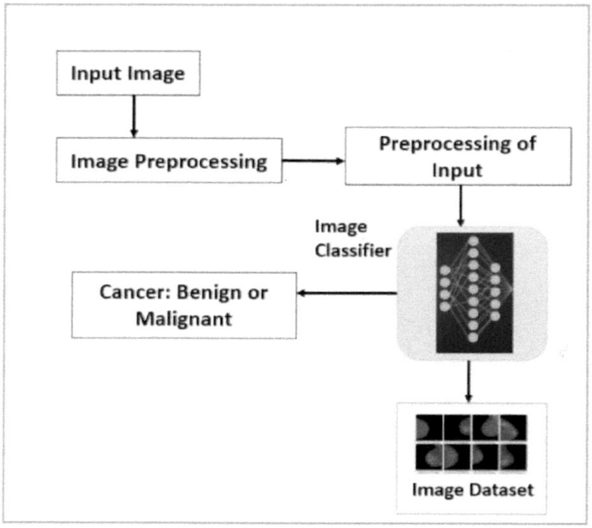

FIGURE 4.3 Deep CNN-based breast cancer detection.

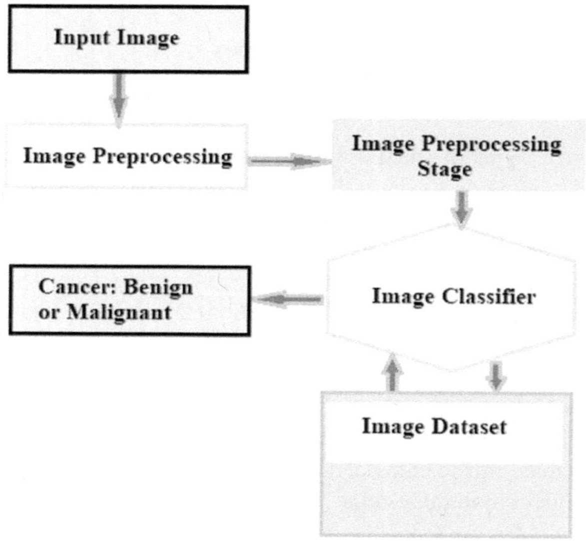

FIGURE 4.4 Breast cancer detection using machine learning.

4.3.1.2.3 Breast Cancer Segmentation with the Help of Multi-Scale CNNs

The authors (Lo & Wang, 2012) in their work have worked on the development of a two-stage segmentation method for breast cancer image segmentation. This could further help in the development of the breast cancer lesion segmentation model. A multi-scale lesion is applied for performing the delineation of the breast images, and then the result is processed using the rectified linear unit. This way, the accuracy of segmentation has significantly improved. The method used in this work has significantly reduced the small area mis-segmentation, giving better results.

Machine learning is well implemented for pattern classification and modeling, as it is possible to perform critical feature filtering and classification tasks. Machine learning methods are highly recommended for clinical methods where decision making and diagnosis are at the critical level. The ML model called support vector regression can be implemented for accuracy in the detection and prediction tasks. Other models, namely extreme learning machines and ensemble learning, have outperformed compared to SVM (Wu & Q, 2022).

4.3.1.2.4 Prediction-Based Approaches for Improving Diagnostic Accuracy

Several authors (Rajaguru & Prabhakar, 2017; Khandezamin et al., 2020) have worked on the improvement of the accuracy of cancer diagnosis with the help of machine learning techniques, which are efficient in classification tasks. They have utilized the machine learning models including support vector machines, random forest, naïve Bayes, and neural networks. The results were compared with the ensemble learning techniques. The aim of the research was to detect the cancer effects and growth in the body early, where accuracy is of the utmost importance. This has made the early start of treatment of the patient possible at the early stage itself. The accuracy of the system is compared with ensemble-based models and found to be effective.

4.3.1.2.5 Nucleus Detection in Breast Cancer using Histopathology Images

Researchers (Xu et al., 2016) identified that deep learning methods are in use recently for classification and big data analysis. The authors used a stacked sparse autoencoder for automated breast cancer tissue grading. In the histopathological images, the Nottingham histologic score system was used to relate the shape and appearance of cancer nuclei. The stacked sparse autoencoder (SSAE) is designed to be able to learn most of the high-level features from pixel intensities in order to find the different features of the nuclei. Th SSAE has outperformed other available methods with greater efficiency. The high-level features captured by this deep learning method can be utilized for detecting multiple nuclei from huge set of histopathological images.

4.3.1.2.6 Breast Cancer Classification Method with Bayesian Linear Discriminants

Researchers (Kamal et al., 2022; Rajaguru & Prabhakar, 2017) have worked on the Bayesian linear discriminant method of artificial intelligence algorithms for breast cancer classification. The machine learning and AI has worked aways in performing the required tasks with greater efficiency and accuracy. The method applied here has exhibited around 91.66% accuracy while performing the classification over the input dataset. The method has utilized benchmark evaluation parameters including perfect classification, false alarm, sensitivity, and specificity to compare and verify the results.

4.3.1.2.7 Applying Logistic Regression and GMDH for Breast Cancer Detection and Classification

Researchers have mentioned that (Bhangu et al., 2020) there is a requirement of a reliable system for breast cancer early detection. The machine learning algorithms have a large set of methods by which the detection of cancer cell largely can be done. In this work, the authors have worked on the development of a model with the help of a logistic regression method and the group method data handling (GMDH) classifier model to do the job of detection and classification. The results of fine needle aspiration have been key to the early detection, whereas the feature selection is done with the help of a machine learning algorithm. The performance of the system is evaluated with metrics including true and false positive rates, accuracy, and F-criteria. The future work could be concentrated on the development of the training set with more proper hospital data in it for improving the accuracy of the method.

4.3.1.2.8 Breast Cancer Survival Prediction Using Machine Learning and Deep Learning

Researchers (Kalafi et al., 2019) have worked on using machine learning and deep learning methods for predicting breast cancer survival. The methods applied here include the multilayer perceptron, random forest method, and decision tree classifier algorithm. All these algorithms have used the tumor size as a critical feature for the prediction. The authors have identified that the parameter configurations and the data transformation have an effect on the accuracy of the designed model. The evaluation parameters include the sensitivity, specificity, precision, and Matthew's correlation coefficient.

4.3.1.2.9 Multiple Compact CNNs for Breast Cancer Classification

Researchers (Zhu et al., 2019) have designed a hybrid model using multiple compact CNNs for the classification of breast cancer images. The model has a local model branch and also a global model branch that together generate the cancer representations. The overfitting problem has been handled with the help of a squeeze excitation pruning channel. The method applied here considers histopathology images for classification. This hybrid CNN can be used for breast cancer auxiliary scenarios and further can reduce the pathology work and allow quality diagnostics.

4.3.1.2.10 Deep Feature Integration and Selection for Breast Cancer Classification

Researchers (Hassan et al., 2023) identified that the capability of deep CNNs could be utilized to classify breast cancer images more appropriately. DL methods have successfully classified the images in many crucial applications. The concept of transfer learning is applied for the same, along with the four schemes of the CNN architecture. The scheme gives better accuracy, as a greater number of CNNs are applied along with a layer of SVM. The system performance is suitable for assisting in the diagnosing and assessing the breast cancer tissues.

4.3.2 GAN in Biomedical Image Segmentation

Authors (Iqbal et al., 2022) have mentioned the potential of GAN in image analysis tasks like segmentation and classification. They have tried to utilize GANs to address the open challenges in biomedical areas. The GAN-based methods for image synthesis are more effective in classification tasks. There are certain GAN-based segmentation methods available for use in image segmentation for various organs of the body with the added advantage of fast processing.

4.3.2.1 Role of F-FDG PET/CT in Early Evaluations

Researchers (Kamal et al., 2022) have highlighted the use of F-FDG PET/CT in the early diagnosis of the disease. The early diagnosis may help in the proper treatment of the disease. In this work, the authors have worked over the F-FDG PET/CT, which results in providing a way to plan the treatment and optimal therapeutic option for each patient condition. This method of evaluation consists of a full-body evaluation for breast cancer. The method has proven to be accurate and efficient for its purpose. It has been simple to manage the patient treatment plan as per the progress in the conditions.

4.4 RECENT DEVELOPMENTS IN TREATMENTS

4.4.1 Big Data Analytics (Qin et al., 2022)

Big data analytics considers a vast amount of medical data to make analyses required in the field. Some technologies, including cross-database and analytical big data, are applicable for breast cancer detection. Mammography is a widely used method for breast cancer screening and has a sensitivity of over 65% in maximum cases. The data obtained from the screening can be utilized for breast cancer prediction and other related statistics. Figure 4.5 shows big data analysis for breast cancer detection.

The third part of Figure 4.5 shows where big data analytics is applied where a set of operations is involved for data enhancement and other data-related issues. After this, the data are classified effectively. A new detection method was identified as predictive analysis, where early-stage breast cancer could be detected with more than 90% accuracy. The big data tools combined with machine learning methods help design an advanced method for detecting breast cancer much earlier to treat the disease at this stage and hence reduce the mortality rate. It is considered that early detection can help treat it well on time, and hence there are options to choose the best way to survive the deadly disease.

4.4.2 Biosensors

Biosensors were developed for analyzing bioanalytical subjects in various fields, including biomedical sciences, chemistry, and others (Mehrotra, 2016). Biosensors comprise a transducer and receptors, which work in coordination in detecting abnormalities in the body areas to detect the disease. The term in medical sciences called biomarkers helps us distinguish whether the test data show any disease. In the case of

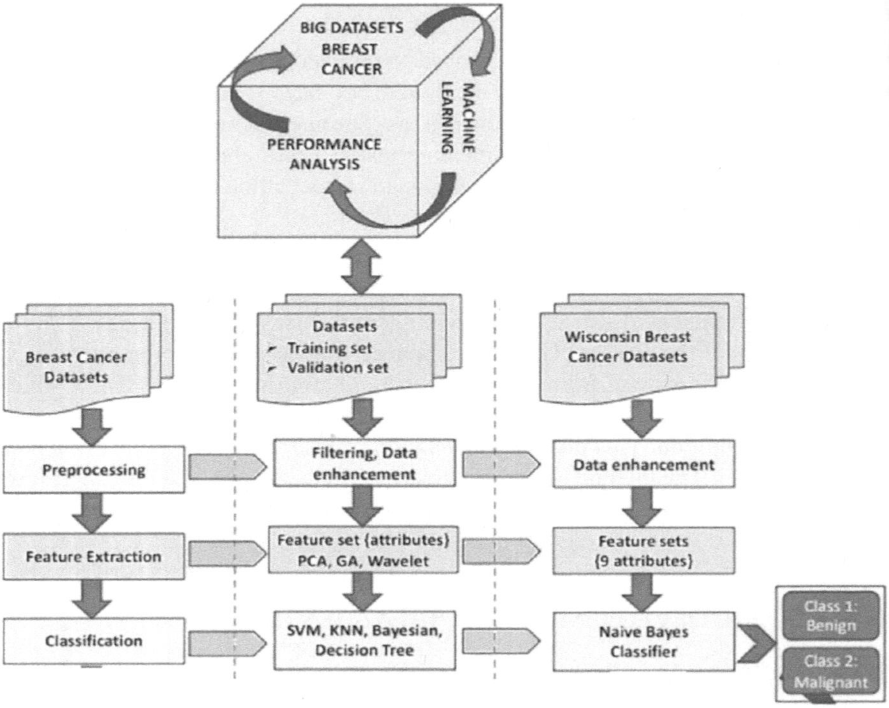

FIGURE 4.5 Big data analytics for breast cancer detection.

breast cancer, biomarkers work by analyzing the tissue samples and indicating a normal or abnormal condition. There are different kinds of biosensors in use, including DNA-based sensors and electrochemical biosensors, which can generate the analysis of body parts with the disease. The biosensors' advantages include simplicity, easy interfaces, high sensitivity, and cost-effectiveness. Surface acoustic wave biosensors are those that are used to indicate the presence of cancer cells. The surface acoustic wave device is developed as a biosensor system for capturing the antibodies and further detecting the abnormalities.

Label-free surface-enhanced Raman spectroscopy biosensors have been researched, where the idea of using human tears and the combination of multivariate identification algorithms is discussed to address breast cancer detection.

4.4.3 Deep Learning Applications for Breast Cancer Risk Prediction

Researchers (Bae & Kim, 2021) implemented the deep learning model mammography-based deep learning, where the tumor size was considered a crucial parameter for training the model. There are certain characteristics in the mammography image that can be considered crucial factors for breast cancer identification. This can be used as an input for the deep learning algorithm to assess the risk of the cancer. The rich information contained in the mammographic image can have detailed information beyond the breast density measure that could be utilized to find the interval as well as screen detected cancers. The image-based risk prediction can be helpful for the proper treatment of the patient at early stages and can also inform about the chances of breast cancer, if any.

4.4.4 Diagnosis of Breast Cancer and Prediction

Researchers (Naji et al., 2021) have concentrated on the treatment aspect of breast cancer, which correlates directly with the early diagnosis of the issue. The machine learning algorithms used in this work are the random forest, logistic regression, decision trees, and the KNN algorithm. The algorithms are made to predict and detect the cancer based on the data inputs, which are evaluated with the confusion matrix and precision parameters. The support vector machine was also employed in to check the accuracy of the system, and it came out to be useful.

4.5 COMPARATIVE ANALYSIS

It is generally better to treat breast cancer at its earliest stages, although prevention of the disease is possible as well. The most important thing when treating breast cancer patients is accurately diagnosing the disease. Data visualization and machine learning methods have been implemented and are being researched more to enhance their capability to detect and predict more accurately, even in complex scenarios. The detection and prediction of breast cancer rely on machine learning and deep learning. These techniques are covered in the analysis herein. The techniques mostly covered are the decision tree, random forest, naive Bayes, k-nearest neighbors, logistic regression, rotation forest, etc. The logistic regression model and support vector machines have shown better accuracy than other techniques, as shown in Table 4.1.

TABLE 4.1
Comparative Analysis

Sr No	Technique	Use	Advantages	Description
1	Logistic regression	One way to perform predictive analysis and build a risk estimation model for breast cancer	Produces better results in terms of specificity and sensitivity	Performed in two stages, including forward propagation and backward propagation
2	k-nearest neighbor	Labels the data before making further predictions	Lazy learning and no assumption	Clustering and regression
3	Naive Bayes classifier	A new classifier based on naive Bayes can be used to classify breast cancer images as benign or malignant using the improved classifier	Requires a small amount of training data	Probability classifier based on Bayes theorem

(Continued)

TABLE 4.1 (*Continued*)
Comparative Analysis

Sr No	Technique	Use	Advantages	Description
4	Random forest	Uses a dual-level randomization procedure	RFs are very efficient in dealing with low-data samples and have low bias	The process is used to achieve more accuracy during the diagnosis using big data classification
5	Decision tree	Uses the highest survival rate and data mining	Discovers hidden data through data mining	Explanatory and confirmatory classification
6	Support vector machine	Uses mammography-based images for classification	Provides better image classification accuracy	Discovers patterns of masked data in the input data for identifying cancer cells

4.6 FUTURE SCOPE

The ability of stakeholders, including medical students, trainee radiologists, licensed radiologists, other doctors, radiographers, computer scientists, data scientists, and data engineers to work together to solve clinically pertinent problems will be crucial for the success of AI and ML applications in radiology in the future. The development of technically sophisticated and clinically applicable AI solutions to meet the unmet requirements in oncology depends on this multidisciplinary discussion, which is essential and necessary. To promote contacts among all stakeholders, locally, nationally, and internationally, there is an obvious need for more multidisciplinary AI gatherings and conferences.

4.7 CONCLUSION

The most common type of cancer is breast cancer. In the early stages, it is curable, but in the later stages, no effective treatment has been found. In this technical era, breast image classification and the use of artificial intelligence, machine learning, and deep learning are being observed to be helpful in facilitating early detection and treatment to increase survival rates for patients. Cancer susceptibility, cancer survival prediction, and cancer recurrence prediction are the three most important aspects of this deadly disease. For these three different aspects, different techniques are being used. The ANN and decision tree-based models are among the most commonly used AI and machine learning tools to predict cancer cells. In breast tissue image classification, support vector machines are used as spectral techniques. Mammographic and demographic image data can be used to train ANN models to predict breast cancer risk. The logistic regression model has worked in resolving breast cancer-related issues.

By carefully planning, executing, selecting data, and exhaustively validating several machine learning algorithms, this chapter shows that it is possible to create an accurate and robust cancer risk assessment tool.

REFERENCES

Abbass, H. A. (2002). An evolutionary artificial neural networks approach for breast cancer diagnosis. *Artificial Intelligence in Medicine*, *25*(3), 265–281. https://doi.org/10.1016/s0933-3657(02)00028-3

Abdolmaleki, P., & Buadu, L. D., & Naderimansh, H. (2001). Feature extraction and classification of breast cancer on dynamic magnetic resonance imaging using artificial neural network. *Elsevier, Cancer Letters*, *171*(2), 183–191. https://doi.org/10.1016/s0304-3835(01)00508-0

Aggarwal, G., & Jain, S. (2019). Analysis of genes responsible for the development of cancer using machine learning. *2019 Third International Conference on Inventive Systems and Control (ICISC)*, 162–167. https://doi.org/10.1109/ICISC44355.2019.9036398

Akay, M. F. (2009). Support vector machines combined with feature selection for breast cancer diagnosis. *Expert Systems with Applications*, *36*(2), 3240–3247. https://doi.org/10.1016/j.eswa.2008.01.009

Andre, T., & Rangayyan, R. M. (2006). Classification of breast masses in mammograms using neural networks with shape, edge sharpness, and texture features. *Journal of Electronic Imaging*, *15*(1). https://doi.org/10.1117/1.2178271

Babu, G. A., Bhukya, S. N., & Sendhil Kumar, R. (2013). Feed forward network with back propogation algorithm for detection of breast cancer. *2013 8th International Conference on Computer Science & Education*. https://doi.org/10.1109/ICCSE.2013.6553907

Bae, M., & Kim, H. (2021). Breast cancer risk prediction using deep learning. *Radiology*, 559–560. https://doi.org/10.1148/radiol.2021211446

Bhangu, K. S., Sandhu, J. K., & Sapra, L. (2020). Improving diagnostic accuracy for breast cancer using prediction-based approaches. *2020 Sixth International Conference on Parallel, Distributed and Grid Computing (PDGC)*, 438–441. https://doi.org/10.1109/PDGC50313.2020.9315815

Bocchi, L., Coppini, G., Nori, J., & Valli, G. (2004). Detection of single and clustered microcalcifi cations in mammograms using fractals models and neural networks. *Medical Engineering & Physics*, *26*(4), 303–312. https://doi.org/10.1016/j.medengphy.2003.11.009

Bosco, J. L. F. (2009). Breast cancer recurrence in older women five to ten years after diagnosis. *Cancer Epidemiology, Biomarkers & Prevention*, *18*(11), 2979–2983. https://doi.org/10.1158/1055-9965.EPI-09-0607

Collins, G. S., Ogundimu, E. O., & Altman, D. G. (2016). Sample size considerations for the external validation of a multivariable prognostic model: A resampling study. *Statistics in Medicine, 35*(2), 214–226. https://doi.org/10.1002/sim.6787

Cruz, J. A., & Wishart, D. S. (2006). Applications of machine learning in cancer prediction and prognosis. *Cancer Informatics*, *2*, 59–77.

Cruz, J. A., & Wishart, D. S. (2007). Applications of machine learning in cancer prediction and prognosis. *Cancer Informatics*, *2*, 59–77.

Guo, H., & Nandi, A. K. (2006). Breast cancer diagnosis using genetic programming generated feature. Pattern recognition. *Pattern Recognition*, *39*(5), 980–987. https://doi org/10.1016/j.patcog.2005.10.001

Hagerty, R. G., Butow, P. N., Ellis, P. M., Dimitry, S., & Tattersall, M. H. N. (2005). Communicating prognosis in cancer care: A systematic review of the literature. *Annals of Oncology*, *16*(8), 1005–1053. https://doi.org/10.1093/annonc/mdi21

Hassan, A., Yahya, A., & Aboshosha, A. (2023). Breast cancer histopathology image classification through assembling multiple compact CNNs. *Neural Computing & Applications*, *2023*. https://doi.org/10.1007/s00521-023-08341-2

Hussain, M., Wajid, S. K., Elzaart, A., & Berbaret, M. (2011). A comparison of SVM kernel functions for breast cancer detection. *2011 Eighth International Conference Computer Graphics, Imaging and Visualization*. https://doi.org/10.1109/CGIV.2011.31

Iqbal, A., & Sharif, M., Yasmin, M., Raza, M., & Aftab, S. (2022). Generative adversarial networks and its applications in the biomedical image segmentation: A comprehensive survey. *International Journal of Multimedia Information Retrieval*, *11*, 333–368. https://doi.org/10.1007/s13735-022-00240-x

Iranpour, M., Almassi, S., & Analoui, M. (2007). Breast cancer detection from FNA using SVM and RBF classifier. *Conference 1st Joint Congress on Fuzzy and Intelligent Systems*.

Janghel, R., Shukla, A., Tiwari, R., & Kala, R. (2010). *Intelligent Decision Support System for Breast Cancer, Advances in Swarm Intelligence, First International Conference, ICSI 2010*, Beijing, China, June 12–15, 2010, Proceedings, Part II, https://doi. org/10.1007/978-3-642-13498-2_46

Kalafi, E. Y., Nor, N. A., Taib, N. A., Ganggayah, M. D., & Town, C. (2019). Detection and classification of breast cancer using logistic regression feature selection and GMDH classifier. *Folia Biologica (Praha)*, *65*(5–6), 212. https://doi.org/32362304

Kamal, A. M., Kamal, O. A., Sakr, H. M., & Ali, S. A. (2022). Role of ^{18}F-FDG PET/CT in evaluation of recently diagnosed breast cancer patients. *Egyptian Journal of Radiology and Nuclear Medicine*, *53*, 178. https://doi.org/10.1186/s43055-022-00866-1

Khandezamin, Z., Naderan, M., & Rashti, M. (2020). Detection and classification of breast cancer using logistic regression feature selection and GMDH classifier. *2nd International Conference on Communication and Electronics Systems (ICCES)*, *111*(103591), 266–269. https://doi.org/10.1016/j.jbi.2020.103591

Krithiga, R., & Geetha, P. (2020). Deep learning based breast cancer detection and classification using fuzzy merging techniques. *Machine Vision and Applications*, *63*, 169–171. https://doi.org/10.1007/s00138-020-01122-0

Lo, C. S., & Wang, C. M. (2012). Support vector machine for breast MR image classification. *Computers & Mathematics With Applications*, *64*(5), 1153–1162. https://doi. org/10.1016/j.camwa.2012.03.033

Maclin, P. S., & Dempsey, J. (1991). Using neural networks to diagnose cancer. *Journal Medical Systems*, *15*(1), 11–19. https://doi.org/10.1007/BF00993877

Markey, M. K., Lo, J. Y., Tourassi, G. D., & Floyd Jr., C. E. (2003). Self-organizing map for cluster analysis of a breast cancer database. *Artificial Intelligence in Medicine*, *27*(2), 113–127. https://doi.org/10.1016/s0933-3657(03)00003-4

McCarthy, J. F., Marx, K. A., Hoffman, P. E., Gee, A. G., O'Nil, P., Ujwal, M. L., & Hotchkiss, J. (2004). Applications of machine learning and high-dimensional visualization in cancer detection, diagnosis, and management. *Annals of New York Academy of Sciences*, *1020*, 239–262. https://doi.org/10.1196/annals.1310.020

Mehrotra, P. (2016). Biosensors and their applications – A review. *Journal of Oral Biology and Craniofacial Research,*https://www.ncbi.nlm.nih.gov/pmc/articles/PMC4862100/ *6*(2), 153–159. https://doi.org/10.1016/j.jobcr.2015.12.002

Naji, M. A., Filali, S. E., Aarika, K., Benlahmar, E. L. H., Abdelouhahid, R. A., & Debauche, O. (2021). Machine learning algorithms for breast cancer prediction and diagnosis. *Procedia Computer Science*, *191*, 487–492. https://doi.org/10.1016/j.procs.2021.07.062

Petricoin, E. F., & Liotta, L. A. (2005). SELDI-TOF-based serum proteomic pattern diagnostics for early detection of cancer. *Current Opinion in Biotechnology*, *15*, 24–30.

Qin, C., Wu, Y., Tian, L., Zhai, Y., Li, F., & Zhang, X. (2022). Joint transformer and multi-scale CNN for DCE-MRI breast cancer segmentation. *Soft Computing*, *26*, 8317–8334. https://doi.org/10.1007/s00500-022-07235-0

Rajaguru, H., & Prabhakar, S. K. (2017a). A comprehensive analysis on breast cancer classification with radial basis function and gaussian mixture model. *16th International Conference on Biomedical Engineering (ICBME), Singapore*, *61*, 21–27.

Rajaguru, H., & Prabhakar, S. K. (2017b). Expectation maximization based logistic regression for breast cancer classification. *2017 International Conference of Electronics, Communication and Aerospace Technology (ICECA)*, 603–606. https://doi.org/10.1109/ICECA.2017.8203608

Rajaguru, H., & Prabhakar, S. K. (2017c). Bayesian linear discriminant analysis for breast cancer classification. *2017 2nd International Conference on Communication and Electronics Systems (ICCES)*, 266–269. https://doi.org/10.1109/CESYS.2017.8321279

Reddy, S. G., & Reddy, K. T. (2014). An SVM based approach to breast cancer classification using RBF and polynomial kernel functions with varying arguments. *International Journal of Computer Science and Information Technologies*, *5*(4), 5901–5904.

Ryu, U., & Chandrasekaran, R. (2007). Breast cancer prediction using the isotonic separation technique. *European Journal of Operational Research*, *181*(2), 842–854. https://doi.org/10.1016/j.ejor.2006.06.031

Sahan, S., Polat, K., Kodaz, H., & Güneş, S. (2007). A new hybrid method based on fuzzy-artificial immune system and k-nn algorithm for breast cancer diagnosis. *Computers in Biology and Medicine*, *37*(3), 415–423. https://doi.org/10.1016/j.compbiomed.2006.05.003

Simes, R. J. (1985). Treatment selection for cancer patients: Application of statistical decision theory to the treatment of advanced ovarian cancer. *Journal Chronic Disease*, *38*(2), 171–186. https://doi.org/10.1016/0021-9681(85)90090-6

Thomas, T., Pradhan, N., & Dhaka, V. S. (2020). Comparative analysis to predict breast cancer using machine learning algorithms: A survey. *2020 International Conference on Inventive Computation Technologies (ICICT)*, 192–196.

Ubeyli, E. D. (2007). Implementing automated diagnostic systems for breast cancer detection. *Expert Systems with Applications*, *33*(4), 1054–1062. https://doi.org/10.1016/j.eswa.2006.08.005

Verma, S. K., Arora, D., & Bhardwaj, R. (2020). Breast cancer survival rate prediction in mammograms using machine learning. *2020 2nd International Conference on Advances in Computing, Communication Control and Networking (ICACCCN)*, 169–171. https://doi.org/10.1109/ICACCCN51052.2020.9362741

Wang, J. X., Zhang, B., Yu, J., Liu, J., Yang, M., & Zheng, S. (2005). Application of serum protein fingerprinting coupled with artificial neural network model in diagnosis of hepatocellular carcinoma. *Chinese Medical Journal*, *118*(15), 1278–1284.

Wolberg, W. H., & Mangasarian, O. L. (1990). Multisurface method of pattern separation for medical diagnosis applied to breast cytology. *Proceedings of the National Academy of Sciences*, *87*(23), 9193–9196. https://doi.org/10.1073/pnas.87.23.9193

Xu, J., Xiang, L., Liu, Q., Gilmore, H., Wu, J., Tang, J., & Madabhushi, A. (2016). Stacked Sparse Autoencoder (SSAE) for nuclei detection on breast cancer histopathology images. *IEEE Transactions on Medical Imaging*, *35*(1), 119–130. https://doi.org/10.1109/TMI.2015.2458702

Zhou, X., Liu, K. Y., & Wong, S. T. C. (2004). Cancer classification and prediction using logistic regression with Bayesian gene selection. *Journal of Biomedical Informatics*, *37*(4), 249–259. https://doi.org/10.1016/j.jbi.2004.07.009

Zhu, C., Song, F., Wang, Y., Dong, D., Guo, Y., & Liu, J. (2019). Breast cancer histopathology image classification through assembling multiple compact CNNs. *BMC Medical Informatics Decision Making*, *198*. https://doi.org/10.1186/s12911-019-0913-x

5 Genetic Diagnosis, Classification, and Risk Prediction in Cancer Using Next-Generation Sequencing in Oncology

Kazeem A. Dauda,†, Kabir O. Olorede*, Alabi W. Banjoko**, Waheed B. Yahya**, and Yusuf O. Ayipo****

*Department of Mathematics and Statistics, Kwara State University, Malate, Nigeria; **Department of Statistics, University of Ilorin, Ilorin, Nigeria; ***Department of Chemistry and Industrial Chemistry, Kwara State University, Ilorin, Nigeria.
†Corresponding Author: kazeem.dauda@kwasu.edu.ng

ABBREVIATIONS

BA	Boruta algorithm
DL	Deep learning
GEO	Gene expression omnibus
GSDRA	Gene selection and dimension reduction algorithm
MID	Mutual information difference
MIM	Mutual information maximization
MIQ	Mutual information quotient
MRMR	Minimum redundancy maximum relevance
NGS	Next-generation sequencing
PRGs	Pyroptosis-related genes
RF	Random forest

5.1 INTRODUCTION

Machine-learning techniques provide important advantages in classifying important biomarkers in clinical oncology in terms of patient genomics and understanding reduced drug toxicity in the treatment of cancer diseases (Buzdin et al., 2020; Zhukov and Tjulandin, 2008; Xiao et al., 2022). The most common malignancy in women is recognized to be breast cancer, which exhibits the fifth highest death rate globally, after

DOI: 10.1201/9781032699882-5

stomach cancer (Sung et al., 2020). Therefore, due to the increase in incidence and mortality, it is very important to evaluate prognosis biomarkers and identify the most appropriate therapeutic regimen for malignant breast cancer tumor patients. In this regard, machine-learning methods such as deep learning methods have become necessary for the efficient and accurate classification of biomarkers and the identification of prognostic factors in gene expression data, either through RNA sequencing or microarray (Rodon et al., 2019). More recently, a new technology known as next-generation sequencing (NGS) has been developed to increase gene expression quantification and allow the investigation of epigenetics on a large scale of genomes (Metzker, 2010; Park et al., 2021).

Analyzing the gene expression data produced by microarray technology or NGS requires two distinct learning approaches, and these approaches are supervised and unsupervised learning. These two machine-learning techniques are purposely mentioned in this chapter since in microarray analysis, the number of genes is significantly greater than the number of samples, thus leading to the need for accurate methodologies (Dauda, 2022; Poplin et al., 2018; Cao et al., 2015). Hence, due to the phenomenon of this curse of dimensionality, researchers have introduced gene selection mechanisms for selecting the most important genes and using them for classification purposes (Mao et al., 2013). Minimizing the number of genes and selecting meaningful ones pose advantages regarding the prediction and classification accuracy of supervised learning, particularly deep learning (Dauda et al., 2021; Cao et al., 2015). Therefore, this chapter is aimed to develop a mechanism that extracts the most informative genes that are associated with breast cancer prognostic progressions. Thus, the chapter considers the use of minimum redundancy maximum relevance (MRMR) (Xie et al., 2022; Alshamlan et al., 2015; Jo et al., 2019) and mutual information maximization (MIM) (Macedo et al., 2022) as filtering processes, followed by the use of the Boruta algorithm (BA) (Dauda et al., 2021), and lastly the implementation of deep learning (DL) (Dauda et al., 2021). The chapter presents an algorithm that utilizes the efficiency of MRMR, MIM, BA, and DL, then termed the MRMRBADL and MIMBADL algorithms, for reliable biomarker selection and classification.

The specific objective of this study is to devise an effective algorithm for identifying and extracting important genes and ignoring noisy, redundant, and irrelevant genes in breast cancer data. The merit of these algorithms (MRMRBADL and MIMBADL) relies on two-component dimension reduction and biomarker classification (Zhang et al., 2019). Precisely speaking, the novelty of this study comes from the process of using three major components of feature selection, and these help our algorithm to be efficient in gene selection and unique in terms of classification since the investigation uses the merit of the deep learning procedure. Finally, the chapter considers the use of five real-life cancer datasets publicly available from the Gene Expression Omnibus (GEO) repository (Barrett et al., 2013).

This chapter has been organized as follows: we begin in section 5.2 by revising some existing approaches to dimension reduction; section 5.3 shows the development of the MRMRBADL and MIMBADL algorithms; section 5.4 describes the novelty of the proposed algorithms on the five real-life data and explains the empirical analysis of the developed algorithm and the results; finally, section 5.5 describes the concluding part of the study.

5.2 BACKGROUND AND DRIVING FORCES

This section briefly explains and introduces some methods applied in the course of dimension reduction for high-throughput profiling data. Both supervised and unsupervised learning algorithms have been adopted to mitigate the challenge of feature selection in next-generation sequencing (NGS) technology. Although these techniques have expanded in the last decade, they still require significant improvement in terms of accuracy and computational time. In early 2017, Ram et al. (2017) considered the use of random forest (RF) to perform dimension reduction on high-dimensional data. However, this study only focused on the selection of genes for diagnosis and effective treatment and ignored other stages of feature selection, which are wrapper and embedded stages. Similarly, Song et al. (2022) considered the use of principal component analysis to distinguish between differentially expressed proptosis-related genes (PRGs) in psoriasis patients and the samples. This study also ignored two of the major components (wrapper and embedded algorithms). Other studies such as Toth et al. (2019), Koul and Manvi (2021), Shukla et al. (2019), and Koppad et al. (2022) have implemented some other measures of feature selection in the line of the filtering procedure using machine-learning techniques. In summary, it is clear that the performance of the dimension reduction methods depends on the three major stages (filtering, wrapper, and embedded), and the stages ensure optimal selection of quality features.

5.3 RESEARCH METHODOLOGY

This section presents the ideas and algorithm procedure of the proposed gene selection method and classification technique. Three main stages (filter, wrapper, and embedded) were involved in this study, and each of them will be thoroughly discussed in the subsequent sections.

5.3.1 Gene Selection and Dimension Reduction Algorithm (GSDRA)

This study proposed two methods of gene selection and dimension reduction (GSDRA) through minimum redundancy maximum relevance (MRMR) and mutual information maximation (MIM) techniques. The procedures of GSDRA consisted of three stages: filter, wrapper, and embedded techniques, as shown in Figure 5.1. The MRMR feature selection method was employed at the filtering stage to remove the possible redundancy, irrelevancy, and noisy genes that might reduce and mislead the prediction accuracy of employed classifier. Afterward, to examine possible dependencies between the gene expression values, the wrapper procedure was adopted through an algorithm called Boruta. The purpose of this second stage is to detect the interaction between the cancer outcome (responder and non-responder) and the gene expression. The last stage consists of implementing and embedding the desired classifier called deep learning. Deep learning was chosen due its capability to classify complex data and ability to train data with linear, non-linear, and interaction effects among the features. The full description of the proposed framework presented in Figure 5.1 is given in Table 5.1.

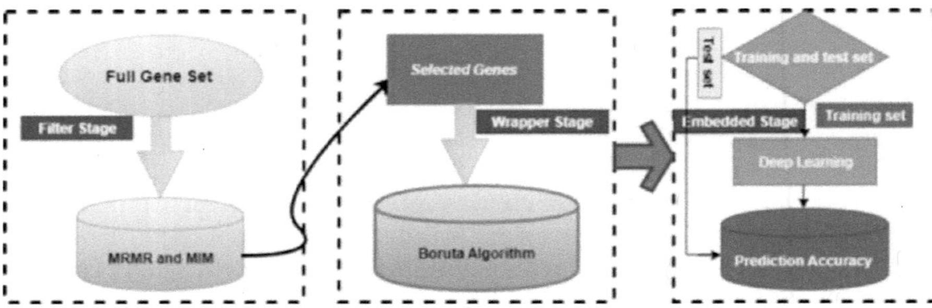

FIGURE 5.1 Proposed framework for gene selection and classification.

TABLE 5.1
Description of the Proposed Framework

Step	Function	Remark
	Filter Stage	
1.	Enter next-generation sequencing data (full gene set)	This study makes use of publicly available data in the GEO repository.
2.	Implement MRMR and MIM algorithms	The most important genes were selected and saved for stage 2.
Wrapper Stage		
3.	Implement Boruta algorithm on the genes selected in stage 1	The most influential genes were selected and saved for stage 3.
Embedded Stage		
4.	Divide the data into training and test sets based on the selected genes in stage 2	The data will be divided into 80% training and 20% test sets.
5.	Train the training set using deep learning	The training set will be trained using deep learning.
6.	Use the test set to validate the trained model	The trained model will be validated using the test set through prediction accuracy.
7.	Finally, compare the prediction accuracy of the proposed model with that of another existing method.	

5.3.2 Filter: Minimum Redundancy Maximum Relevance (MRMR) and Mutual Information Maximation (MIM)

Selecting the most influential genes from high-dimensional data involves the filtering process. This chapter considers the use of MRMR and MIM, and the details are given in the next sections.

5.3.2.1 Filter: Minimum Redundancy Maximum Relevance (MRMR)

The MRMR was purposely designed to reduce the irrelevant features during the feature selection procedure, as was suggested by Ding and Peng (2005). The MRMR also tried to observe the redundancy and relevancy of the features and class of vectors containing a set of given features. This was achieved by using mutual information provided in Equation (1) through feature space x and target response y.

$$I(x \mid y) = \sum_{i,j} \log \frac{p(x_i, y_j)}{p(x_i)\,p(y_j)} \tag{1}$$

Where $p()$ denotes probability. Let S be a set of given features and h a class of random variables. Thus, the redundancy (w_i) of S can be measured using the quantity in Equation (2). Subsequently, the relevancy (V_I) of S will be measured using Equation (3).

$$w_i = \frac{1}{|S|^2} \sum_{i,j \in s} I(i, j), \tag{2}$$

$$V_I = \frac{1}{|S|} \sum_{i \in s} I(h, j). \tag{3}$$

Therefore, S will then be evaluated using the any of the quantities in below:

MIQ (mutual information quotient): $V_I - w_i$

MID (mutual information difference): $\frac{V_I}{w_i}$

In the subset of all features S cannot be tested in a given dataset, then the MRMR algorithm is adopted for implementation (for full details see Jo et al., 2019).

5.3.2.2 Filter: Mutual Information Maximation (MIM)

The second filter method considered in this study was MIM, initially developed by Lewis (1992). In recent years, the application of MIM has attracted the attention of many computational scientists due to its ability to accurately select influential features with the class label using information theory. In the MIM procedure, each feature in the dataset is independent of other features, and the specific formula is presented in Equation (4) as follows:

$$J(x_k) = I(x_k; y). \tag{4}$$

Where x_k is the candidate feature and y denotes the class label.

5.3.3 Wrapper: Boruta Algorithm (BA)

The Boruta algorithm (BA) is an extension of knowledge that determines important genes by comparing the importance of all real genes to random probes (Kursa and Rudnicki, 2010). The BA was purposely developed to identify all relevant genes in the realm of classification learning algorithms. The main concept behind the BA is to compare the important genes with those of randomly chosen shadow genes using statistical tests and random forests.

5.3.3.1 Proposed BA Working Structure (MRMR+BA and MIM+BA)

This section presents the implementation of the filter method within the realm of BA. In the same vein, we combine filter and wrapper techniques as a single algorithm, as presented in Algorithm 1.

Algorithm 1 BA Working Structure

```
1: Recall the most relevant gene from filtering methods (MRMR and MIM)
2: Implement wrapper using BA structure ;
3: Return the best and the optimal genes subset;
4: Recall the best and the optimal genes selected by the BA;
5: Implement embedded method
```

5.3.4 Embedded: Deep Learning (DL)

The machine-learning technique that uses multiple layers of neural networks to build the processing data and perform large computations on a large amount of data is known as deep learning (Dauda et al., 2021). The working structure of deep learning is based on the function of the human brain with the capability of learning without a human supervisor. The functional form of DL consists of three layers, as shown in Figure 5.2, and these include input, hidden, and output layers. The input layer contains the input features, which are known in this study to be gene expression, while the hidden layers is just like training the brain through the hidden million neurons. The output layer consists of a set of target values that the study wants to classify or predict based on the available information. The full details of DL can be found in the study of Poplin et al. (2018).

5.3.4.1 Proposed MRMRBADL and MIMBADL Algorithm

This method relies on the efficiency of the filtering, wrapper, and embedded techniques, as presented in the previous section. The procedure involves selecting the most influential genes through the filtering and wrapper and then implementing the embedded method (DL) at the final stage of Algorithm 2, as presented. The next section presents the various results generated through the proposed algorithm and the existing methods.

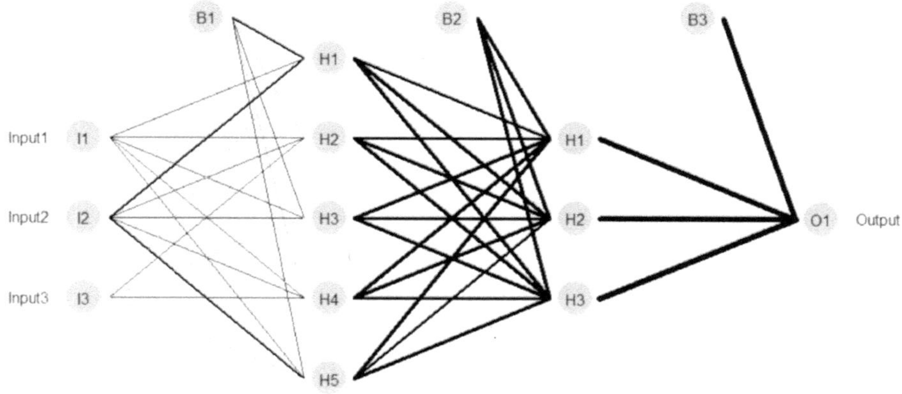

FIGURE 5.2 DL algorithm architecture.

Algorithm 2 MRMRBADL and MIMBADL Working Structure.

Recall the most relevance gene from filtering methods (MRMR and MIM)
Implement wrapper using BA structure ;
Return the best and the optimal genes subset;
Recall the best and the optimal genes selected by the BA;
Implement embedded method

5.3.5 Measures of Indices

In an attempt to ensure the efficiency of the proposed model and compare the performance of this method, this study aims at using some promising methods of evaluation. These methods include the prediction accuracy and misclassification error rate together with a number of genes selected at each stage of our proposed algorithms. In computing the prediction accuracy and misclassification error rate, we let

TP = true positive, FP = false positive, TN = true negative, and FN = false negative. Thus,

$$\text{Prediction Accuracy} = \frac{TP + TN}{TP + TN + FP + FN}$$

$$\text{Misclassification Error} = \frac{FP + FN}{TP + TN + FP + FN}$$

5.4 RESULTS AND DISCUSSION

This section presents the results of the proposed algorithms on the five real-life datasets extracted from the next-generation sequencing dataset in oncology. The five datasets were publicly available and can be downloaded through the Gene Expression Omnibus (GEO) repository (Barrett et al., 2013). The datasets were mainly from patients with breast cancer, and the dataset IDs, therapies, and experimental platforms are presented in Table 5.2. The full description of these genomic datasets can be found in the literature as presented and cited in the last column of Table 5.2.

5.4.1 Filter: Gene Selection Results

At the first stage of this study, the MRMR and MIM were implemented on the five real-life datasets to filter out irrelevant genes that might not be associated with responders to cancer chemotherapy. Therefore, the filter stage only retains genes that of importance to the prediction of cancer chemotherapy response. This stage has successfully enhanced the correlation between genes and cancer chemotherapy responders while reducing the potential correlation between different genes during the implementation process. The results of this section are presented in Table 5.3, and the results revealed that the chosen procedures for the filtering process (MRMR and MIM) selected viewer genes more than the conditional mutual information maximization (CMIM) method by Fleuret (2004). This filtering stage is very important since nuisance genes might reduce the performance of the machine-learning algorithm at the final stage of our proposed algorithm. The next section contains the results of stage 2, as shown in Figure 5.1.

TABLE 5.2
Overview of the Five Selected Transcriptomic Datasets of Responders/Non-Responders to Cancer Chemotherapy, Responders (R) vs Non-Responders (NR)

Dataset ID	Therapy	Experimental Platform	References
GSE18728	Docetaxel, capecitabine	Affymetrix Human Genome U133 Plus 2.0 Array	Korde et al., 2010
GSE41998	Neoadjuvant doxorubicin + cyclophosphamide, followed by paclitaxel	Affymetrix Human Genome U133 Array	Horak et al., 2013
GSE50948	Paclitaxel + doxorubicin followed by cyclophosphamide + methotrexate/fluorouracil followed by trastuzumab	Affymetrix Human Genome U133 Plus 2.0 Array	Prat et al., 2020
GSE20181	Letrozole	Affymetrix Human Genome U133A Array	Miller and Larionov, 2010
GSE37946	Trastuzumab	Affymetrix Human Genome U133A Array	Liu et al., 2012

5.4.2 Wrapper: MRMR+BA and MIM+BA Results

The second stage of this investigation involved the implementation of a wrapper procedure based on the results generated through the filtering process, as shown in the flowchart (see Figure 5.1). This stage used the Boruta algorithm to further select the most influential and important genes through the efficiency of this algorithm. The power of this procedure contends in the number of genes selected and computational time against some with the existing methods in the literature (Almazrua and Alshamlan, 2022; Zhao et al., 2019). The investigation also considers the use of prediction accuracy and misclassification error rate to further investigate the performance of the proposed method over the existing techniques.

The results in Table 5.4 reveal the performance of the proposed methods over the existing method in terms of the number of selected genes and the computational

TABLE 5.3
Comprehensive Comparison between the State-of-the-Art Mutual Information Methods in Terms of the Number of Selected Genes for the Five Benchmark Microarray Gene Expression Datasets

Dataset	#Sample Size	#Gene	MRMR	CMIM	MIM
GSE18728	60	16383	**3564**	4377	5141
GSE41998	279	16383	**8191**	8193	8192
GSE50948	156	16383	**8191**	8193	8192
GSE20181	176	16383	**8191**	8193	8192
GSE37946	50	16383	**8190**	8197	8192

The **bold results** denote optimal performance over the unbolded values.

TABLE 5.4
Comparison of MRMR+BA and MIM+BA against Some Existing Methods in Terms of the Number of Genes Selected and Computational Time

	Proposed Methods				Existing Methods			
	MRMR+BA		MIM+BA		CMIM+RF (Almazrua and Alshamlan, 2022)		MRMR+RF (Zhao et al., 2019)	
Dataset	# of Genes	Time*	# of Genes	Time*	# of Genes	Time*	# of Genes	Time*
GSE18728	**5**	37.40	10	**21.70**	195	343.20	182	147.21
GSE41998	8	**1.94**	8	95.23	530	444.11	529	110.92
GSE50948	8	**78.04**	**5**	99.01	423	49.81	401	54.30
GSE20181	**6**	47.64	20	**38.65**	534	43.89	562	66.70
GSE37946	**1**	33.01	10	**29.54**	154	39.51	159	38.48

The **bold results** denote optimal performance over the unbolded values.

time. The two proposed methods (MRMR+BA and MIM+BA) compete favorably based on the number of genes selected and the computational time. However, the MRMR+BA approach appears to be more consistent and selects more viewer genes than the MIM+BA approach, all achieved with very little computational time. Nevertheless, both developed methods outperformed the existing methods irrespective of the indices. Subsequently, this chapter further presents the selected genes from the oncology datasets using boxplots, as shown in Figures 5.3 and 5.4. The figures reveal the most prominent and common genes associated with cancer chemotherapy status.

In other to investigate more on how the proposed methods performed over the existing methods, we considered the use of prediction accuracy and error rate; the corresponding results are presented in Table 5.5. The results also revealed that MRMR+BA and MIM+BA compete favorably irrespective of the evaluation methods, and both of them outperform the existing methods.

5.4.3 Embedded: MRMRBADL and MIMBADL Algorithm Results

The last stage of this investigation included the implementation of MRMRBADL and MIMBADL algorithms. The selected genes from stage 2 of our flowchart were then progressed to the embedded method, and in this stage, only the most important genes selected from stage 2 were used to train the algorithm. This study evaluates the performance of the developed algorithms against the existing method using prediction accuracy, and the results are presented in Table 5.6. The results in Table 5.6 reveal that the proposed methods (MRMRBADL and MIMBADL) outperformed the existing method.

5.4.4 Future Prospects and Limitations

The most critical and challenging task in machine learning in the realm of next-generation sequencing is dimension reduction. Dimension reduction tries to obtain a valuable and high-quality feature subset while maintaining the initial critical characteristics of the data. Thus, in the course of obtaining the quality features, this investigation simultaneously engaged and developed three machine-learning algorithms through filtering, wrapper, and embedded. The results highlight the contribution of the three machine-learning algorithms in feature selection based on next-generation sequencing data. More importantly, they reveal the superiority of the developed methods over the existing techniques. Besides the achievements of the proposed methods mentioned above, the following limitations should be noted: a limited number of filtering, wrapper, and embedded techniques were considered, and the investigation has not employed a wide range of other techniques. Therefore, we suggest that future studies should include a wide range of filtering, wrapper, and embedded techniques.

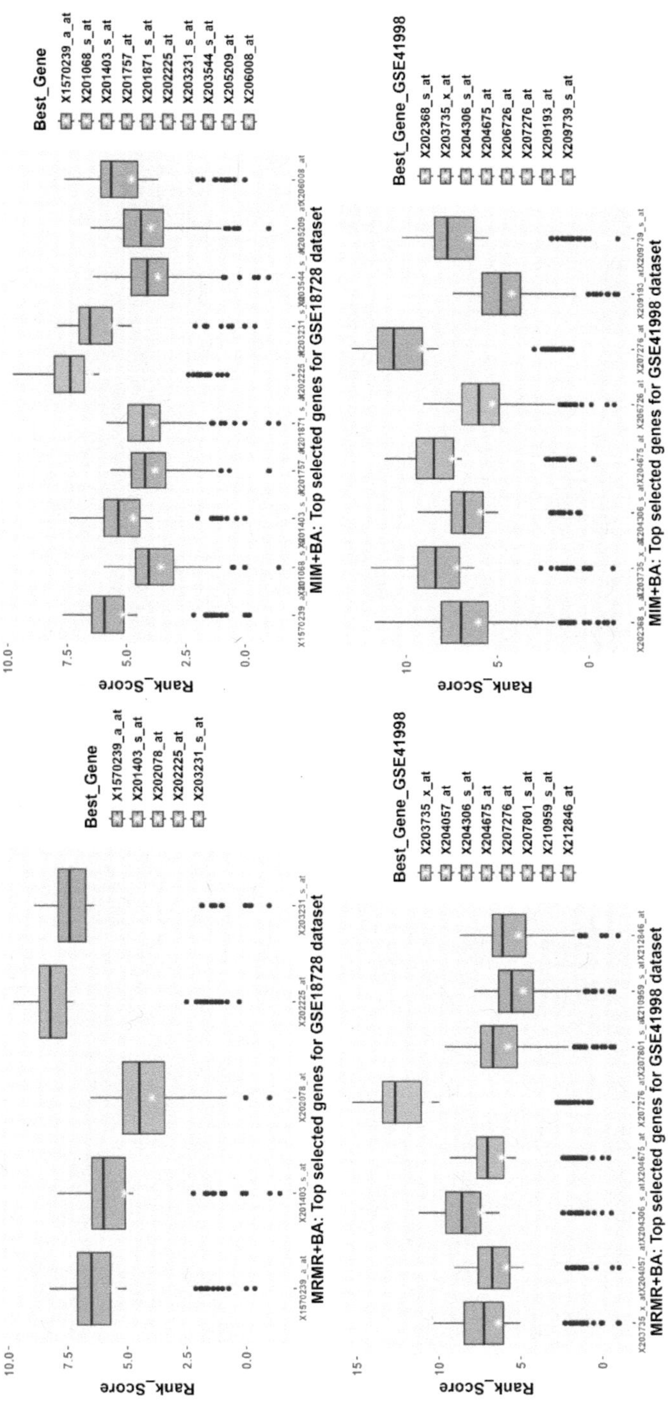

FIGURE 5.3 MRMR+BA and MIM+BA selected genes for GSE18728 and GSE41998 datasets.

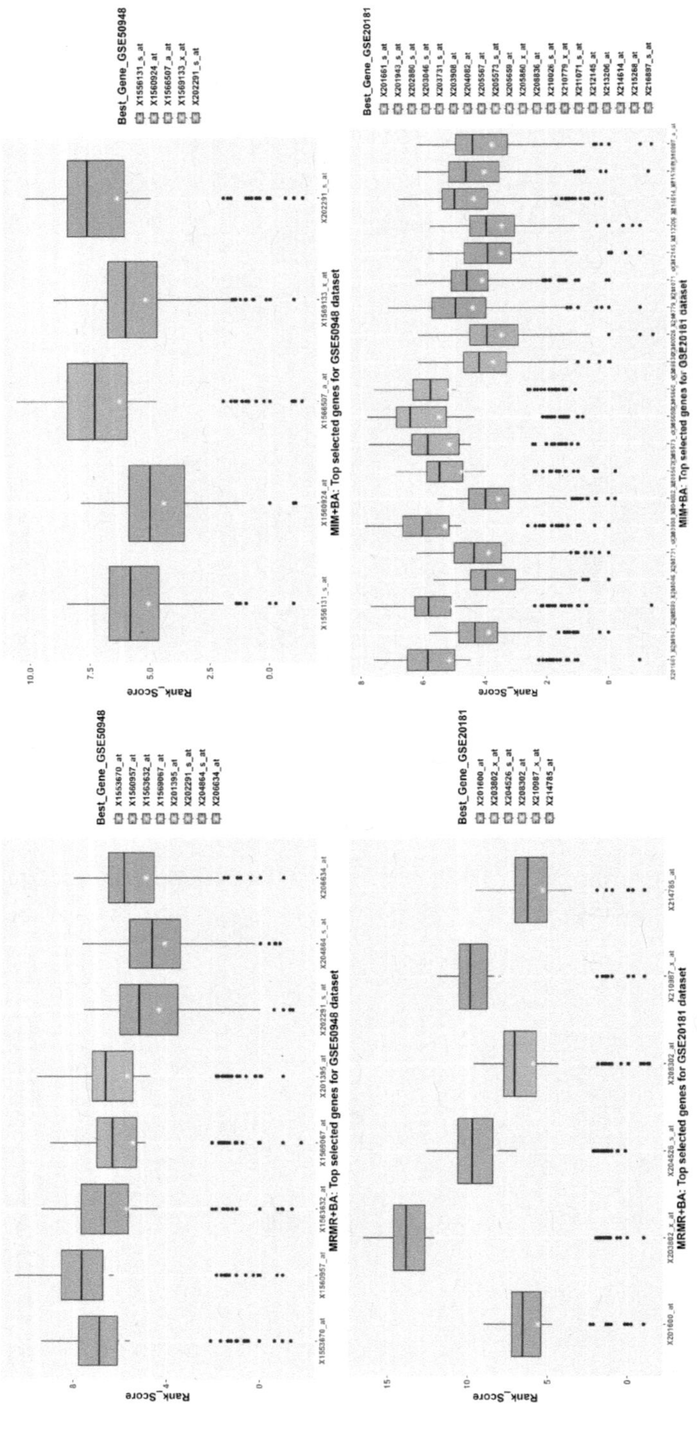

FIGURE 5.4 MRMR+BA and MIM+BA selected genes for GSE50948 and GSE20181 datasets.

TABLE 5.5
Comparison of MRMR+BA and MIM+BA against Some Existing Methods in Terms of Prediction Accuracy and Error Rate

	Proposed Methods				Existing Methods			
	MRMR+BA		MIM+BA		CMIM+RF		MRMR+RF	
Dataset	Accuracy	Error Rate	Accuracy	Error Rate	Accuracy	Error Rate	Accuracy	Error Rate
GSE18728	**1.0000**	**0.0000**	0.8689	0.1311	0.7049	0.2951	0.5574	0.4426
GSE41998	0.8495	0.1505	**0.8638**	**0.1362**	0.8244	0.1756	0.8387	0.1613
GSE50948	**0.7949**	**0.2051**	0.6979	0.3021	0.6731	0.3269	0.6591	0.3526
GSE20181	0.7614	0.2386	**0.9205**	**0.0795**	0.7443	0.2557	0.6591	0.3409
GSE37946	0.5600	0.4400	**0.8800**	**0.1200**	0.5600	0.4400	0.3400	0.6600

The **bold results** denote optimal performance over the unbolded values.

TABLE 5.6
Comparative Performance of the Proposed MRMRBADL and MIMBADL against CMIM+GA+SV based on Model Prediction Accuracy

	Proposed Methods		Existing Method
Dataset	MRMR+BA+DNN	MIM+BA+DNN	CMIM+GA+SVM (Almazrua and Alshamlan, 2022)
GSE18728	0.8033	**0.8689**	0.6230
GSE41998	0.6165	**0.8354**	0.8351
GSE50948	**0.7500**	0.6731	0.6603
GSE20181	0.6818	**0.6989**	0.6250
GSE37946	0.5421	**0.7800**	0.5400

The **bold results** denote optimal performance over the unbolded values.

5.5 CONCLUSION

In this chapter, we proposed applying filter (MRMR and MIM), wrapper (BA), and embedded (DL) methods to the next-generation sequencing microarray gene expression profiling oncological dataset. In addition, we proposed two new algorithms called MRMRBADL and MIMBADL to efficiently select and identify relevant and informative genes and solve dimension reduction problems in the realm of high-dimensionality microarray datasets. Furthermore, the proposed methods can also be used to solve classification problems that deal with high-dimensionality datasets. In evaluating the two propped algorithms, extensive experiments were conducted using five microarray gene expression profiling datasets. The proposed algorithms were compared to some existing methods, and results showed that the proposed algorithms achieved superior results over those of the existing methods. Moreover, these algorithms also selected viewer genes and identified the genes X202078_at, X201403_s_at, X203231_s_at, X1570239_a_at, and X202225_at as most relevant and informative genes in cancer chemotherapy. Finally, this chapter has revealed the efficiency of using filter and wrapper methods as tools for dimension reduction in microarray gene expression.

REFERENCES

Almazrua H, Alshamlan H. A comprehensive survey of recent hybrid feature selection methods in cancer microarray gene expression data. *IEEE Access*. 2022;10:71427–71449. https://doi.org/10.1109/ACCESS.2022.3185226

Alshamlan H, Badr G, Alohali Y. mRMR-ABC: A hybrid gene selection algorithm for cancer classification using microarray gene expression profiling. *Biomed Res Int*. 2015;2015:604910. https://doi.org/10.1155/2015/604910

Barrett T, Wilhite SE, Ledoux P, Evangelista C, Kim IF, Tomashevsky M, Marshall KA, Phillippy KH, Sherman PM, Holko M, Yefanov A, Lee H, Zhang N, Robertson CL, Serova N, Davis S, Soboleva A. NCBI GEO: Archive for functional genomics data sets–update. *Nucleic Acids Res*. 2013;41(Database issue):D991–D995. https://doi.org/10.1093/nar/gks1193

Buzdin A, Sorokin M, Garazha A, Glusker A, Aleshin A, Poddubskaya E, et al. RNA sequencing for research and diagnostics in clinical oncology. *Semin Cancer Biol*. 2020;60:311–323.

Cao J, Zhang L, Wang B, Li F, Yang J. A fast gene selection method for multi-cancer classification using multiple support vector data description. *J Biomed Inform*. 2015;53:381–389. https://doi.org/10.1016/j.jbi.2014.12.009

Dauda KA. Development and modeling of decision tree for survival data with multiple events using deviance and cox-snell residuals within node homogeneity techniques. *Int J Adv Health Sci Technol*. 2022;2(3).

Dauda KA, Olorede KO, Aderoju SA. A novel hybrid dimension reduction technique for efficient selection of bio-marker genes and prediction of heart failure status of patients. *Sci Afr*. 2021:e00778, ISSN 2468–2276. https://doi.org/10.1016/j.sciaf.2021.e00778

Ding C, Peng H. Minimum redundancy feature selection from microarray gene expression data. *J Bioinform Comput Biol*. 2005;3:185–205. 9 MRMR homepage. Available online: http://home.penglab.com/proj/mRMR/ (accessed on 28 January 2019).

Fleuret F. Fast binary feature selection with conditional mutual information. *J Mach Learn Res*. 2004;5:1531–1555.

Horak CE, Pusztai L, Xing G, Trifan OC, Saura C, Tseng L-M, et al. Biomarker analysis of neoadjuvant doxorubicin/cyclophosphamide followed by ixabepilone or paclitaxel in early-stage breast cancer. *Clin Cancer Res Off J Am Assoc Cancer Res*. 2013;19:1587–1595.

Jo I, Lee S, Oh S. Improved measures of redundancy and relevance for mRMR feature selection. *Computers*. 2019;8(2):42. https://doi.org/10.3390/computers8020042

Koppad S, Basava A, Nash K, Gkoutos GV, Acharjee A. Machine learning-based identification of colon cancer candidate diagnostics genes. *Biology*. 2022;11:365. https://doi.org/10.3390/biology11030365

Korde LA, Lusa L, McShane L, Lebowitz PF, Lukes L, Camphausen K, et al. Gene expression pathway analysis to predict response to neoadjuvant docetaxel and capecitabine for breast cancer. *Breast Cancer Res Treat*. 2010;119:685–699.

Koul N, Manvi SS. Cancer classification using ensemble feature selection and random forest classifier. *IOP Conf Ser: Mater Sci Eng.* 2021;1074:012004.

Kursa MB and Rudnicki WR. Feature selection with the Boruta package. *J Stat Softw.* 2010;36(11):1–13. Available online: www.jstatsoft.org/v36/i11/

Lewis DD. Feature selection and feature extraction for text categorization. In Speech and Natural Language: Proceedings of a Workshop Held at Harriman, February 23–26, New York, 1992:93.

Liu JC, Voisin V, Bader GD, Deng T, Pusztai L, Symmans WF, et al. Seventeengene signature from enriched Her2/Neu mammary tumor-initiating cells predicts clinical outcome for human HER2+: ERα-breast cancer. *Proc Natl Acad Sci U S A.* 2012;109:5832–5837.

Macedo F, Valadas R, Carrasquinha E, Oliveira MR, Pacheco A. Feature selection using decomposed mutual information maximization. *Neurocomputing.* 2022;513:215–232. https://doi.org/10.1016/j.neucom.2022.09.101. ISSN 0925-2312

Mao Z, Cai W, Shao X. Selecting significant genes by randomization test for cancer classification using gene expression data. *J Biomed Inform.* 2013;46:594–601. https://doi.org/10.1016/j.jbi.2013.03.009

Metzker ML. Sequencing technologies—the next generation. *Nat Rev Genet.* 2010;11(1):31–46.

Miller WR, Larionov A. Changes in expression of oestrogen regulated and proliferation genes with neoadjuvant treatment highlight heterogeneity of clinical resistance to the aromatase inhibitor, letrozole. *Breast Cancer Res.* 2010;12: R52.

Park Y, Heider D, Hauschild A-C. Integrative analysis of next-generation sequencing for next-generation cancer research toward artificial intelligence. *Cancers.* 2021;13:3148. https://doi.org/10.3390/cancers13133148

Poplin R, Chang PC, Alexander D, Schwartz S, Colthurst T, Ku A, et al. A universal snp and small-indel variant caller using deep neural networks. *Nat Biotechnol.* 2018;36:983–987. https://doi.org/10.1038/nbt.4235

Prat A, Bianchini G, Thomas M, Belousov A, Cheang MCU, Koehler A, et al. Research-based PAM50 subtype predictor identifies higher responses and Borisov et al. BMC Medical Genomics 2020, 13(Suppl 8):111 Page 8 of 9 improved survival outcomes in HER2-positive breast cancer in the NOAH study. *Clin Cancer Res Off J Am Assoc Cancer Res.* 2014;20:511–521.

Ram M, Najafi A, Shakeri MT. Classification and biomarker genes selection for cancer gene expression data using random forest. *Iran J Pathol.* 2017;12(4):339–347.

Rodon J, Soria J-C, Berger R, Miller WH, Rubin E, Kugel A, et al. Genomic and transcriptomic profiling expands precision cancer medicine: The winther trial. *Nat Med.* 2019;25:751–758.

Shukla AK, Singh P, Vardhan M. A new hybrid feature subset selection framework based on binary genetic algorithm and information theory. *Int J Comput Intell Appl.* 2019;18(3):Art. no. 1950020.

Song J-K, Zhang Y, Fei X-Y, Chen Y-R, Luo Y, Jiang J-S, Ru Y, Xiang Y-W, Li B, Luo Y, Kuai L. Classification and biomarker gene selection of pyroptosis-related gene expression in psoriasis using a random forest algorithm. *Front Genet.* 2022;13:850108. https://doi.org/10.3389/fgene.2022.850108

Sung H, Ferlay J, Siegel RL, Laversanne M, Soerjomataram I, Jemal A, Bray F. Global cancer statistics 2020: GLOBOCAN estimates of incidence and mortality worldwide for 36 cancers in 185 countries. *CA Cancer J Clin.* 2021;71:209–249. https://doi.org/10.3322/caac.21660. PMID:33538338

Toth R, Schiffmann H, Hube-Magg C, et al. Random forest-based modelling to detect biomarkers for prostate cancer progression. *Clin Epigenet.* 2019;11:148. https://doi.org/10.1186/s13148-019-0736-8

Xiao Y, Bi M, Guo H, Li M. Multi-omics approaches for biomarker discovery in early ovarian cancer diagnosis. *EBioMed.* 2022;79:104001. https://doi.org/10.1016/j.ebiom.2022.104001

Xie S, Zhang Y, Lv D, et al. A new improved maximal relevance and minimal redundancy method based on feature subset. *J Supercomput.* 2022. https://doi.org/10.1007/s11227-022-04763-2

Zhang L, Thapa I, Haas C, et al. Multiplatform biomarker identification using a data-driven approach enables single-sample classification. *BMC Bioinform.* 2019;20:601. https://doi.org/10.1186/s12859-019-3140-7

Zhao H-S, Huang X-Y, Huang Y. An ensemble forecast method of rainstorm based on mRMR and random forest algorithms *IOP Conf. Ser.: Earth Environ. Sci.* 2019;237:022006.

Zhukov NV, Tjulandin SA. Targeted therapy in the treatment of solid tumors: Practice contradicts theory. *Biochem Biokhimiia.* 2008;73:605–618.

6 AI and ML in the Treatment of Cardiovascular Diseases

Reena Thakur, Pradnya Borkar**, and Madhavi Wairagade**

*Jhulelal Institute of Technology, Nagpur, India;
**Symbiosis Institute of Technology, Symbiosis International (Deemed University), Pune, India

ABBREVIATIONS

AI and ML Artificial Intelligence and Machine Learning

6.1 INTRODUCTION

6.1.1 Early Medical Information Systems and Computer Algorithms

Since the 1960s, scientists have been researching the potential application of early AI information systems, computers, and algorithms in medical problems, particularly in decision-making for clinical research. Figure 6.1 shows how the majority of reasoning, thinking, and cognitive processes occur in the brain's neocortex. This region's neuronal activity can now be imitated by machine learning and deep learning programs. This is especially true given recent advancements in AI. Currently, supercomputers like IBM's Watson can analyze terabytes of data to detect patterns. Major corporations, including Facebook, Apple, and Amazon, widely employ these machines for picture, voice, and speech recognition. In the challenging Chinese game of Go, the best human player in the world has already been defeated by these self-taught deep learning AI systems (LeCun et al., 2015; Silver & Schrittwieser, 2017).

The authors of Warner et al. (1964) and Gorry and Barnett (1968) conducted one of the earliest studies evaluating computer algorithms and mathematical programs in cardiovascular care in 1963 and 1968, respectively. They investigated the possibility of diagnosing congenital cardiac disease using mathematical methods. A mathematical model based on Baye's theorem of probability was presented by Warner et al. for the clinical diagnosis of congenital cardiac disease. With the aid of their technique, congenital heart disease can be accurately identified with the same level of precision as a physician and refined using symptom and physical sign refinement data matrices for diseases (Warner et al., 1964). Unfortunately, using diagnosis support systems had several drawbacks.

DOI: 10.1201/9781032699882-6

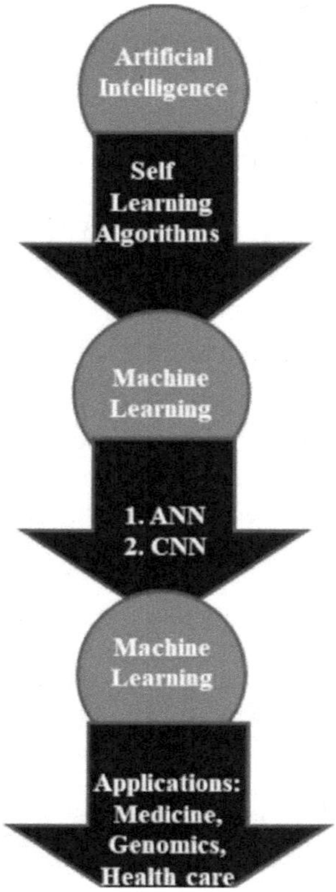

FIGURE 6.1 Relationships between AI, ML, and DL.

The diagnostic capacities were examined by Berner et al. in their 1994 study. They recommended that only doctors who can effectively use the data offered by these systems should use these tools. They expressed concern that crucial diagnoses might occasionally be missed, prompting unnecessary and wasteful investigations in the hands of untrained personnel (Berner et al., 1994). Early artificial intelligence systems assisted in the interpretation of test results in addition to providing clinical decision support. Researchers created the first computer algorithm to evaluate pulmonary function testing in individuals with lung illness. Reports were produced utilizing electronic patient data to determine the existence and severity of lung disease (Aikins et al., 1983).

There were several drawbacks in clinical research to the use of computers. First, most of these systems use the "if this occurs, take this action" tenet before using arithmetic to calculate the likelihood of various events. Clinical issues, however, are complex, multivariate, random, and related to the actual world. For instance, A 40-year-old American man and a 25-year-old Caucasian woman may have the same or a different cause of fever and stomach pain. Many options could arise due to socioeconomic considerations, prior medical/surgical history, travel history, drug use, and personal habits, further complicating the scenario. Several people may experience distinct symptoms and indicators of the same disease. Moreover, diseases may present differently when a range of intrinsic and extrinsic elements are present. As a result, it is challenging to construct algorithms and clinical decision support systems. Such technologies supporting clinical decisions also need more clinical perception, reasoning, and understanding. However, there are issues with these systems' validity, dependability, usefulness, reproducibility, and safety (Berner et al., 1994; Szolovits et al., 1988).

6.1.2 Machine Learning (ML)

A computer system built on a collection of algorithms that makes an effort to evaluate enormous amounts of data received from various sources is called a subfield of AI. A computer may be designed to make intelligent decisions in various ways, but employing the appropriate algorithms for each task is crucial. One of the most popular AI methods for processing massive data is machine learning (ML). It provides a self-adaptive mechanism that, with practice and new data, offers ever-better analysis and patterns. The digital age has brought about the development of several methodologies, which has caused an explosion of data of all types from around the world. Big data, also called vast amounts of data, is easily accessible, frequently used, and may be shared through services like cloud computing.

Without explicit instructions, machine learning (ML) uses statistical techniques to automatically gain knowledge from experience and data. It has seen a sharp increase in popularity in recent years. In particular, a method called deep learning (DL) has achieved ground-breaking outcomes in a number of significant issues, such as picture categorization and speed recognition.

The rise of deep learning is primarily responsible for the recent increase in interest in and initiatives to integrate AI into a variety of businesses. Convoluted neural networks (CNNs), also known as deep neural networks, are a type of machine learning that accesses more complex information from an image by employing several layers of data, such as many layers of image processing. This AI function, which mimics how the brain analyses data and creates patterns that may be used in decision-making, is modeled after the neurons in the brain of a human being. It has the ability to learn from data unsupervised. Deep or complicated neural networks are the most popular ML methods in the biomedical field. These connected artificial neural networks adhere to mathematical models. In genomics and molecular biology, handling "big data" is made possible by their broad range of applications. They are most frequently used for visual image analysis.

Artificial intelligence (AI) recognizes patterns utilizing various neural networks through deep learning-based data repositories available for use. The procedure is affordable, and access to computing power is simple. The Internet of Things (IoT), remote sensors, digital cameras, image scanners, and electrical appliances can all be used by neural networks to obtain data quickly. AI can acquire knowledge from both labeled and unstructured data. Artificial neural networks organized in a hierarchy carry out the machine learning process. As previously indicated, artificial neural networks utilized in AI are constructed using neuron nodes connected in a web-like pattern, much like the human brain. In contrast, conventional computer programs construct analyses with data linearly. Machines may analyze data nonlinearly thanks to the hierarchical design of deep learning systems (Farnell et al., 2020).

It could take years or even decades to sift, comprehend, and extract usable information from large amount of data because it is frequently unstructured and so large.

The human brain needs help to analyze such vast data sets meaningfully. As a result, it is essential to find patterns and connections and make forecasts using computers. Companies from all industries embrace AI systems quickly, as they realize the enormous potential of utilizing this wealth of data. The exponential growth of computers, data storage, and sensor technology is creating a new world where enormous amounts of data can be gathered and analyzed.

6.1.3 Applications of ML in Healthcare

ML has several uses in the medical industry. It may simplify challenging, time-taking work in this field. Modern healthcare can be improved due to the advancement of faster processors, machine learning (ML), and accessibility to digital health data. These innovative technologies improve therapeutic results, reduce expenses, and quicken finding the right drugs. The major companies in the healthcare industry are currently drawn to machine learning (Alsuliman et al., 2020). In general, there are three types of ML applications in the medical field:

- First Category: Enhancing Current Medical Facilities. These are simple ML applications in the medical industry. It will be helpful to enhance the functionality of already-built structures (Kandhway et al., 2020; Zerouaoui & Idri, 2021). For typical applications like simulation and data confirmation, these ML-based solutions specify specialized, rule-based jobs. The classification of digital medical images is one of the uses of machine learning in healthcare. It increases the precision of conventional image processing methods. Radiological images can also be examined using machine learning to see if a particular disease is present. Moreover, ML can also be applied for the evaluation of retinal images and to identify patients who may be vulnerable to visual threats. For instance, the medical startup Aindra uses artificial intelligence and machine learning (Natarajan, 2023). It classifies medical photos using a platform with machine learning. Its goal is to more quickly and accurately diagnose tumors.
- Second Category: Modernizing Medical Facilities. These machine learning applications provide structures with new powers. They move closer to becoming individuals. One of these ML applications is precision medicine (Handelman et al., 2018; Vatandsoost & Litkouhi, 2019). It is a type of medical care that concentrates on a person's unique requirements based on their features (for example, the genetic arrangement of the person). iCarbonx is one business that is pushing in the direction of personalized healthcare services (Wang, 2021). Artificial intelligence, biotechnology, and large databases are all used in this.
- Third Category: Independent Medical Structures. This category is expanding. ML-based models will be created to perform their tasks autonomously based on pre-established objectives (Himidan & Kim, 2015). One of the fields of healthcare potential future uses is the construction of hospitals without doctors (Assaf et al., 2021; De Bruyne et al., 2021). Thus, we must

> prepare for a robotic future that relies on AL and ML. Hence, we need to prepare for the possibility of future robots being used in hospitals. All medical treatments, from diagnostics to surgery, will soon be performed by robots. Today, in wealthy nations, robots help surgeons (Rahmani et al., 2021; Lee et al., 2021). This new technology is still in its infancy and needs improvement despite its various downsides and shortcomings. The Mayo Clinic, for instance, is getting closer to being a hospital without doctors. Currently, it works with its components. Nonetheless, these parts should undergo thorough testing by applicable regulations. Surgeons now use robots to enhance their surgical methods (Tao et al., 2021; Alizadehsani et al., 2019).

Deep learning is the current name for the artificial intelligence technique formerly known as neural networks. Two professors (McCulloch & Pitts, 1943) first proposed this area of artificial intelligence in 1943. They provided the first mathematical depiction of artificial neural networks in a ground-breaking research paper in the Journal of Mathematical Biophysics. They explained how brain neurons could interact with one another and use an analogy of the "and," "or," and "not" gates in physics to construct incredibly complex patterns using the necessary information from sensory inputs. Also, they discussed the brain's role as an "information processor." In essence, scientists concluded that neurons function as logic gates, integrating multiple inputs to produce a single output (McCulloch & Pitts, 1943), which tremendously impacted our knowledge of how the brain operates.

In artificial neural networks (ANNs), the complete structure is built up of interconnected "nodes" that process input and generate an output; artificial neural network (ANN) nodes are like biological neurons in this regard. In artificial neural networks, there are three types of nodes: input, hidden, and output (Figure 6.2). The input nodes act like sensory neurons in the central nervous system, bringing in a data stream for processing. The hidden nodes process the data in the data set, and the output nodes ultimately interpret it. The convolutional neural network (CNN) is a kind of ANN that "learns" using various techniques, such as "backpropagation," and has layers of hidden nodes for processing input (Dilsizian & Siegel, 2018). The characteristics of "parameter sharing" and "pooling," which lower the amount of processing power needed, enhance picture processing, and advance data processing, are unique to CNNs (Zerouaoui & Idri, 2021; Handelman et al., 2018; Vatandsoost & Litkouhi, 2019). By effectively allowing networks to learn from their errors (backpropagation) or internal relationships, these machine learning (ML) techniques reduce the complexity of the data/images (parameter sharing and pooling) (Dilsizian & Siegel, 2018). Deep learning networks require a hierarchical representation of data in multilayered networks, where each layer is a representation that is a high-level abstraction of the representation from the previous layer of the neural networks, in contrast to machine learning algorithms, which almost always require structured data (Figure 6.2). Hence, deep learning techniques benefit from voice and sound identification, complex image analysis, and visual interpretation.

ML/AI has many applications in cardiovascular medicine, including pharmacological therapy, pharmacogenomics, managing heart failure, cardiovascular imaging, and

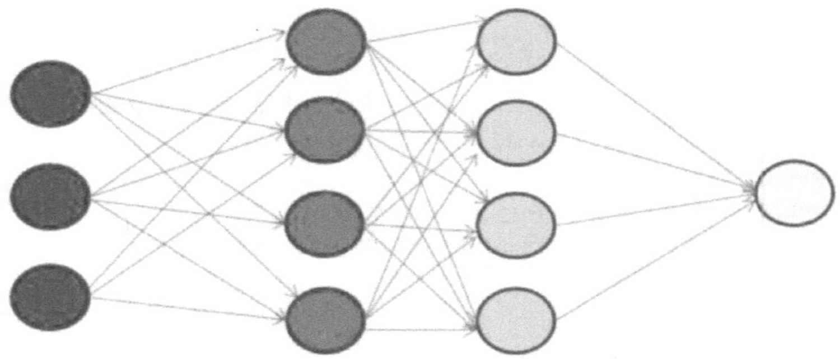

FIGURE 6.2 One to several layers in hidden layers.

diagnostics. In cardiovascular medicine, AI facilitates methods for utilizing extensive data and precision medicine, enhancing cardiologist capability. AI/ML systems can accurately predict and classify a wide range of clinical data without making any assumptions. So, applying AI to cardiovascular care has potential benefits. Following is a brief discussion about how AI influences various facets of cardiovascular treatment here.

6.1.4 Clinical Uses of AI in Cardiovascular Drug Therapy

Drug therapy was one of the first areas of AI in cardiovascular care (Figure 6.3). Population genetics uses of AI have advanced precision medicine. The applications of precision medicine, big data, and AI are helping to identify effective medicines while lowering the likelihood of side effects in a given patient. These technologies have significantly influenced the creation of newer pharmaceuticals. (Dilsizian & Siegel, 2018; Kalinin et al., 2018; Cavallari & Weitzel, 2015). As prospective therapeutic targets, several cardiovascular drugs are being researched (Sibbing et al., 2019; Kitzmiller et al., 2016).

Interestingly, as demonstrated in randomized clinical studies (Sibbing et al., 2019; Kitzmiller et al., 2016), pharmacogenomics and precision medicine have already significantly impacted the dose of warfarin in a range of patient populations. Those getting pharmacogenetically based warfarin doses spent longer in the therapeutic range of their international normalized ratios (INRs) than those receiving standard care, according to (Sibbing et al., 2019). Researchers (Tao et al., 2021) discovered comparable outcomes in a warfarin-treated Asian patient population. After a heart valve replacement, the research discussed in (Pirmohamed et al., 2013) used the backpropagation neural network model to estimate the warfarin maintenance dose. Deep learning-based AI systems could benefit from precision medicine, individualized drug therapy, and drug discovery (Sibbing et al., 2019).

Heart failure treatment is a recently emerging use of AI in cardiovascular medicine and illness management. AI has made it feasible to develop new cardiovascular pharmacological medicines for the management of hypertension, a novel technique for

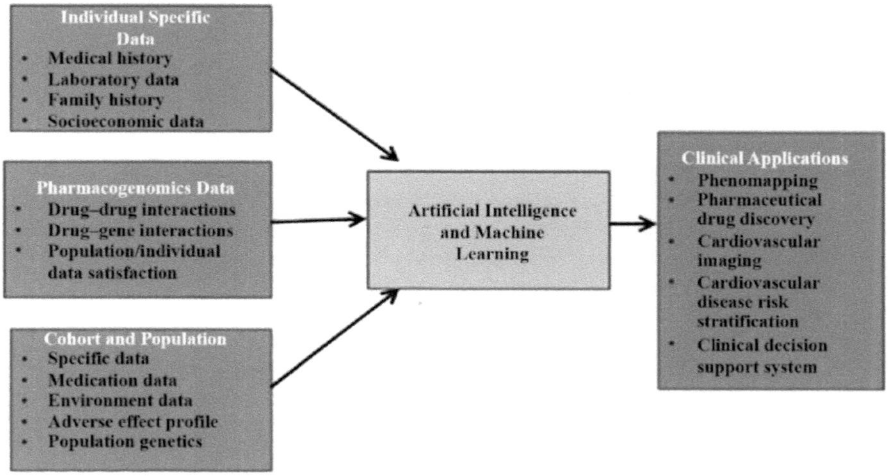

FIGURE 6.3 Artificial intelligence's use in cardiovascular research and medicine.

heart failure phenotyping and cardiovascular risk stratification, and enhanced medical medication therapy (Syn et al., 2018; Li et al., 2020; Shah, 2017; Shameer et al., 2018; Zellweger et al., 2018). Samuel et al. (1959) developed a distinct category of heart failure with preserved ejection fraction (HFpEF) to comprehend the etiology of heart failure. The basis for this particular classification was "phenomapping," a method that used unsupervised deep learning algorithms powered by artificial intelligence (AI) to analyze extensive clinical, laboratory, echocardiography, and imaging data (Li et al., 2020).

Researchers (Li et al., 2020; Shah, 2017) utilized three categories to classify HFpEF. The individuals in pheno-group 1 (natriuretic peptide deficiency syndrome phenotype) had the most significant outcomes despite being the youngest and most obese. They also had the fewest heart problems and low brain natriuretic peptide (BNP) levels. The worst left ventricular relaxation (lowest e' velocity) was seen in patients in pheno-group 2, which also had the highest prevalence of diabetes and obesity and increased BNP levels (obesity-cardiometabolic phenotype). The worst outcomes were shown in pheno-group 3, or the cardiorenal phenotype, which had the highest prevalence of renal, electrocardiographic, and echocardiographic dysfunction (Li et al., 2020). Identifying patients who react to various targeted drug therapies and creating brand new targeted drug therapies may benefit from the phenotyping of HFpEF patients (Syn et al., 2018).

In order to investigate the relationship between exercise intolerance and left ventricular systolic reserve function in HFpEF patients, the research in (Zellweger et al., 2018) applied ML. They discovered a connection between weakened left ventricular systolic capacity and inadequate reserve capacity. In the end, AI has already started to profoundly affect how we treat various cardiac conditions and apply pharmacological therapy. The feasibility of AI with precision medicine has been shown in studies on warfarin doses (Pirmohamed et al., 2013) and heart failure applications (Syn et al., 2018; Li et al., 2020; Zellweger et al., 2018). AI has thus opened up new avenues for pharmacological and cardiovascular therapy.

TABLE 6.1
Summary of Algorithms Commonly Used in Machine Learning

Name of Method	Observation
Artificial neural networks (ANNs)	An ANN comprises several nodes, often known as "neurons," arranged in layers (input, hidden, and output) connected by weighted edges. Each network layer gradually processes input feature vectors using non-linear transformations until the last layer generates an output (such as a class label). The edge weights are gradually adjusted using the backpropagation process to account for any errors that the ANN's output may exhibit during training. Deep learning is based on ANNs.
Support vector machine (SVM)	By utilizing mappings known as kernels to project training data onto a higher-dimensional space, the SVM classifier is created. A boundary is subsequently established in this new area to maximize class separation. Then, the previously learned boundary is applied to identify new samples as they are projected into this higher-dimensional environment.
Decision tree	The most fundamental tree-based machine learning model is the decision tree. Iteratively creating a tree structure that, given an input feature vector, can accurately assign labels by constructing the proper "splits" is known as recursive partitioning. The objective is to develop a tree structure that can do this. It is essential because ensemble learning can be combined with trees to create robust classifiers like boosted trees and random forests.
k-nearest neighbors (KNN)	Each item that needs to be classified in a KNN algorithm is compared using a distance function to the k training examples closest to it, where k is an integer, and a majority vote determines its label.

6.1.5 Cardiovascular Imaging Applications of ML

Table 6.1 shows the standard summary of algorithms used in ML.

6.2 PRESENT AND FUTURE USE OF AI IN MEDICINE

AI systems can now replicate several medical procedures that need human expertise with accuracy levels comparable to or higher than those attained by human experts because of advancements in ML algorithms. Deep learning systems are increasingly trained in medicine using sizable annotated data sets, freeing up medical professionals' attention for other, more productive jobs and initiatives. AI in medicine has boundless potential and has the potential to significantly enhance clinical practice's delivery of healthcare.

Goldenberg et al. claim that by taking over challenging activities presently handled by humans, the future of medicine could be transformed by computer-based decision support systems based on machine learning. The clinical process can be improved, diagnosis accuracy can be increased, throughput efficiency can be increased, human resource costs can be reduced, and therapy options can be improved with ML systems (Goldenberg et al., 2019).

However, you must possess synergistic cross-disciplinary talents to effectively use AI in medicine. Despite recent encouraging biology and biomarker results, personalized medicine is still a long way off, and novel drugs that come out of preclinical trials are rarely assessed for their diagnostic and therapeutic potential. The discrepancy between experimental data on new anticancer molecules and their actual use in diagnosis and therapy is caused by several factors, including biological differences between human disease and animal models, inconsistent experimental methodologies, incorrect interpretation of experimental results, and a lack of validation of such data by pathologists with extensive experience in animal cancer models, etc. For instance, integrating the complementary approaches of nuclear medicine, radiology, and surgical pathology is essential to give individualized care for cancer. Each field contributes to the diagnosis, prognosis, and evaluation of therapy responses. Creating a medical paradigm that acknowledges the uniqueness of every human being can be sped up by a structural model of collaboration between various professions. A recent study examined fifteen articles on cutting-edge AI applications for the accurate and early identification of breast, lung, prostate, and lymphoma. One example involved using a deep neural network to identify abnormalities in aggressive breast cancer mammograms. The researchers of this study were persuaded that information they examined provided the scientific rationale for additional translational medical research using a combination of surgical pathology, imaging, and nuclear medicine (Bonanno et al., 2019).

ML is pioneering a new paradigm for scientific investigation. In research, the traditional "hypothesis testing" methodology is applied, in which data analysis yields explanatory mechanisms that suggest additional tests, yielding classic findings. However, because of the rapid development of technology, many studies today gather a ton of data and are "hypothesis-generating." Examples include studies on genomics and other omics. The development of picture digitization has resulted in experiments that produce massive amounts of data, such as gigabytes or terabytes. Deep learning advancements make it possible to extract crucial information from photos, putting molecular analysis and visual observation on an equal footing. Deep learning makes it possible to combine and understand image-based data with genomic information, allowing for using this data to provide new and correct knowledge. Genomic analysis makes excellent use of deep learning. Using this hypothesis-generating pattern, we can search for significance in a heavy data set despite logically progressing from an observation to a better explanation one step at a time. Deep learning has changed the research direction as a result (Cohen & Furie, 2019).

6.2.1 AI and ML Applications in Cardiovascular Imaging

The discipline of cardiovascular medicine could be entirely transformed by artificial intelligence and machine learning. AI has found use in predicting aberrant fractional flow reserve in patients undergoing coronary computed tomography angiograms (CCTA), determining left ventricular ejection fraction, diagnosing obstructive coronary artery disease, and reducing readmission rates in heart failure patients (Tables 6.2 and 6.3). Recently, the research mentioned in (Zellweger et al., 2014; Lee et al., 2017) investigated the application of AI as a noninvasive tool for

TABLE 6.2
Basic Terminologies in AI

Artificial Intelligence	Basic Terms
Machine learning	According to its definition, it is a multidisciplinary field that applies statistical methods to help computers learn from data sets without being explicitly programmed.
Deep learning	It involves using algorithms in multilayered neural networks to process raw data.
Supervised learning	Data sets with well-known outcomes can be used to discover patterns in artificial intelligence.
Unsupervised learning	In artificial intelligence, patterns can be extracted from unlabeled data sets.
Artificial neural networks (ANNs)	Multiple machine learning algorithms can be coordinated and processed together with this framework.
Convolutional neural networks (CNNs)	These are artificial neural networks (ANNs) that may "learn" through several techniques and aid in the analysis of complex data and images.

TABLE 6.3
Summary of Various Studies to Explore the Role of AI in Cardiovascular Medicine

Findings	Name of Method
Warfarin maintenance dose prediction using AI (Li et al., 2020)	Model for a backpropagation neural network
The grouping of HFpEF into various categories (Shah, 2017)	Phenomapping and big data
Using artificial intelligence to diagnose coronary artery disease noninvasively (Zellweger et al., 2018)	AI-based mimetic algorithm (MPA)
Classification of echocardiograms based on the apical view automatically (Khamis et al., 2017)	Classification in stages and supervised learning
Identifying physical hypertrophy and hypertrophic cardiomyopathy with different signs and symptoms in athletes (Narula et al., 2016)	Artificial neural networks, support vector machines, and random forests
Left ventricular function in patients with heart failure and a preserved ejection fraction (Sanchez-Martinez et al., 2018)	Unsupervised machine learning methods
Machine learning to differentiate restrictive cardiomyopathy from constrictive pericarditis (Sengupta et al., 2016)	Machine learning using associative memory classifier
Cardiovascular contractility and myocardial infarction: spatial-temporal effects (Tabassian et al., 2017)	Analyzing the principal components and automatically classifying
Using echocardiography images to assess mitral regurgitation (Moghaddasi & Nourian, 2017)	Template matching, linear discriminant analysis, and support vector machines
Using cardiac MRI images to differentiate acute from chronic myocardial infarction (Larroza et al., 2017)	Support vector machines (SVM) using Polynesia kernels, random forest
Measuring right ventricular function using cardiac MRI in three dimensions in patients with pulmonary hypertension (Dawes et al., 2017)	Instruction under the supervision and principal component analysis
Using AI-based learning techniques to identify asymptomatic left ventricular dysfunction (Attia et al., 2019)	Convolution neural networks
Calculator based on machine learning (ML) to predict cardiovascular risk (Kakadiaris et al., 2018)	Support vector machine

detecting coronary artery disease. Researchers noticed that the Framingham risk score was inadequate in detecting individuals with angiographically confirmed coronary artery disease (CAD); thus, they utilized an AI-based mimetic pattern-based algorithm (MPA). They found that the modified MPA had a 98% and 95% positive predictive value for the exclusion of CAD in the "training" and "test" populations, respectively (Zellweger et al., 2014; Lee et al., 2017).

6.2.2 Use of AI and ML in CVD

AI is being used in science by programming the machines so that they respond rapidly to the clinical emergency and have better treatment. It can be used in detecting CVD, coronary heart diseases, and strokes. There is a range of equipment and science which are that can assist us by giving the fast facts about risks.

There are more than a few improvements which can assist in CVD, including:

- It can be used to predict the hazard in embolic stroke condition.
- It can be used to detected arrhythmia with the aid of monitoring the heartbeat.

Nowadays, managing coronary heart failure, pharmacogenomics, cardiovascular imaging, and diagnostics are just a few areas where ML/AI has observed a vast range of applications. The effectiveness of the cardiologist can be increased by using AI to provide tools for monitoring precision medication and vast amounts of information on cardiovascular medication.

In addition to any assumptions, AI/ML algorithms can accurately analyze extremely diverse clinical information for prediction and categorization. Hence, incorporating AI will benefit cardiovascular treatment. Here, we have discussed how AI affects several cardiovascular care areas. The basic terminologies in AI have been described in Table 6.2. A summary of various studies to explore the role of AI in cardiovascular medicine has been given in Table 6.3, and Figure 6.4 shows the supervised and unsupervised learning.

Possibilities and opportunities for cardiovascular medicine and artificial intelligence are represented in Table 6.4 and problems and dangers with cardiovascular medicine and artificial intelligence are shown in Table 6.5.

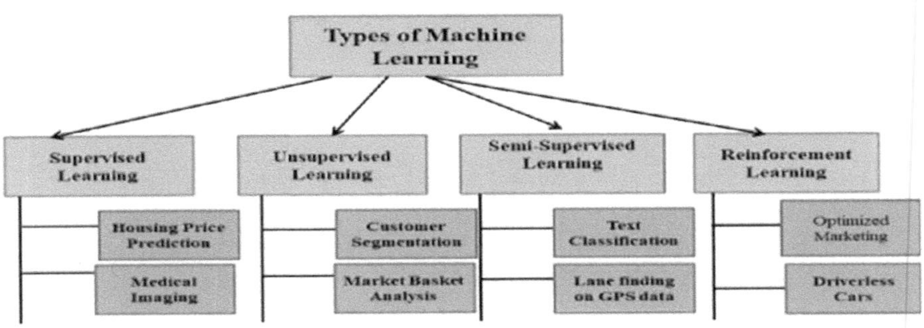

FIGURE 6.4 Unsupervised and supervised learning.

TABLE 6.4
Possibilities and Opportunities for Cardiovascular Medicine and Artificial Intelligence

- AI and machine learning can aid in improved cardiovascular risk ratings in CAD with angiographical documentation (Zellweger et al., 2014)
- Echocardiography, cardiac CT/MRI, AI-based cardiovascular diagnosis, medical education, (Kalinin et al., 2018) separating acute from chronic myocardial infarction, (Pirmohamed et al., 2013), and understanding myocardial contractile activity are only a few of the applications of AI-based systems that are already accessible.
- AI and big data have changed population health and cardiovascular risk stratification, making precision treatment possible (Dawes et al., 2017; Al'Aref et al., 2019; Peng et al., 2016).
- Heart failure phenotyping and genomics are also applications of AI and big data (Syn et al., 2018).
- Health care outcomes can be improved and systems-based practices can be developed with the help of artificial intelligence systems (Dawes et al., 2017).

TABLE 6.5
Cardiovascular Medicine and Artificial Intelligence: Problems and Dangers

- Dichotomy and incorrect calibration are recognized issues with machine learning techniques based on artificial intelligence (AI) (Cohen & Furie, 2019).
- There is a need to address data privacy concerns with AI-based systems (Krittanawong et al., 2018; Przewlocka-Kosmala et al., 2019), and there is a requirement for comprehensive data protection regulations in the US, comparable to the General Data Protection Regulation (GDPR) in the EU (Larroza et al., 2017; Van Rosendael et al., 2018).
- To avoid selection bias, historical bias, and stereotypes when collecting and analyzing data, AI-based systems should maintain data integrity (Kakadiaris et al., 2018; Van Rosendael et al., 2018).
- AI-based systems should refrain from using flawed methods to stop the encoding of discrimination in automated systems and avoid using assumptions such as conflating correlation and causality (Kakadiaris et al., 2018; Van Rosendael et al., 2018).
- In addition to lack of standardization, suitability, reproducibility issues, and legal responsibilities, AI-based systems face other challenges (Van Rosendael et al., 2018; Al'Aref et al., 2019).

6.2.3 Problems and Unsolved Issues

The constraints and difficulties encountered when developing ML-based approaches are discussed in this section.

- Data Accessibility: Training ML-based models frequently necessitates access to sizable databases. When the datasets are large, these models perform well and make few errors. To address this issue, developing new systems for electronically recording medical data is vital.
- Data Quality: Another critical issue is that every inaccuracy made when recording data, whether unintentional or intentional, increases the error

rate. Data quality is, therefore, a significant issue. When choosing how to classify data samples, medical professionals can make mistakes that lead to these problems. These problems can be significantly reduced, and data preparation techniques can improve the dataset's quality.

- Healthcare real-time datasets are quite dimensional. This issue lengthens learning time, makes models more complex, and causes overfitting. So, this problem should always be taken into account by ML-based approaches. There are some methods for lowering dimensionality that works well. For instance, feature extraction and feature selection efficiently address this issue. More research in this field is necessary to develop more effective strategies for lowering dimensionality.
- Efficiency: When ML-based models in healthcare successfully address a pressing issue, they are advantageous. Sometimes, it is optional to utilize machine learning techniques to tackle an issue; instead, the problem can be solved successfully using already available techniques. When datasets are highly dimensional, all parameters are not readily predicted; it takes a long time to infer the proper findings, or when conventional methods are ineffective for resolving this problem, ML-based methods are required. So, researchers must employ current and authentic machine learning methods.
- Privacy: Patients' privacy must be considered when developing ML-based models because patients may be identified using anonymous data. When conducting more research to solve this issue, researchers should consider patient privacy's importance.

6.3 FUTURE OF AI AND ML IN THE TREATMENT OF CARDIOVASCULAR DISEASE

International morbidity and mortality continue to be significantly influenced by cardiac disorders. Patient outcomes are improved on time and with excellent diagnosis, therapy, and follow-up, and excellent use of fitness resources is ensured. Due to the data-driven approach used to treat many complex heart problems and the extensive use of cardiac imaging modalities, including ECG, echocardiography, CT, and nuclear imaging, cardiovascular medicine is thankfully a research topic for AI. As with other interventions, medical trials are the foundation for showing scientific utility. As a result, most research up to this point has been created in a computer employing homogenous single-center research groups. There will always be a change from multicenter clinical trials for internal validation to exploratory validation studies for external validation. In order to comprehend how AI-ECG algorithms can be used in real-world settings, the first potential scientific trial for AI-ECG was previously published (Moghaddasi & Nourian, 2017). The study indicated that the control arm had lower diagnostic accuracy and employed an AI-ECG algorithm to identify LV dysfunction in addition to giving the 120 primary care groups in the control arm access to the AI algorithm (Moghaddasi & Nourian, 2017). Published cardiac content is primarily restricted to contexts of ongoing research rather than therapeutic utilization, except for AI applications in ECG. Due to growing funding for AI research projects, a sharp rise in medical databases, scientific smartphone features, and wearable technology, a favorable environment exists for learning more about AI platforms in cardiology.

6.4 CONCLUSION

The chapter describes early medical information systems and computer algorithms. Machine learning and its applications in healthcare are explained in detail. Furthermore, cardiovascular imaging applications are explained. Future prospects, issues, and uses are explained in detail.

REFERENCES

Aikins, J. S., Kunz, J. C., Shortliffe, E. H., Fallat, R. J. PUFF: An expert system for interpretation of pulmonary function data. *Comput Biomed Res.* 1983;16:199–208.

Al'Aref, S. J., Anchouche, K., Singh, G. Clinical applications of machine learning in cardiovascular disease and its relevance to cardiac imaging. *Eur Heart J.* 2019;40:1975–1986. https://doi.org/10.1093/eurheartj/ehy404.

Alizadehsani, R., Roshanzamir, M., Abdar, M., Beykikhoshk, A., Khosravi, A., Panahiazar, M., Koohestani, A., Khozeimeh, F., Nahavandi, S., Sarrafzadegan, N. A database for using machine learning and data mining techniques for coronary artery disease diagnosis. *Sci Data.* 2019;6:1–13.

Alsuliman, T., Humaidan, D., Sliman, L. Machine learning and artificial intelligence in the service of medicine: Necessity or potentiality? *Curr Res Transl Med.* 2020;68:245–251.

Assaf, D., Rayman, S., Segev, L., Neuman, Y., Zippel, D., Goitein, D. Improving pre-bariatric surgery diagnosis of hiatal hernia using machine learning models. *Minim Invasive Ther Allied Technol.* 2021:1–7.

Attia, Z. I., Kapa, S., Lopez-Jimenez, F. Screening for cardiac contractile dysfunction using an artificial intelligence-enabled electrocardiogram. *Nat Med.* 2019;25:70–74. https://doi.org/10.1038/s41591-018-0240-2.

Berner, E. S., Webster, G. D., Shugerman, A. A., Jackson, J. R., Algina, J., Baker, A. L., Ball, E. V., Cobbs, C. G., Dennis, V. W., Frenkel, E. P. Performance of four computer-based diagnostic systems. *N Engl J Med.* 1994;330:1792–1796. www.openclinical.org/aisp_puff.html. Accessed 12 April 2020.

Bonanno, E., Toschi, N., Bombonati, A., Muto, P., Schillaci, O. Imaging diagnostic and pathology in the Management of Oncological-Patients. *Contrast Media Mol Imaging.*2019;2019:2513680.

Cavallari, L. H., Weitzel, K. Pharmacogenomics in cardiology—genetics and drug response: 10 years of progress. *Future Cardiol.* 2015;11:281–286.

Cohen, S., Furie, M. B. Artificial intelligence and pathobiology join forces in the American journal of pathology. *Am J Pathol.*2019;189(1):4–5.

Dawes, T. J. W., de Marvao, A., Shi, W. Machine learning of three-dimensional right ventricular motion enables outcome prediction in pulmonary hypertension: A cardiac MR imaging study. *Radiology.* 2017;283:381–390. https://doi.org/10.1148/radiol.2016161315.

De Bruyne, S., Speeckaert, M. M., Van Biesen, W., Delanghe, J. R. Recent evolutions of machine learning applications in clinical laboratory medicine. *Crit. Rev. Clin. Lab. Sci.* 2021;58:131–152.

Dilsizian, M. E., Siegel, E. L. Machine meets biology: A primer on artificial intelligence in cardiology and cardiac imaging. *Curr Cardiol Rep.* 2018;20:139. https://doi.org/10.1007/s11886-018-1074-8.

Farnell, D. A., Huntsman, D., Bashashati, A. The coming 15 years in gynaecological pathology: Digitisation, artificial intelligence, and new technologies. *Histopathology*. 2020; 76(1):171–177. https://doi.org/10.1111/his.13991.

Goldenberg, S. L., Nir, G., Salcudean, S. E. A new era: Artificial intelligence and machine learning in prostate cancer. *Nat Rev Urol*.2019;16(7):391–403. https://doi.org/10.1038/s41585-019-0193-3.

Gorry, G. A., Barnett, G. O. Sequential diagnosis by computer. *JAMA*. 1968;205:849–854.

Handelman, G., Kok, H., Chandra, R., Razavi, A., Lee, M., Asadi, H. Machine learning and the future of medicine. *J Intern Med*. 2018;284:603–619.

Himidan, S., Kim, P. The evolving identity, capacity, and capability of the future surgeon. In *Seminars in Pediatric Surgery*; W. B. Saunders, Elsevier: Amsterdam, The Netherlands, 2015; Volume 24, pp. 145–149.

Kakadiaris, I. A., Vrigkas, M., Yen, A. A., Kuznetsova, T., Budoff, M., Naghavi, M. Machine learning outperforms ACC/AHA CVD risk calculator in MESA. *J Am Heart Assoc*. 2018;7:e009476. https://doi.org/10.1161/JAHA.118.009476.

Kalinin, A. A., Higgins, G. A., Reamaroon, N. Deep learning in pharmacogenomics: From gene regulation to patient stratification. *Pharmacogenomics*. 2018;19:629–650.

Kandhway, P., Bhandari, A. K., Singh, A. A novel reformed histogram equalization based medical image contrast enhancement using krill herd optimization. *Biomed Signal Process Control*. 2020;56:101677.

Khamis, H., Zurakhov, G., Azar, V., Raz, A., Friedman, Z., Adam, D. Automatic apical view classification of echocardiograms using a discriminative learning dictionary. *Med Image Anal*. 2017;36:15–21.

Kitzmiller, J. P., Mikulik, E. B., Dauki, A. M., Murkherjee, C., Luzum, J. A. Pharmacogenomics of statins: Understanding susceptibility to adverse effects. *Pharmgenomics Pers Med*. 2016;9:97–106.

Krittanawong, C., Bomback, A. S., Baber, U., Bangalore, S., Messerli, F. H., Tang, W. W. Future direction for using artificial intelligence to predict and manage hypertension. *Curr Hypertens Rep*. 2018;20:75.

Larroza, A., Materka, A., López-Lereu, M. P., Monmeneu, J. V., Bodí, V., Moratal, D. Differentiation between acute and chronic myocardial infarction by means of texture analysis of late gadolinium enhancement and cine cardiac magnetic resonance imaging. *Eur J Radiol*. 2017;92:78–83.

LeCun, Y., Bengio, Y., Hinton, G. Deep learning. *Nature*. 2015;521:436–444. https://doi.org/10.1038/nature14539.

Lee, K. T., Hour, A. L., Shia, B. C., Chu, P. H. The application and future of big database studies in cardiology: A single-center experience. *Acta Cardiol Sin*. 2017;33:581–587.

Lee, S. W., Ali, S., Yousefpoor, M. S., Yousefpoor, E., Lalbakhsh, P., Javaheri, D., Rahmani, A. M., Hosseinzadeh, M. An energy-aware and predictive fuzzy logic-based routing scheme in flying ad hoc networks (fanets). *IEEE Access*. 2021;9:129977–130005.

Li, Q., Wang, J., Tao, H., Zhou, Q., Chen, J., Fu, B., Qin, W., Li, D., Hou, J., Chen, J. The prediction model of warfarin individual maintenance dose for patients undergoing heart valve replacement, based on the back propagation neural network. *Clin Drug Investig*. 2020;40:41–53.

Mathur, P., Srivastava, S., Xu, X., Mehta, J. Artificial intelligence, machine learning, and cardiovascular disease. *Clin Med Insight Cardiol*. 2020;14:1179546820927404. https://doi.org/10.1177/1179546820927404.

McCulloch, W. S., Pitts, W. A. Logical calculus of the ideas immanent in nervous activity. *Bull Math Biophys*. 1943;5:115–133.

Moghaddasi, H., Nourian, S. Automatic assessment of mitral regurgitation severity based on extensive textural features on 2D echocardiography videos. *Comput Biol Med.* 2017;73:47–55. https://doi.org/10.1016/j.compbiomed.2016.03.026.

Narula, S., Shameer, K., Salem Omar, A. M., Dudley, J. T., Sengupta, P. P. Machine-learning algorithms to automate morphological and functional assessments in 2D-echocardiography. *J Am Coll Cardiol.* 2016;68:2287–2295. https://doi.org/10.1016/j.jacc.2016.08.062.

Natarajan, A. *The Medical Startup Aindra Uses Artificial Intelligence and Machine Learning,* 2023. https://www.aindra.in. Retrieved March 11, 2023, from https://aindra.in/

Peng, P., Lekadir, K., Gooya, A., Shao, L., Petersen, S. E., Frangi, A. F. A review of heart chamber segmentation for structural and functional analysis using cardiac magnetic resonance imaging. *MAGMA*. 2016;29:155–195.

Pirmohamed, M., Burnside, G., Eriksson, N. A randomized trial of genotype-guided dosing of warfarin. *N Engl J Med.* 2013;369:2294–2303.

Przewlocka-Kosmala, M., Marwick, T. H., Dabrowski, A., Kosmala, W. Contribution of cardiovascular reserve to prognostic categories of heart failure with preserved ejection fraction: A classification based on machine learning. *J Am Soc Echocardiogr.* 2019;32:604–615.

Rahmani, A. M., Ali, S., Yousefpoor, M. S., Yousefpoor, E., Naqvi, R. A., Siddique, K., Hosseinzadeh, M. An area coverage scheme based on fuzzy logic and shuffled frog-leaping algorithm (sfla) in heterogeneous wireless sensor networks. *Mathematics.* 2021;9:2251.

Samuel, L. A. Some studies in machine learning using the game of checkers. *IBM J Res Dev.* 1959;3:210–229.

Sanchez-Martinez, S., Duchateau, N., Erdei, T., et al. Machine learning analysis of left ventricular function to characterize heart failure with preserved ejection fraction. *Circ Cardiovasc Imaging.* 2018;11:e007138.

Sengupta, P. P., Huang, Y. M., Bansal, M., et al. Cognitive machine-learning algorithm for cardiac imaging: A pilot study for differentiating constrictive pericarditis from restrictive cardiomyopathy. *Circ Cardiovasc Imaging.* 2016;9:e004330.

Shah, S. J., Katz, D. H., Selvaraj, S., Burke, M. A., Yancy, C. W., Gheorghiade, M., Bonow, R. O., Huang, C.-C., Deo, R. C. Phenomapping for novel classification of heart failure with preserved ejection fraction. *Circulation.* 2015;131:269–279.

Shah, S. J. Precision medicine for heart failure with preserved ejection fraction: An overview. *J Cardiovasc Transl Res.* 2017;10:233–244.

Shameer, K., Johnson, K. W., Glicksberg, B. S., Dudley, J. T., Sengupta, P. P. Machine learning in cardiovascular medicine: Are we there yet? *Heart.* 2018;104:1156–1164.

Sibbing, D., Aradi, D., Alexopoulos, D. Updated expert consensus statement on platelet function and genetic testing for guiding P2Y12 receptor inhibitor treatment in percutaneous coronary intervention. *JACC Cardiovasc Interv.* 2019;12:1521–1537.

Silver, D., Schrittwieser, J. Mastering the game of Go without human knowledge. *Nature.* 2017;550:354–359.

Syn, N. L., Wong, A. L., Lee, S. C., et al. Genotype-guided versus traditional clinical dosing of warfarin in patients of Asian ancestry: A randomized controlled trial. *BMC Med.* 2018;16:104.

Szolovits, P., Patil, R. S., Schwartz, W. B. Artificial intelligence in medical diagnosis. *Ann Intern Med.* 1988;108:80–87.

Tabassian, M., Alessandrini, M., Herbots, L., et al. Machine learning of the spatio-temporal characteristics of echocardiographic deformation curves for infarct classification. *Int J Cardiovasc Imaging.* 2017;33:1159–1167.

Tao, W., Concepcion, A. N., Vianen, M., Marijnissen, A. C., Lafeber, F. P., Radstake, T. R., Pandit, A. Multiomics and machine learning accurately predict clinical response to adalimumab and etanercept therapy in patients with rheumatoid arthritis. *Arthritis Rheumatol.* 2021;73:212–222.

Van Rosendael, A. R., Maliakal, G., Kolli, K. K. Maximization of the usage of coronary CTA derived plaque information using a machine learning based algorithm to improve risk stratification; insights from the CONFIRM registry. *J Cardiovasc Comput Tomogr.* 2018;12:204–209.

Vatandsoost, M., Litkouhi, S. The future of healthcare facilities: How technology and medical advances may shape hospitals of the future. *Hosp Pract Res.* 2019;4:1–11.

Wang, J. *iCarbonx is one business that is pushing in the direction of personalized healthcare services* (2021, January). https://www.icarbonx.com/en. Retrieved March 10, 2023, from https://www.icarbonx.com/en

Warner, H. R., Toronto, A. F., Veasy, L. G. Experience with Baye's theorem for computer diagnosis of congenital heart disease. *Ann N Y Acad Sci.* 1964;115:558–567.

Zellweger, M. J., Brinkert, M., Bucher, U., Tsirkin, A., Ruff, P., Pfisterer, M. E. A new memetic pattern based algorithm to diagnose/exclude coronary artery disease. *Int J Cardiol.* 2014;174:184–186.

Zellweger, M. J., Tsirkin, A., Vasilchenko, V., Failer, M., Dressel, A., Kleber, M., Ruff, P., März, W. A new non-invasive diagnostic tool in coronary artery disease: Artificial intelligence as an essential element of predictive, preventive, and personalized medicine. *EPMA J.* 2018;9:235–247.

Zerouaoui, H., Idri, A. Reviewing machine learning and image processing based decision-making systems for breast cancer imaging. *J Med Syst.* 2021;45:1–20.

7 Role of Big Data, AI, and Machine Learning in Decisions for Disease Diagnosis and Treatment

J. Suji Priya, R. Thirumalaisamy**,†, S. Aruna*, and R. Sarulatha**

*Department of Master of Computer Applications, Sona College of Technology, Salem, Tamil Nadu, India; **Department of Biotechnology, Sona College Arts and Science, Salem, Tamil Nadu, India

†Corresponding Author: tmalaisamy@gmail.com

ABBREVIATIONS

AI	Artificial intelligence
CDS	Clinical decision support
CT	Computed tomography
CTA	Computed tomography angiography
CNN	Convolutional neural network
EHR	Electronic health records
GAN	Generative adversarial networks
HIT	Health information technology
IoT	Internet of Things
LRP	Layer-wise relevance propagation
ML	Machine learning
MPM	Medical practice management
NLP	Natural Language Processing

7.1 INTRODUCTION

Currently, data analytics, machine learning, and data mining made it possible for early disease identification and treatment (Istepanian and Al-Anzi, 2018). The exponential growth of AI in the last decade is evidenced to be the potential platform for optimal decision-making by super-intelligence, where the human mind is limited to process huge data in a narrow time range (Iqbal et al., 2021). For instance, it may require a few

DOI: 10.1201/9781032699882-7

minutes for a radiologist to look at a computed tomography (CT) scan, which comprises 50 images approximately. However, an artificial intelligence (AI)-based Big Data analytics application might perform the same in just a few seconds (Khan et al., 2021). Therefore, with the aid of these technologies, doctors and clinicians can diagnose diseases at earlier stages more effectively and efficiently. Similarly, cardiovascular imaging is now integrated with pathology and Big Data from eHealth records to identify patients' conditions better and provide them special attention (Karatas et al., 2022). Researchers at the Massachusetts Institute of Technology and Massachusetts General Hospital have developed a system that uses a wearable device to collect data about the movement of a user's vocal cords and uses machine learning to detect subtle signs of abnormal speech that could indicate a person has a voice disorder called muscle tension dysphonia (MTD) (Castro and New, 2016). Correspondingly, by understanding the biology of tumors, AI-based precision medicine can be implemented in order to assist the doctors to classify cancer patients based on their tumor's molecular changes (Porumb et al., 2020). Big Data in the healthcare sector makes reference to plentiful health data accumulated from various sources such as health records in electronic form, a digital form of patient's medical chart; medical imaging, a process of imaging internal parts of the body for clinical analysis and medical intervention; genome sequencing to determine the order of DNA nucleotides or bases in a genome; and wearable healthcare devices. Using AI-based Big Data analytics solutions, patients' clinical data can be analyzed in light of the 3 V's of volume, velocity, and variety, which sets it apart from traditional medical records. Consequently, informed decisions can be made regarding patients' diagnosis, treatment, and prevention of diseases (Porumb et al., 2020).

7.2 DISEASE DIAGNOSIS AND TREATMENT

Why is diagnosis important in the healthcare industry? As we all know, early diagnosis and treatment are essential to avoid long-term complications for the infected patient, and it is a never-ending challenge in the medical field. Diagnosis is simply a prior identification of the nature of an illness by some examinations or symptoms. It can improve the effectiveness of treatments, too. The prevalence of infectious diseases has grown significantly in recent years because of pathogenic microorganisms such as bacteria, viruses, parasites, and fungi; contagious diseases pose a greater challenge today than in the past two decades.

7.3 UNDERSTANDING THE HEALTHCARE SYSTEM

Several healthcare industries, including biology, genetics, medical equipment, medical tourism and other sectors, started adopting future technologies like Big Data, machine learning (ML), and artificial intelligence (AI) for addressing all sorts of challenges, including disease diagnosis and treatment (Myszczynska et al., 2020). In these recent years, India has excelled at healthcare. We are aware that during the past ten years, the healthcare sector has experienced one of the fastest economic growth rates. As the world enters the levelling coronavirus pandemic, it is most important to have a robust public healthcare system (Ngiam et al., 2019).

The healthcare system differs among geographical locations around the world. The complete methodologies of treating patients and the cost or the method of charging them vary. Developed nations employ a variety of strategies to offer universal coverage, considering that a single-payer system is a response to the government. Several countries rely on private insurers, while a third group, including the United States, uses a combination of the two.

Artificial intelligence has entered unlimited applications and fields. Among these areas are the development of computer applications in medical diagnosis (Aggarwal et al., 2022). Recent advances enable healthcare providers to reach effective diagnoses more quickly, improving patient outcomes and lowering associated healthcare costs. In this chapter, we will discuss the role of Big Data analytics in healthcare; among the vast benefits of AI and ML in the field of diagnosis, we will see fewer of the challenges in AI healthcare and more about future research and possibilities (Cammarota et al., 2020).

7.4 CONCEPTUAL ROLE OF AI AND BIG DATA IN HEALTHCARE

The entire world is moving ahead over advanced techniques like AI, machine learning, and Big Data. According to Acumen Research and Consulting, the global market will hit $8 billion by 2026. The vast skills in AI and Big Data will be used for optimized information processing to solve real-world problems and to address several healthcare-related issues and improve advancements.

Some of them are:

- Giving the best self-service for a patient with chatbots
- With more efficient computer-aided design, diagnosing patients
- The process of discovering a drug's molecular structure by analysis of picture data
- The analysis and diagnosis of patients by radiologists
- Using more understanding clinical data to customize therapies

7.5 EMERGING FIELD OF BIG DATA ANALYTICS IN HEALTHCARE

To understand the need for Big Data analytics, we need to look at the glimpses of Big Data. As the name indicates, Big Data is a massive amount of data. We all use smart phones. Have we ever wondered how much data gets generated in the form of text, phone calls, and music that we constantly add to our playlists? It is approximately 40 exabytes of monthly data for a single smart phone user; think of 5 million users around us. It is quite a massive right. As data grows daily, handling such data is typically hard with a traditional method. In order to derive useful information from large amounts of data, Big Data analytics is a new, innovative way to analyze and utilize data. The prime objective of the BDA is cost reduction with the help of BDA technologies Hadoop and cloud-based analytics. It enables faster and better decision making for any organization (Maheshwari et al., 2021).

One example of Big Data is the New York Stock Exchange, which produces one terabyte of new trading data every day. Another example is Facebook's databases, which receive over 500 terabytes of new data every day. In a similar vein, 1000 flights per day generate many petabytes of data.

Big Data comes in a variety of forms. Data is referred to as "structured" when it can be stored, accessed, and processed in a fixed format. Unstructured data is difficult to deconstruct because it is not organized in relational databases. Such data include text, video files, audio files, mobile activity, social media posts, satellite imagery, surveillance imagery, and many more. Semi-structured data contains both the forms of the aforementioned types of data.

Characteristics of Big Data are best understood by factors such as volume, variety, velocity, variability, etc.

Big Data analytics refers to data mining techniques in this context. The data mining technique can be used for the heterogeneous healthcare datasets needed for diagnosis and treatment, such as anomaly detection, clustering, and classification, which call for summarizing and visualizing those Big Data sets. Improved illness prevention, telemedicine after processing essential real-time data, and better diagnosis context using massive patient data are the results of applying these Big Data approaches (Kumari et al., 2019).

Analysis of those huge data involves "Big Data analytics". Furthermore, it can be categorized into different analytics, like:

a. Descriptive analytics: This type of analytics is where our data are summarized in a human-understandable form. It is used to gain awareness of the current business situation for the betterment of the company's growth, profit, and more.
b. Diagnostic analytics: This type of analytics is performed to understand what causes the problem. It provides an in-depth search insight into a particular problem. Diagnostic analytics is helpful for getting at the root of an organizational issue.
c. Predictive analytics: This type of analytics investigates the previous historical and current data to make predictions about the future. It uses data mining, AI, and machine learning for making prediction.
d. Prescriptive analytics: This type of analytics is all about prescription, prescribing the solution for the problem by analyzing the sufficient data that we have already.

Although the models and methods utilized in each of the four types of analytics—descriptive, predictive, prescriptive, and discovery—are different, many applications use all four. A common workflow for Big Data analytics in the healthcare system is presented in Figure 7.1.

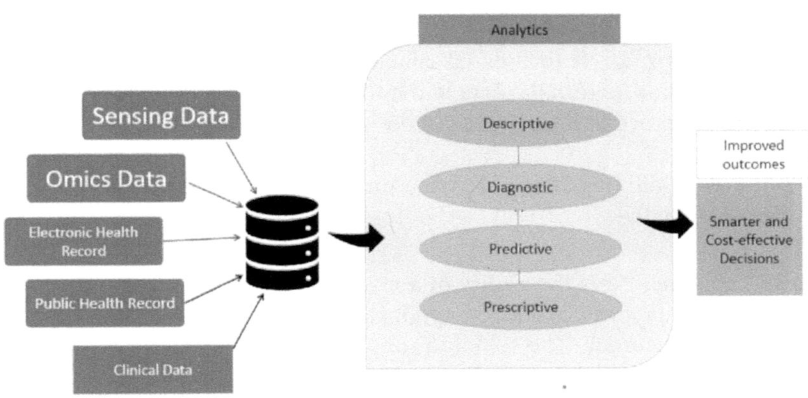

FIGURE 7.1 Workflow of Big Data analytics in the healthcare system.

The workflow of Big Data analytics in healthcare typically involves the following steps:

a. Data collection: Data is collected from various sources such as electronic health records (EHRs), medical devices, wearables, and other sources such as social media.
b. Data integration: The collected data is integrated and stored in data warehouses, which are designed to handle massive amounts of data.
c. Data pre-processing: The data is pre-processed to ensure consistency and accuracy and to remove any irrelevant or redundant data.
d. Data analysis: Advanced analytics tools such as machine learning and artificial intelligence are used to analyze the data and identify patterns, trends, and correlations.
e. Insights and predictions: The insights gained from the analysis are used to make predictions and inform healthcare decisions.
f. Reporting and visualization: The insights are presented in a meaningful and understandable way through reporting and visualization tools.
g. Action: The insights and predictions are used to inform clinical decisions and improve patient outcomes.

Overall, the goal of Big Data analytics in healthcare aims to use data-driven insights and predictions to provide more innovative and affordable healthcare options.

7.6 GLIMPSES OF ARTIFICIAL INTELLIGENCE

Artificial intelligence (AI) is the simulation of human intelligence by machines in computer systems. AI aims to create a system that can function intelligently and independently. Among its specific applications are expert systems, natural language processing, speech recognition, and machine vision. A learning process, a reasoning process, and a self-correcting process are involved:

- Learning process: It focuses on acquiring data and creating rules (algorithms) for how to turn the data into information.
- Reasoning process: It focuses on choosing the algorithm to reach a desired outcome.
- Self-correction: It is designed to fine-tune algorithms and provide accurate data continually.

As we know that AI is the ability of a machine to imitate human intelligence, that is, cognitive process, AI-based applications execute tasks intelligently, creating enormous accuracy. The six main subsets of AI are machine learning, deep learning, robotics, neural networks, natural language processing, and genetic algorithms.

7.7 GLIMPSES OF MACHINE LEARNING

Machine learning is one of the subsets of AI that is actually a computer program which increases the ability to learn, improve the quality of identifying the pattern, and make decisions to predict the future with minimal human intervention. It allows the computer to learn, respond, and adjust to the human behavior. The way the ML learns and responds is categorized into three types:

a. Supervised learning: This is the type of learning that uses the previous statistics and data to predict the future results.
b. Unsupervised learning: This type of learning is studying sampling input data; in this case, we do not know the actual output, but it finds the prediction of it.
c. Reinforcement learning: This type enables the system to study the previous benefits and results of its activities. This kind of machine learning is usually purely focused on the boosted effectiveness of the function.

The objective here is to consider its ability for diagnosing. However, ML applications are not limited to diagnosis and can be used in any sector as well. Let us return to our topic of using these concepts and technologies of AI and ML in diagnosing the treatment or disease. Types of machine learning and their algorithms are presented in Table 7.1.

TABLE 7.1
Types of Machine Learning and Algorithms

Types of Learning	Classification of Learning	Examples
Hybrid learning	Semi-supervised learning	Generative models, low-density separation, Laplacian regularization
	Self-supervised learning	Contra positive SSL, non-contrastive SSL
	Multi-instance learning	Standard assumption, GMIL assumption, boosting
Statistical inference	Inductive learning	Decision trees, covering algorithms
	Deductive learning	Neural guided deductive search
	Transductive learning	Partitioning transduction, agglomerative transduction, manifold transduction
Learning techniques	Multitask learning	Non-convex penalties, non-separable kernels
	Active learning	Stream based selective sampling, pool-based sampling
	Online learning	Linear least squares, batch learning
	Transfer learning	Kernel mean matching, Kullback–Leibler
	Ensemble learning	Bagging, random forest
Learning problems	Supervised learning	Decision trees, support vector machines
	Unsupervised learning	Principle component analysis, K-means clustering, independent component analysis
	Reinforcement learning	Montecarlo, Q-learning state-action-reward-state-action (SARSA)

7.8 ROLE OF BIG DATA IN DISEASE DIAGNOSIS AND TREATMENT

In recent years, innovative technologies have been built to collect healthcare digital data processes like medical data, dental data, surgical data, behavioral data, protein therapeutics data, genetic mutation data, and clinical trial data aimed at evaluating a medical, surgical, or behavioral intervention. To regulate medical procedures and transmit telemetry data for real-time and other types of analytics, new medical gadgets are constantly being developed. This is conceptually represented by the following action:

- Adapt the analysis and decision-making process to take advantage of Big Data in order to make more informed decisions.

7.9 ROLE OF AI IN DISEASE DIAGNOSIS AND TREATMENT

7.9.1 Prediction of Heart Attacks

Fat and cholesterol, among other substances, are present in the bloodstream and contribute to the formation of plaque. Over time, atherosclerotic plaque can cause arteries to narrow and harden, much like a clogged sink drain. When this happens in the arteries, it can obstruct blood flow and lead to serious conditions such as heart attacks or strokes.

To accurately measure the amount of plaque in an artery, doctors previously required 25 to 30 minutes using a coronary computed tomography angiography (CTA). However, researchers at Cedars Sinai have developed an AI system that can perform the same task in just a few seconds (Rauch, 2023). The researchers provided 900 coronary CTA images that had already been professionally analyzed to the computer, which was able to accurately recognize and measure plaque in the images.

In a separate study with 1611 participants, the AI algorithm's metrics effectively predicted the incidence of heart attacks within five years (Cedars-Sinai Medical Center, 2022).

7.9.2 Heart Disease Diagnosis Methodology

The technology was created for the purpose of detecting cardiac disease. Using a few chosen characteristics, the effectiveness of several machine learning classifiers for HD identification has been evaluated. The typical, most recent feature algorithm selection consists of relief, RMR, LASSO, and LLBFS. For feature selection, the author (Karthikeyan et al., 2021) also put forth the FCMIM algorithm. The effectiveness of the classifiers was assessed on certain feature sets that were chosen using the proposed FCMIM algorithm and state-of-the-art FS methods.

The proposed FCMIM method and state-of-the-art FS techniques were used to test the performance of the classifiers on particular feature sets. Cross-validation using the LOSO method was also used to choose the best model. Accuracy, specificity, sensitivity, MCC, and processing time were performance indicators for the model that were automatically calculated for classifier assessment.

They were utilized for the selection of suitable characteristics, including relief, MRMR, LASSO, and LLBFS. The developed FS algorithm was then used for the selection of features in the second phase of the studies. The performance of the classifiers was then assessed using a subset of characteristics.

7.10 ELECTRONIC HEALTH RECORDS (EHRS)

These are the most significant use of Big Data in healthcare. Every person receives a digital profile that includes information about their past, medical history, allergies, results of blood tests, etc. Through secure information systems, government and industry service providers can access and share records. Clinicians can make adjustments over time without having to submit additional paperwork or worry about data replication because each record is made up of a single editable file.

When a patient needs new lab work, EHRs may send notifications and reminders, and they can also keep track of prescriptions to ensure that patients are taking their drugs as prescribed by a doctor.

7.10.1 New Generation of EHRs

As patients continue to generate terabytes of data through the continuous monitoring of various health factors, physicians may be overwhelmed with the information they need to analyze. This requires the development of a new generation of electronic health records (EHRs) that serve as diagnostic aids as well as digital folders. In order to facilitate decision making, companies like Roche-Flatiron have already begun incorporating predictive and analytical tools into their EHRs. Be that as it may, these devices should be straightforward, versatile, and auditable to forestall possible inclinations and guarantee patient wellbeing. Patients may also request access to machine learning models to generate clinical decisions to gain greater insight and guard against malpractice. The design of a new generation of electronic health records for patient in hospital is presented in Figure 7.2.

In order to create the next generation of EHRs that are user-friendly and efficient, it will be necessary to work together with doctors, patients, providers, and insurance companies. Because it developed its own electronic health record (EHR), the Veterans Administration (VA)'s strategy can serve as an instructive model for the National Health Service (NHS). Nonetheless, the VA's answer was not broadly taken on because of an absence of help for ceaseless upkeep and charging. The NHS should also take note of private EHRs, which gained prominence by providing personalized support for providers. In Denmark, EHR implementation benefited from private competitors implementing regional solutions, striking a balance between competition and standardization. Therefore, designing the next generation of EHRs will require a collaborative effort that considers the needs of all stakeholders while maintaining a balance between competition and standardization.

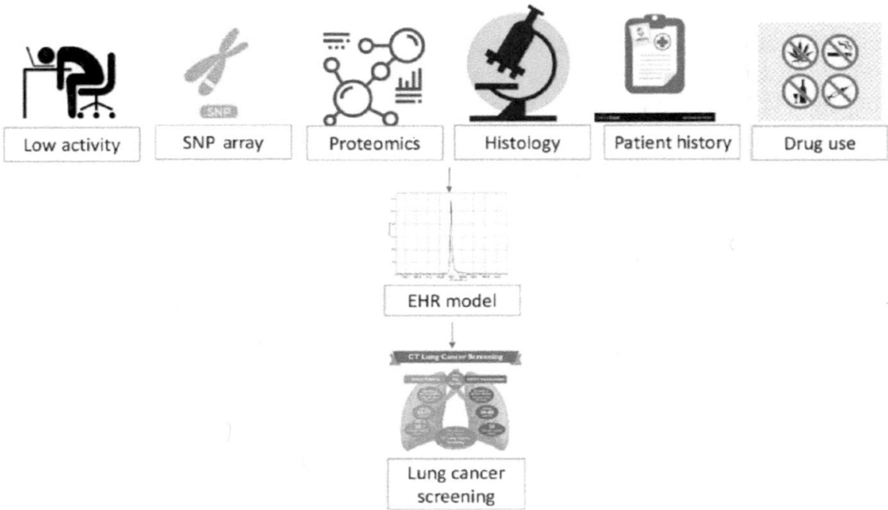

FIGURE 7.2 Designing a new generation of electronic health records.

7.10.2 Digitization of Healthcare and Big Data

Electronic medical records (EMRs) and electronic health records (EHRs) are important components of healthcare data management, along with personal health records (PHRs), medical practice management software (MPM), and other technologies. Together, they have the potential to enhance the quality, efficiency, and cost-effectiveness of healthcare services while also reducing medical errors. Healthcare data encompasses a wide range of information, including data from EMRs, pharmacy records, insurance records, genomics-driven experiments, and internet of things (IoT) devices. While the adoption of EHRs was initially slow, it has grown significantly since 2009, with healthcare data management increasingly reliant on information technology. The development of wellness monitoring devices and software has also gained traction, enabling real-time monitoring of health status and sharing of health data with healthcare providers. These devices generate vast amounts of data that can be analyzed to provide real-time medical care and improve health outcomes while controlling costs. The use of Big Data in healthcare holds great promise for transforming the delivery of healthcare services.

7.11 ENHANCING PATIENT ENGAGEMENT AND SAFETY

Data analytics in healthcare heavily relies on real-time alerts. In hospitals, clinical decision support (CDS) software rapidly analyses patient data and provides recommendations to healthcare workers as they make decision-making directives.

In order to save money on pricey in-house treatments, doctors urge patients to avoid visiting hospitals. Data analytics is one of the business intelligence buzzwords for 2021 and can be implemented into a new strategy (Bourke et al., 2020).

Wearables will be used to continuously gather and send patient health information to the cloud. Thanks to access to the database on the health of the general public, doctors can compare this data in a socioeconomic context and modify the delivery plans as appropriate. With the help of cutting-edge tools, institutions and care managers will keep an eye on this massive data stream and respond whenever the results are distressing.

7.12 DISEASE DIAGNOSIS AND TREATMENT RECOMMENDATION SYSTEM

7.12.1 Standardization Process for Medical Data

In today's healthcare landscape, different hospitals may use different standards for specific inspection tasks, and what is acceptable at one hospital may not meet the standards of another (Shilo et al., 2020). Unfortunately, only some hospitals use uniform criteria for inspection reports, which can lead to inconsistencies in the medical datasets collected across various institutions. A method of standardization is required to address this issue.

Extensive historical medical datasets are collected from cooperating hospitals. Prior to the data-gathering process, sensitive patient information such as ID codes, patient names, phone numbers, and addresses are filtered out to protect patient privacy. Before doing the clustering and association analysis, the inspection datasets must first go through a number of standardization-related tasks, including data integration and cleaning. This standardization process ensures that the medical datasets are consistent and can be analyzed accurately, providing valuable insights into disease diagnosis and treatment.

7.12.2 Pre-Processing of Patient Inspection Data

Inspection datasets are used as the data source for disease symptom clustering, benefiting from accurate tools and quantifiable data. Inspection datasets are gathered during the pre-processing stage from various hospitals and departments. The inspection data are in numerous data formats, such as numeric, text, and image formats, due to the variety of their contents.

a. Inspection data in numeric format: The datasets for routine blood inspections, routine urine inspections, and routine bone marrow analyses are some inspection-task-generated report datasets maintained in numeric format. There could be more than one inspection. Figure 7.1 shows the workflow for what should be tested during each inspection task, such as disease diagnosis and treatment recommendations.
b. Text-based inspection data: Together with the aforementioned inspection responsibilities, there is another class of inspection chores known as imaging tasks. Examples of these tasks include CT scanning, MRI scanning, X-ray scanning, type-B sonography, and color Doppler ultrasound. The symptom descriptions for these inspection tasks are delivered verbally or

visually. The patient inspection data's feature variables are determined by the patient's information and any associated symptom outcomes from each inspection task.

7.12.3 Pre-Processing of Disease Diagnosis and Treatment Data

a. Disease diagnosis-scheme data: The diagnosis-scheme data refers to the in-depth diagnoses of diseases that doctors have documented, not just the straightforward definitions of the disorders. During various stages of the same disease's treatment, various diagnosis approaches are offered. These plans are written down in text format by medical professionals or their helpers.
b. Disease treatment-scheme data: Injections, intravenous infusions, surgical procedures, needle therapy, cupping therapy, and physical therapy are all available therapeutic options at hospitals. Depending on the results of the most recent inspection, the medical practitioner may modify the patient's treatment plans during the course of treating a condition. In the case of an illness, a critical condition is advised for treatment plan A, a moderate condition for scheme B, and a light condition for scheme C. In other words, a particular treatment plan or a mix of treatment plans is used for the disease's present stage of therapy.

After data pre-processing, we involve the existing work in the processes that include DPCA-based disease symptom clustering, disease diagnosis, and treatment recommendations, that is, association analysis of disease diagnosis and treatment schemes.

7.13 EXISTING DISEASE PREVENTION METHODOLOGIES

Even though they are among the most prevalent and expensive health issues, chronic illnesses are also the most avoidable. Early detection and prevention are the best and most cheap methods to lower morbidity and death and help people live better lives.

7.13.1 Nutrients, Foods, and Medicine

Diet plays a crucial role in maintaining, preventing, and treating illness. It is a lifestyle element that can aid in the prevention of illnesses like diabetes, cancer, cardiovascular disease, metabolic syndrome, and obesity. A poor diet combined with a sedentary lifestyle can have serious consequences. Developing countries often suffer from nutritionally deficient diets, leading to chronic diseases.

Each person can lower their risk of chronic disease by improving their diet and lifestyle. Tobacco use, poor diet, and inactivity are often linked to chronic diseases. Studies show that a healthy diet and regular exercise not only affect current health but also reduce morbidity.

Food and nutrition treatments can benefit each stage of prevention. In early stages, such as obesity, food and nutrition interventions can be employed to prevent disease. Even if an illness has already been diagnosed, diet can still help lessen the impact of the condition. The author (White, 2020) has discussed that opportunities for prevention arise at every stage in the process, and three main levels are described: primary, secondary, and tertiary. Prevention strategies include health promotion focused on determinants, clinical prevention to reduce modifiable risk factors, case finding, screening, and addressing functional outcomes relevant to quality of life. Diet can be used to lessen a disease's symptoms in its secondary stage, and it can also lessen its effects in its tertiary stage, such as preventing stomach ulcers.

7.13.2 Policy, Systems, and Environmental Change

Following years of concentrating on the person, policies, systems, and environmental improvements represent a new way of thinking about raising the standard of care in the healthcare industry. At the same time, it impacts substantial portions of the global populace. If we create an atmosphere that encourages a population to embrace a healthy lifestyle, adequate diet, and drugs, disease prevention will be much simpler. Promoting social, environmental, policy, and systems approaches to support a healthy lifestyle is common in developed countries. Examples include low-fat menu options in restaurants, smoking bans, higher tobacco product prices, nutritional food restrictions for all students, and infrastructure design encouraging a lifestyle change, i.e., more physical activity.

7.13.3 Information Technologies

The main objective of health information technology (HIT) is to utilize the power of information technology in the healthcare sector to enhance efficiency and reduce costs. Through the use of advanced patient information processing, HIT provides benefits to patients, healthcare organizations, and governments. In the healthcare and IT industries, a number of electronic techniques are used to enhance the quality of clinical and preventative services, such as early disease diagnosis, risk reduction, and complication management. Healthcare transactions generate vast amounts of data. With the advent of medical record databases and the increasing connectivity between doctors, patients, and health records, researchers have developed effective disease prevention systems. Therefore, there is a need to utilize creative, team-based, and cost-effective informatics and information technology to transform health data into information. IT adds strategic value to enhance health outcomes and quality by transforming this enormous amount of data into information. The healthcare industry continues to be interested in computer-based disease control and prevention.

7.14 APPLICATIONS OF MACHINE LEARNING IN HEALTHCARE

a. Cardiac disease: Most researchers and practitioners use machine learning (ML) approaches to identify cardiac disease (Battineni et al., 2020). For instance, some offered an automated technique based on neuro-fuzzy integrated systems for identifying coronary heart disease that reaches an accuracy of about 89%. One of the study's significant weaknesses is the absence of a thorough description of how the suggested technique will function in various situations, including multiclass classification, extensive data analysis, and imbalanced class distribution. Additionally, the model's accuracy and credibility are not explained, despite current medical domains strongly advocating for it, especially to make the approach more understandable to users from non-medical domains.

b. Kidney disease: Kidney affliction, often known as renal ailment, refers to nephropathy or kidney damage. The National Kidney Foundation estimates that 10% of the world's population suffers from chronic kidney disease (CKD), and millions die each year because they do not have access to affordable treatment. Predictive analysis using machine learning techniques such as Random Forest, Support Vector Machine and Decision Tree can be helpful through an early detection of CKD for efficient and timely interventions (Debal and Sitote, 2022).

c. Parkinson's disease: Parkinson's disease is one condition from the environment for which ML data has been extensively considered. This is a neurological condition with sluggish but constant progression. People struggle to express themselves, write, march, and perform other mental actions when dopamine-bearing neurons in specific areas of the brain are injured or die. Various ML-based classification algorithms such as Multilayer perceptron, Support Vector Machine, and K-Nearest Neighbor have been discussed on benchmark voice dataset to know which of these classifiers are most efficient for Parkinson's disease prediction (Pahuja and Nagabhushan, 2021).

iv. Alzheimer's disease: Alzheimer's disease affects 60–70% of those who are diagnosed with senility and frequently begins mildly but worsens with time. Language problems, confusion, mood swings, and increased worry about behavioral abnormalities are all signs of Alzheimer's disease. Body functions evenly deteriorate, and the common longevity is three to nine years after the diagnosis. Early detection, on the other hand, can assist in preventing and taking necessary actions to engage in the appropriate situation as soon as possible, raising the feasibility of longevity. Detecting Alzheimer's disease patients throughout their lifespan has demonstrated encouraging results through machine learning and deep learning. Some of the ML algorithms like SVM and DT are used to detect single-subject Alzheimer's disease and mild cognitive impairment (MCI) prediction.

7.15 ROLE OF MACHINE LEARNING IN PRECISION MEDICINE

Precision medicine is a novel approach to diagnosing diseases and patient care. It is used to prescribe medicine to an individual according to their genomic appearance for disease prevention and treatment. In order to diagnose and treat the disease, personal information about the patient, genetic data, environmental factors, and lifestyle are analyzed. The collected data are considered multi-modal because they are taken from multiple domains. In precision medicine, patient care integrates individuals' multi-modal or multi-omics data to make patient-tailored decisions, emphasizing understanding and treating disease. This method enables doctors and researchers to forecast treatment and prevention strategies for a specific ailment that may be tested on subpopulations with varying disease risks, prognoses, and responses to therapy as a result of variations in underlying biology and other factors. With the help of various algorithms, artificial intelligence has successfully classified problems and resolved problems related to precision medicine, such as precise disease diagnosis, disease detection and prediction, and therapy optimization. AI now offers additional ways to dynamically change medicine dosage for only one or dual therapy for individual patients utilizing patient-specific data gathered over time and predicting patient reactions to therapies. Applications of ML in precision medicine are outlined in Figure 7.3.

The evaluation of multiple patient datasets, including clinical, genomic, metabolomics, imaging, claims, experimental, nutritional, and lifestyle data, is one of the most recent developments in the application of ML algorithms in precision medicine. Healthcare practitioners now have the chance to find and share data using machine learning algorithms in precision medicine. This can either affirm or modify the direction of a medical decision from one based on the evidence for the average

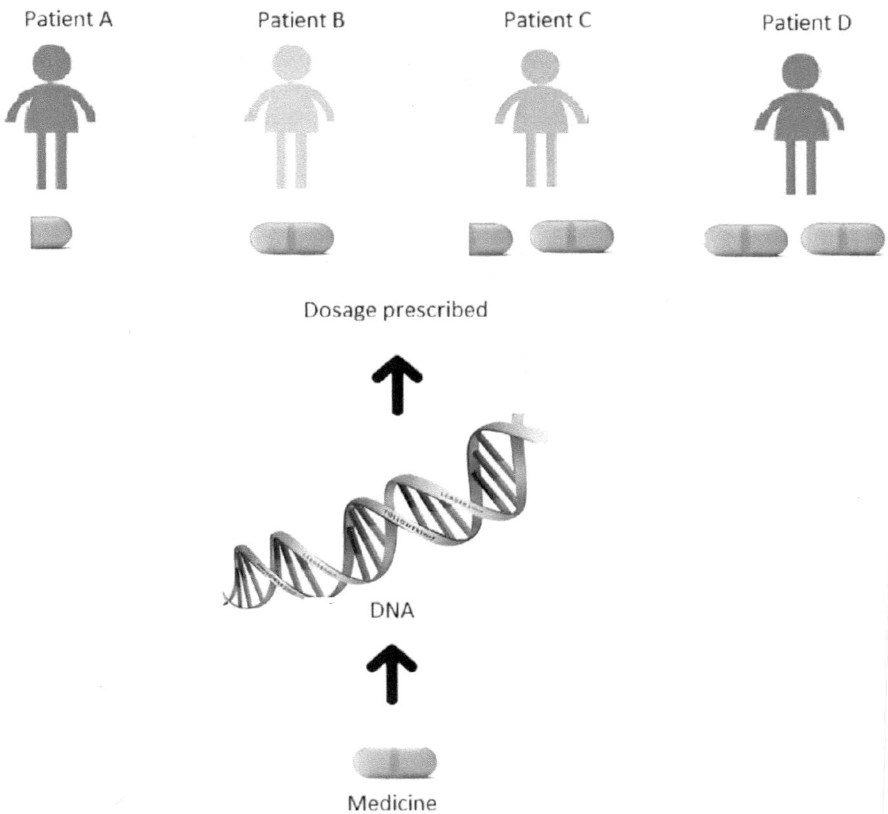

FIGURE 7.3 Machine learning in precision medicine.

patient to one based on the unique qualities of the individual. It makes it simpler for a doctor to give each patient individualized care.

7.15.1 Some Use Cases of Adopting AI in Disease Diagnosis and Treatment

To help with cancer diagnosis and treatment in the era of precision medicine, let us create a thorough understanding of artificial intelligence. The general process flow for precision medicine using machine learning for all diseases is presented in Figure 7.4.

Applying the machine learning algorithm to the genomic dataset of a patient to predict various diseases like cancer, neurological disorders, and lung and heart diseases reduces the burden of healthcare professionals. Large datasets can be more thoroughly analyzed with multi-modal data, which greatly advances the understanding of human health and disease. The machine learning algorithm is applied to train the clinical data set for disease prediction. The categories of the machine learning algorithm are classification, clustering, and regression. Algorithms for supervised learning include classification and regression, whereas unsupervised learning techniques include clustering. Classification is used to predict the disease, clustering is used for segmentation of data, and regression is used to evaluate potential high risk and also identify the patients' survival rate. The relationship between artificial intelligence, machine learning, and deep learning and their common algorithm representation is displayed in Figure 7.5.

We use AI as a whole, including ML and DL. Artificial intelligence (AI) has contributed to the decision of several clinical problems, such as cancer. Deep learning (DL), a subfield of AI, is characterized by its capability to operate computerized characteristic extraction and has extraordinary strength in assimilating and contrasting large amounts of complex data.

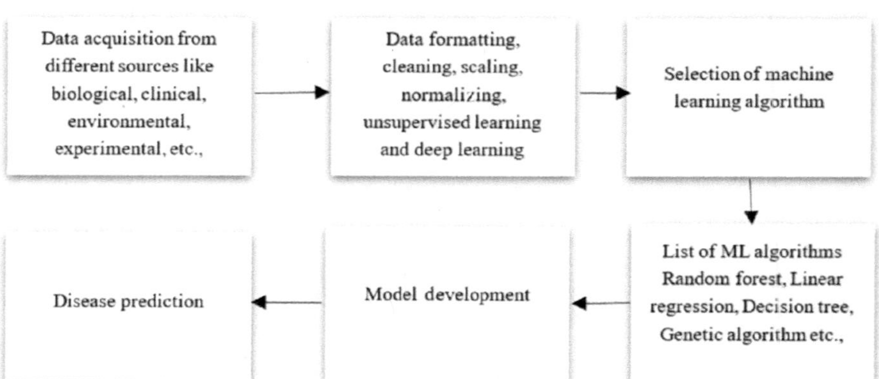

FIGURE 7.4 Process flow for precision medicine using machine learning.

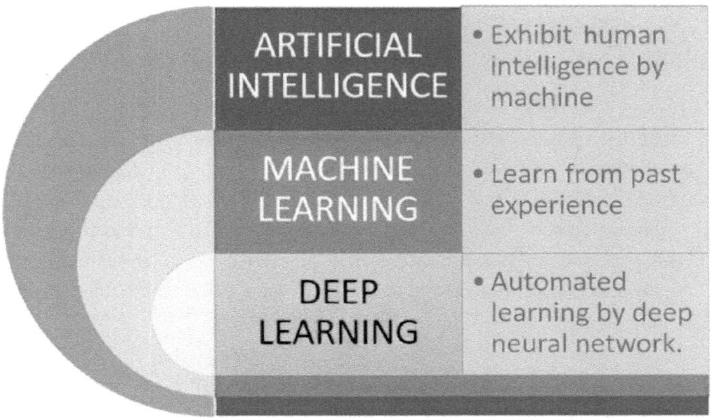

FIGURE 7.5 The relationship between artificial intelligence, machine learning, and deep learning, with commonly used algorithms as examples. CNN, convolutional neural network.

Usually, the process for handling cancer will be progressing. Steps of cancer include: cancer screening, diagnosis, classification, and grading.

The treatment choices and patient outcomes include early cancer detection by screening, accurate cancer diagnosis, categorization, and grading. The awareness of AI applications in these sectors has grown over the last few years. These applications frequently offer performance compared to human professionals and advantages in scalability and time saving. More importantly, AI has shown that it can solve complicated problems that make it difficult for humans. Cancer screening has helped certain common cancers have lower fatality rates. Automation is being used to increase the effectiveness of cancer screening due to the need for high throughput technologies and quick turnaround.

They have created a DL classifier based on biopsy-based gold standard slides. Compared to conventional colonoscopy, AI-assisted colonoscopy considerably enhanced adenoma detection rates and the mean number of adenomas discovered per patient for colorectal cancer screening. This was due to the discovery of more tiny adenomas. This is crucial since a 1% increase in the adenoma detection rate is linked to a 3% decline in the incidence of colorectal cancer. CNN-based models have the potential to revolutionize lung cancer screening when they achieve classification accuracies of 80% to 95% in several successful models. Preclinical investigations and clinical trials have demonstrated that AI mammography improves breast cancer screening. Artificial Intelligence has established a breast cancer screening. AI system employing a combination of three CNN-based models. The AI system's AUC was 11.5% higher than the six radiologists' average AUC, according to a separate study. It is noteworthy that this AI system can generalize from training data to multicenter data (Chen et al., 2018). Artificial intelligence and its applications in the medical field are presented in Table 7.2.

TABLE 7.2
Artificial Intelligence and Its Applications in the Medical Field

User Group	Category	Example of Applications	Technology
Patient	Health monitoring/Risk assessment	Devices, Wearables, Smart phone	Machine learning, Natural language processing (NLP)
	Disease prevention and management	Obesity reduction. Emotional and mental health support	Coversational AI, NLP, Speech recognition, chatbots
	Medication management	Medication adherence	Robotic home telehealth
Clinician care teams	Early detection, prediction and diagnostic tools	Imaging for cardiac arrhythmia detection, retinopathy. Early cancer detection (eg. melanoma)	Machine learning
	Surgical procedures	Remote controlled robotic surgery, AI supported surgical roadmaps	Robotic, machine learning
	Precision medicine	Personalized chemotherapy treatment	Supervised machine learning, reinforcement learning
	Patient safety	Early detection of sepsis	Machine learning

The concept of adapting care for each patient is referred to as precision medicine. Immunotherapy medications have received approval for treating metastatic melanoma, lung cancer, and other cancers.

7.16 PATIENT PROGNOSIS, RESPONSE TO THERAPY, AND PRECISION MEDICINE

Radiology text data was used to create a DL model that accurately predicts the best overall approach and progression-free survival for NSCLC patients receiving a programmable cell death protein-1 inhibitor. Precision medicine refers to the customization of treatment for specific individuals (Ho et al., 2020). Big Data and AI can be used in tandem to fulfill this demand. About 35% of locally advanced cancer patients experienced a pathologic comprehensive response after receiving NAC, which was linked to a higher survival rate. A poor reply to NAC, however, was linked to a poor prognosis.

Therefore, reliable therapeutic response prediction is important in order to prevent undue toxicity and surgical delays. The key challenge in precision medicine is to link health-related data of an individual to functional outcomes in their response to specific treatments. The standard approach is to use person-specific data derived from genomics, transcriptomics, imaging, biomarkers, and biometrics, followed by longitudinal studies with statistical and computational analysis to identify which patients respond to which treatments (Van Den Berg et al., 2019). AI now offers additional ways to dynamically change medicine dosage for single or dual therapy for individual patients utilizing patient-specific data gathered over time in addition to predicting patient reactions to therapies.

7.17 QUALITY AND BIG DATA ANALYTICS

Healthcare and medical data are categorized as Big Data because of their complexity, timeliness, and enormous volume and quantity. Examples of patient-related data include electronic health records (EHRs) for patients, diagnostic reports, physician prescriptions, medical pictures, pharmacy records, and research data from medical magazines. To improve the quality of service, identify illnesses early to lower risk factors, and manage hospital information systems more efficiently, it is critical to digitize the data generated by the healthcare sector today. Big Data analytics have a huge potential to boost healthcare's effectiveness and standard of treatment. Medical data analysis insights may presumably be used to enhance clinical models and realize efficiency via sensible delivery.

7.18 DEEP LEARNING IN CANCER RESEARCH

DL methods have been used in a variety of areas of cancer research, including the development of anti-cancer therapies, the study of molecular foundations, and the execution of randomized controlled trials (Lemaire et al., 2021). Studies have employed DL to evaluate the link among genotypes and phenotypes to elucidate the molecular pathways underlying cancer, with a significant number of successes previously documented. These genetic variations' identification identifies pertinent biological pathways and proposes potential drug research targets (Corti et al., 2022). Additionally, ML techniques have been used to speed up the early identification of possible anti-cancer medicines.

Identifying molecules with good on-target and limited off-target effects is a crucial component of the drug discovery process.

One of the most difficult components of conducting trials is thought to be successfully attracting the right patients. Matching complicated eligibility requirements to possible subjects is a tiresome, time-consuming, and challenging activity. It received an 84% overall micro-F1 rating. RCTs must be carried out effectively; top enrolling investigator selection is crucial.

7.19 REVOLUTIONIZING HEALTHCARE USING AI

7.19.1 Microscopy-Based Assessment of Cancer Using Deep Learning

The traditional way to diagnose cancer is through histopathology or AI in healthcare for disease prevention, detection, diagnosis, and treatment. Revolutionizing healthcare using AI cytopathology involves visually inspecting patient samples under a microscope to identify tumor cells and characterize their features. This process can be time-consuming and subjective, but a deep convolutional neural network (CNN) that is able to extract features from high-resolution image data is excellent. Studies have shown that deep CNNs can be as effective as pathologists in grading different types of cancer, including prostate, breast, and colon cancers and lymphoma. Additionally, explainability methods like layer-wise relevance propagation (LRP) can help pathologists validate the predictions made by deep learning models. The semantic segmentation approach uses generative adversarial networks (GANs). These can be used to localize particular regions of interest on histopathological images. A CNN-based generator, for instance, can be trained to separate cancer tissue, enabling a CNN-based classifier to grade prostate cancer with an accuracy on par with that of anatomical pathologists. These results imply that decision making and cancer diagnosis could be enhanced by DL models.

7.19.2 Cancer Survival and Prognosis

Predicting prognosis and patient survival in clinical oncology is crucial for informing treatment decisions. Deep learning (DL) applied to various types of data, such as genomic and transcriptomic data, can potentially enhance prognosis prediction. While the Cox proportional hazard regression model (Cox-PH) is the most commonly used method for survival prediction, its linear nature can overlook complex nonlinear relationships between features. On the other hand, DL models are inherently nonlinear and can capture complex molecular interactions using their flexible architecture, making them promising for predicting prognosis. Incorporating biological pathways into DL models has allowed the identification of key survival drivers among thousands of features. Advanced DL models, such as PASNET and Cox-PASNet, have shown promising results in identifying clinically actionable genetic traits in cancers such as glioblastoma multiforme and ovarian cancer. The survival of different malignancies has also been predicted using CNN models trained on histopathological images. MesoNet uses a feature contribution explainability algorithm called CHOWDER to identify stromal cells as important contributors to survival predictions. Multi-modal DL analysis that integrates histopathology images and omics data can potentially stratify patients into prognostic groups better and suggest personalized treatments. Combining multi-modal and explainability methods such as PathME shows particular promise in this area.

In conclusion, by enhancing precision, speed, and consistency in diagnosis, prognosis, and prediction, deep learning has the potential to revolutionize microscopy-based cancer evaluation. However, further research is needed to optimize these algorithms for different types of cancer and ensure their effectiveness and safety in clinical settings.

7.20 CHALLENGES AND FUTURE IMPLICATIONS

Understanding the challenges and difficulties in implementing the ideas in the real world is also essential.

- Generalizability and practical relevance: Due to the large differences in medical data between institutions, DL models' performance tends to suffer when utilized at several hospitals; as a result, external validation sets may be required to confirm their effectiveness (Peterson et al., 2006). In order to reproduce actual clinical circumstances, future studies should create a multi-modal DL model that includes both the aforementioned data and imaging data.

- The black box issue with interpretability: DL has come under fire for being a "black box" that doesn't clarify how the model turns given inputs into outputs. However, several initiatives have already been made to increase the transparency of this black box. These ground-breaking studies improve the use and applicability of DL technologies in clinical oncology conditions.
- Medical ethics and data access: Overfitting insufficient training data is a modeling error in statistics that may happen when a function is too closely aligned to a limited data set. Medical data are frequently the property of particular institutions due to privacy concerns around patient information, and there are not any protocols to share data among institutions. Fortunately, this challenge is starting to be overcome thanks to multicenter data-sharing agreements and distributed DL that protects privacy. The Cancer Imaging Archive, which combines medical images from numerous hospitals and institutes, is a prominent illustration of data sharing. It may help encourage based biometric studies.

Governments and businesses should create a reputable framework in the future to realize secure data sharing. DL is a recently created AI approach for oncology that is advancing quickly. Cancer diagnosis and therapy could be made more accurate and effective using medical data, algorithm development, and DL approaches. Future studies should concentrate on reproducibility and understandability to make DL approaches more practical to realize clinical deployment.

7.21 CONCLUSION

AI-driven Big Data analytics approach helps clinicians to make faster and better data-driven decisions that improve the efficiency and accuracy of diagnosing various disease conditions of the patients. Intelligent health care systems and patient care in general can both benefit from artificial intelligence. The broad and diverse field of artificial intelligence (AI) is made up of deep learning, neural networks, analytics, data, and insights. It is constantly expanding and evolving to satisfy the needs of the healthcare industry and its clients. For the diagnosis of diseases, the development of new treatments, and the identification of patient risk factors, artificial intelligence techniques, ranging from machine learning to deep learning, are widely used in the healthcare sector. For artificial intelligence technologies to efficiently diagnose diseases, a variety of medical data sources, including ultrasound, magnetic resonance imaging, mammography, genomics, computed tomography scans, etc., are needed. Aside from that, AI has essentially improved hospital visits and sped up the process of getting patients ready to continue their recovery at home.

The chapter is also helpful to know about recent innovations and future perspectives of biomedical engineering and its application in the medical field. It is evident that our improvements in AI, machine learning, and Big Data prove good growth in healthcare industries; the growth is not limited to any of the extents. As we discussed above, we need all the new technologies to enhance our living standards and save the valuable lives on this earth. There is also a shortage of healthcare professionals that will reach 10 million by 2030. Overall, we know healthcare is becoming too expensive and exclusive that is really designed for a different world (Munoz-Gama et al., 2022). Utilizing this kind of artificial intelligence can give everyone access to better and timely quality health care services at reasonable cost.

REFERENCES

Aggarwal, Karan, Maad M. Mijwil, Abdel-Hameed Al-Mistarehi, Safwan Alomari, Murat Gök, Anas M. Zein Alaabdin, and Safaa H. Abdulrhman. 2022. Has the future started? The current growth of artificial intelligence, machine learning, and deep learning. *Iraqi Journal for Computer Science and Mathematics* 3.1: 115–123.

Battineni, Gopi, Getu Gamo Sagaro, Nalini Chinatalapudi, and Francesco Amenta. 2020. Applications of machine learning predictive models in the chronic disease diagnosis. *Journal of Personalized Medicine* 10: 21.

Bourke, Alison, William G. Dixon, Andrew Roddam, Kueiyu Joshua Lin, Gillian C. Hall, Jeffrey R. Curtis, Sabine N. van der Veer, et al. 2020. Incorporating patient generated health data into pharmacoepidemiological research. *Pharmacoepidemiology and Drug Safety* 12: 1540–1549.

Cammarota, Giovanni, Gianluca Ianiro, Anna Ahern, Carmine Carbone, Andriy Temko, Marcus J. Claesson, Antonio Gasbarrini, and Giampaolo Tortora. 2020. Gut microbiome, big data and machine learning to promote precision medicine for cancer. *Nature Reviews Gastroenterology & Hepatology* 17.10: 635–648.

Castro, D., and J. New. 2016. The promise of artificial intelligence. *Center for Data Innovation* 115.10: 32–35.

Cedars-Sinai Medical Center. Artificial intelligence tool may help predict heart attacks. *ScienceDaily*, 22 March 2022. www.sciencedaily.com/releases/2022/03/220322221827.htm

Chen, J., Li, K., Rong, H., Bilal, K., Yang, N. and Li, K. 2018. A disease diagnosis and treatment recommendation system based on big data mining and cloud computing. *Information Sciences*, 435, pp. 124–149.

Corti, Chiara, Marisa Cobanaj, Edward C. Dee, Carmen Criscitiello, Sara M. Tolaney, Leo A. Celi, and Giuseppe Curigliano. 2022. Artificial intelligence in cancer research and precision medicine: Applications, limitations and priorities to drive transformation in the delivery of equitable and unbiased care. *Cancer Treatment Reviews*: 102498.

Debal, D. A., and T. M. Sitote. 2022. Chronic kidney disease prediction using machine learning techniques. *Journal of Big Data* 9.1: 1–19.

Ho, Dean, Stephen R. Quake, Edward R. B. McCabe, Wee Joo Chng, Edward K. Chow, Xianting Ding, Bruce D. Gelb, et al. 2020. Enabling technologies for personalized and precision medicine. *Trends in Biotechnology* 38.5: 497–518.

Iqbal, M. J., Z. Javed, H. Sadia, I. A. Qureshi, A. Irshad, R. Ahmed, K. Malik, S. Raza, A. Abbas, R. Pezzani, and J. Sharifi-Rad. 2021. Clinical applications of artificial intelligence and machine learning in cancer diagnosis: Looking into the future. *Cancer Cell International* 21.1: 1–11.

Istepanian, R. S., and T. Al-Anzi. 2018. m-Health 2.0: New perspectives on mobile health, machine learning and big data analytics. *Methods* 151: 34–40.

Karthikeyan, N., P. Padmanaban, A. Prasanth, and D. Ragunath. 2021. Machine learning based classification models for heart disease prediction. *Journal of Physics: Conference Series* 1916.1: 012092.

Karatas, Mumtaz, Levent Eriskin, Muhammet Deveci, Dragan Pamucar, and Harish Garg. 2022. Big Data for healthcare industry 4.0: Applications, challenges and future perspectives. *Expert Systems with Applications*: 116912.

Khan, Tanveer, Antonis Michalas, and Adnan Akhunzada. 2021. Fake news outbreak 2021: Can we stop the viral spread? *Journal of Network and Computer Applications* 190: 103112.

Kumari, Aparna, Sudeep Tanwar, Sudhanshu Tyagi, and Neeraj Kumar. 2019. Verification and validation techniques for streaming big data analytics in internet of things environment. *IET Networks* 8.3: 155–163.

Lemaire, Vincent, Colby S. Shemesh, and Anand Rotte. 2021. Pharmacology-based ranking of anti-cancer drugs to guide clinical development of cancer immunotherapy combinations. *Journal of Experimental & Clinical Cancer Research* 40.1: 311.

Maheshwari, S., P. Gautam, and C. K. Jaggi. 2021. Role of big data analytics in supply chain management: Current trends and future perspectives. *International Journal of Production Research* 59.6: 1875–1900.

Munoz-Gama, Jorge, Niels Martin, Carlos Fernandez-Llatas, Owen A. Johnson, Marcos Sepúlveda, Emmanuel Helm, Victor Galvez-Yanjari, et al. 2022. Process mining for healthcare: Characteristics and challenges. *Journal of Biomedical Informatics* 127: 103994.

Myszczynska, Monika A., Poojitha N. Ojamies, Alix M. B. Lacoste, Daniel Neil, Amir Saffari, Richard Mead, Guillaume M. Hautbergue, Joanna D. Holbrook, and Laura Ferraiuolo. 2020. Applications of machine learning to diagnosis and treatment of neurodegenerative diseases. *Nature Reviews Neurology* 16.8: 440–456.

Ngiam, Kee Yuan, and Wei Khor. 2019. Big data and machine learning algorithms for healthcare delivery. *The Lancet Oncology* 20.5: e262–e273.

Pahuja, G., and T. N. Nagabhushan. 2021. A comparative study of existing machine learning approaches for Parkinson's disease detection. *IETE Journal of Research* 67.1: 4–14.

Peterson, Eric D., Matthew T. Roe, Jyotsna Mulgund, Elizabeth R. DeLong, Barbara L. Lytle, Ralph G. Brindis, Sidney C. Smith, et al. 2006. Association between hospital process performance and outcomes among patients with acute coronary syndromes. *Jama* 295.16: 1912–1920.

Porumb, Mihaela, Saverio Stranges, Antonio Pescapè, and Leandro Pecchia. 2020. Precision medicine and artificial intelligence: A pilot study on deep learning for hypoglycemic events detection based on ECG. *Scientific Reports* 10.1: 170.

Rauch, S. Case studies: The growing role of big data in healthcare. September 2023. https://www.cedars-sinai.org/newsroom/artificial-intelligence-tool-may-help-predict-heart-attacks/

Shilo, Smadar, Hagai Rossman, and Eran Segal. 2020. Axes of a revolution: Challenges and promises of big data in healthcare. *Nature Medicine* 26.1: 29–38.

Van Den Berg, Albert, Christine L. Mummery, Robert Passier, and Andries D. Van der Meer. 2019. Personalised organs-on-chips: Functional testing for precision medicine. *Lab on a Chip* 19.2: 198–205.

White, F. 2020. Application of disease etiology and natural history to prevention in primary health care: A discourse. *Medical Principles and Practice* 29.6: 501–513.

8 Artificial Intelligence in Drug Research—A New Wave of Innovation in Drug Discovery

Puja Ghosh, Muhasina K. M.*, Akey Krishna Swaroop**, Esakkimuthukumar M.**, Rana Pratap Singh***, Ramveer Singh****, Antony Justin*,†, Jubie Selvaraj**, and Duraiswamy Basavan*,†*

*Department of Pharmacology, JSS College of Pharmacy, JSS Academy of Higher Education & Research, Ooty, Nilgiris, Tamilnadu, India; **Department of Pharmaceutical Chemistry, JSS College of Pharmacy, JSS Academy of Higher Education & Research, Ooty, Nilgiris, Tamilnadu, India; ***Department of Pharmaceutical Regulatory Affairs, JSS College of Pharmacy, JSS Academy of Higher Education & Research, Ooty, Nilgiris, Tamilnadu, India; ****Department of Botany and Microbiology, Gurukula Kangri University, Haridwar, India

†Corresponding Authors: bdurais@jssuni.edu.in; justin@jssuni.edu.in

ABBREVIATIONS

ACT	Artemisinin-based combined treatment
AI	Artificial intelligence
ANN	Artificial neural network
CBR	Case-based reasoning
DL	Deep learning
DT	Digital twin
ES	Expert system
FL	Fuzzy logic
GA	Genetic algorithms
KronRLS	Kronecker-regularized least squares
LMCS	Ligand maximal common substructure

DOI: 10.1201/9781032699882-8

QSAR	Quantitative structure–activity relationship
QSPR	Quantitative structure–property relationship
RF	Random forest
SEA	Similarity ensemble approach
SVM	Support vector machine

8.1 INTRODUCTION

The most potent and effective analytical tool for humanity now available is artificial intelligence (AI) (Silver et al., 2017). Computer-aided drug development has made extensive use of machine-learning techniques (Vamathevan et al., 2019). Artificial neural networks with numerous hidden processing layers, or "deep learning" techniques, have recently received more attention because of their capacity to use the input data to automatically extract features that can represent nonlinear input–output correlations.

These deep learning idea characteristics complement more conventional machine-learning strategies, which depend on created molecular targets (Walters & Barzilay, 2020). Deep learning has seen a comparatively late renaissance of interest in the field of drug discovery (Schneider, 2019), which has already sparked an unparalleled boom of novel modelling techniques and applications (Wu et al., 2018).

Statisticians and bioinformaticians, rather than data scientists, are needed for many health-related investigations. There is a necessity to create better tools to distinguish individual situations from the general inclination of the volume of information in the setting of omics, which generates several data points for gene expression, gene polymorphisms, proteomics metabolomics, and lipidomics (Agrebi & Larbi, 2020). Recent research has demonstrated the value of using machine learning to

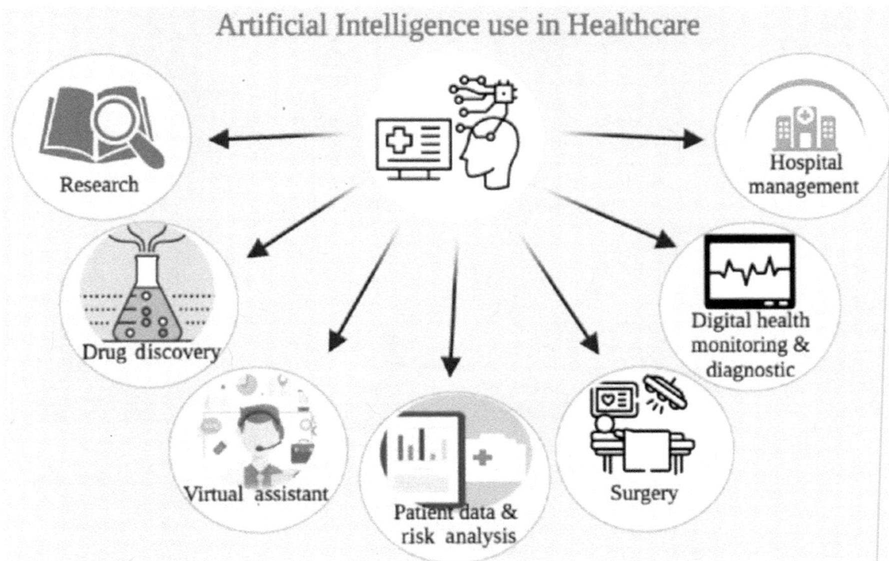

FIGURE 8.1 Uses of AI in healthcare.

enhance image processing when traditional technologies are unable to detect early indicators of illnesses (J. H. Chen & Asch, 2017). This is especially the case in cancer, where AI techniques frequently aid in management and therapy (Boon et al., 2018). This holds even in underdeveloped nations when a lack of resources, high healthcare costs, and other restrictions make it impossible to provide the best care possible. A team recently demonstrated the potential to create a lower-cost lymphoma diagnostic point of care depending on basic imaging and deep learning (Im et al., 2018). AI is used in many healthcare systems, which are shown in Figure 8.1.

According to AI, there are presently more than 7 billion linked items in continuous use throughout the universe, and utilizing this would significantly increase the chances to improve our livelihood. To better diagnose infectious diseases; identify the processes of infections, treatment resistance, and transmission; and modify vaccine designs, these datasets and traditional healthcare datasets are being employed (Figure 8.2) (Agrebi & Larbi, 2020).

With a sensitivity for virological failure diagnosis of >95%, machine learning can reduce the need for viral impact loading, in this case by 1/3, helping to save time, resources, and lives without compromising safety. These machine-learning applications combined, as shown in Figure 8.3, have significantly enhanced the treatment of infectious diseases. Although this demonstrates the immense ability of AI, many elements still require improvement to fully make use of its ability to assist remove undesirable infections, lessen the impact of seasonal viruses, and better comprehend the relationships between humans and pathogens.

Many pharmaceutical corporations have invested in and formed partnerships with AI businesses to provide better healthcare solutions, especially in the years

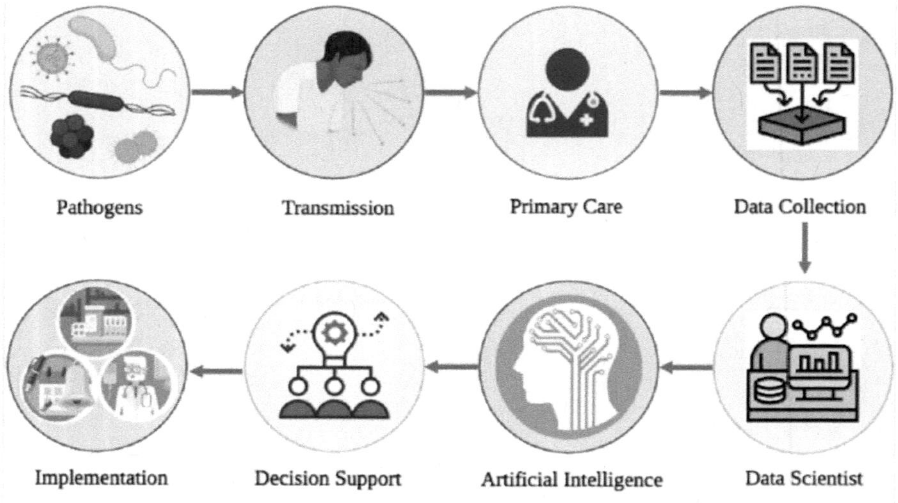

FIGURE 8.2 Essential ideas in the prevention and treatment of infectious illnesses. The sequence presents the crucial elements to prevent transmission and enhance control through preventive measures (vaccination and cleanliness). In this approach, the AI ecosystem plays a crucial role.

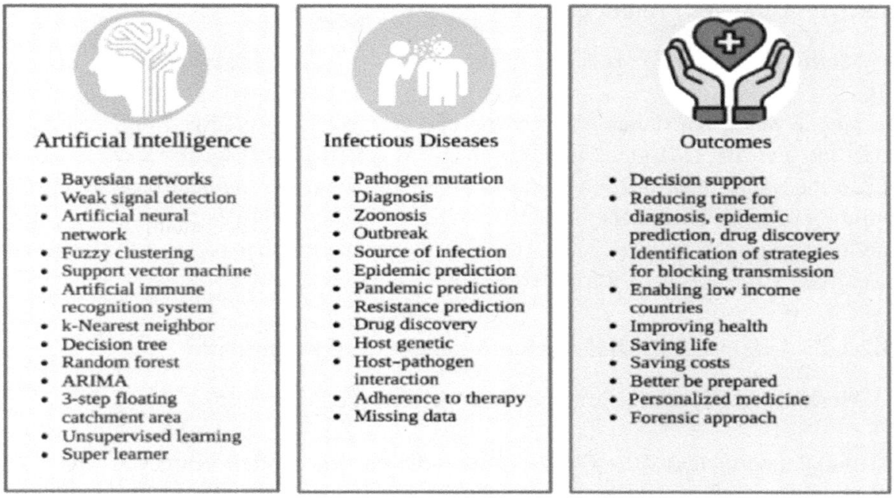

FIGURE 8.3 Artificial intelligence aids involved in drug discovery.

2016 and 2017 (Mak & Pichika, 2019). With the switch from traditional medicine to contemporary medicine, AI healthcare is based on data (Krittanawong, 2018).

This chapter explains the role of artificial intelligence in diagnosis, management, medication development, and drug discovery, including natural products, and also in the prevention of major diseases. The chapter continues with the prediction of targets using AI and the implementation of AI-based drugs in drug repurposing. The chapter concludes by mentioning the computational tools databases in the drug discovery process and the future perspectives and limitations of AI applications.

8.2 ROLE OF ARTIFICIAL INTELLIGENCE IN DISEASE MANAGEMENT

8.2.1 Diabetes Management Using AI

Despite the quick advancements in science and technology in healthcare, diabetes is still a chronic, incurable disease. The conversion of clinical and genetic data into useful knowledge has advanced significantly thanks to artificial intelligence (AI) technology. Given its advantages in fostering individualization and full-course education intervention based on the distinctive images of various persons, the application of AI technology in disease training would be quite advantageous. Substantial benefits of AI-based teaching include cost savings, simple implementation, high penetration, variable physician interaction, prevention of repetitive attempts, decreased burden for medical staff, and improved performance. The majority of the current AI tools used in diabetes education are focused on complications monitoring, self-management, blood sugar monitoring, lifestyle advising, and insulin injection guidance. Here, we make an effort to provide the most thorough illustration of the current AI approaches that have been used in the management of diabetes from multiple angles (Li et al., 2020).

8.2.1.1 Diabetes Prediction

Method: SVM (support vector machine), ML (machine learning)

In recent years, SVM has emerged as one of the most well-liked and adaptable machine learning (ML) techniques used. SVM is being used, for instance, to investigate the viability of utilizing data acquired in electronic medical records for the building of efficient models for diabetes risk prediction and to extract relevant information from huge databases. However, a reasonable number of false positives are tolerated by the approach (Noble & Valdes, 2011).

8.2.1.2 Exercise and Diet Advice Assessment of Retinopathy

Method: ANN (artificial neural network), DL (deep learning)

Artificial neural networks (ANNs) represent the most often employed methods. Interconnected neurons, or the way the human brain works, form the foundation of ANN. A deep learning (DL) algorithm is an evolution of an artificial neural network (ANN). For example, a regression model based on ANN techniques was later proposed and was able to analyze the actual exercise level of individuals carrying accelerometer sensors and heart monitors in addition to monitoring the differences in blood glucose concentrations that happened while the patients were exercising (Marlow & McLain, 2011).

8.2.1.3 Dosage Advice for Insulin

Method: CBR (case-based reasoning)

CBR is involved to produce an individual bolus of insulin using an insulin intravenous bolus estimator and to help patients maintain optimum blood glucose levels while receiving the best possible care. CBR gains knowledge from previous similar eating experiences that were documented in cases using a couple of criteria (e.g., meal time, exercise). Nevertheless, there are a few drawbacks to CBR because it frequently takes too long to apply and requires a big sample size (Nimri et al., 2017).

8.2.1.4 Checking Blood Sugar to Predict Foot Ulcers

Method: GA (genetic algorithms)

By generating a group of individuals' answers to optimization issues, GA mimics natural selection. Recently, this method has been used to identify foot ulcers early. Segmentation, geometric transformation, and asymmetry analysis make up this method's three phases (Walsh et al., 2015).

8.2.1.5 Hypoglycaemia Detection Peripheral Neuropathy

Method: FL (fuzzy logic) ES (expert system)

Systems with the capacity to record expert thinking and facts are referred to as ES. One of the most popular ES utilized in the study of diabetes is fuzzy systems. It is a new version of expert systems that process data using fuzzy logic and learns on its own (Nimri et al., 2017).

8.2.1.6 Diabetes Management

Method: DT (digital twin)

DT is often developed using supervised learning. The incorporation of DL in the platforms can integrate both patient and doctor support systems for the objective of modifying the illness by capturing data on food, exercise, medication use, and blood sugar levels (Quinn et al., 2011).

8.2.2 Role of AI in COVID-19

The medical world is searching for cutting-edge strategies to monitor and restrain the COVID-19 (coronavirus) pandemic's progress in the middle of the current global health crisis. On the other hand, a method known as artificial intelligence makes it simple to monitor the spread of this virus, identifies people who are especially vulnerable, and helps with actual infection management. By carefully examining the patients' history data, it can also accurately forecast the likelihood of mortality. Figure 8.4 illustrates how AI may provide extensive testing, health care, warning, and infection control solutions to aid in the fight against this disease (Haleem, Javaid et al., 2020).

8.2.2.1 AI's Use in the COVID-19 Epidemic

Artificial intelligence (AI) can quickly spot anomalous findings and other "red flags," notifying people and the right healthcare institutions (Aminian et al., 2020). It makes decision making quicker and more cost effective. helps in the creation of an innovative assessment and improved performance for COVID-19 instances using workable algorithms. AI assists in the detection of infected instances by using diagnostic imaging technology like computer tomography (CT) and magnetic resonance imaging (MRI) scans of a person's body organs (Luo et al., 2020).

8.2.2.2 Maintaining a Record of the Treatment

AI is capable of creating a sophisticated framework for continuously tracking and forecasting the spread of this virus. A neural network can be used to filter out the visual characteristics of this disease, which will aid in the careful observation and care of those who have been affected. It can provide ongoing health updates on the patient and guidance on how to stop the COVID-19 epidemic (Haleem, Vaishya et al., 2020).

8.2.2.3 Finding the Individuals' Contacts

Artificial intelligence (AI) has the potential to successfully seek down contacts for people and keep an eye on them by identifying groups and "hot spots," as well as by assessing the virus's level of transmission. It can predict the development and likely reappearance of this condition in the future (Haleem, Javaid et al., 2020).

8.2.2.4 Case and Mortality Projections

Utilizing information on the dangers of transmission and the virus's anticipated spread from social media, AI can monitor and predict the characteristics of the virus. Furthermore, it can forecast the number of confirmed cases and fatalities in any location. AI can assist in identifying the countries, communities, and regions that are most vulnerable so that appropriate action may be taken (Haleem, Javaid et al., 2020). Even during the development of the vaccine, AI is helpful for clinical studies and expedites the discovery of medicines and vaccines (Chen et al., 2020).

8.2.2.5 Creation of Pharmaceuticals and Vaccines

AI is used for medication development by looking at the COVID-19 data that is currently available. It can be useful for designing and creating drug delivery systems. This technology helps to significantly speed up the process compared to traditional testing, which is time-consuming and could not be feasible for a person to accomplish (Biswas et al., 2021). AI can help in the search for efficient drugs to treat COVID-19 patients. It has grown into a powerful tool for creating vaccines and designs for diagnostic tests (Sohrabi et al., 2020).

8.2.2.6 Lowering the Workload for Healthcare Professionals

During the COVID-19 epidemic, patient numbers increased dramatically and suddenly, placing a heavy burden on healthcare workers. AI was employed in this case to lighten the workload of healthcare professionals (Gozes et al., 2020). With the aid of technology resources and data science, AI helps in earlier detection and prompt therapy of this new ailment, giving students and professionals the finest education possible. AI can enhance patient care in the future and address more possible issues, which will relieve some of the pressure on physicians (Gupta et al., 2020).

8.2.2.7 Disease Prevention

Through the application of actual data assessment, AI can also offer current information that is important for preventing this sickness. It can estimate the likely areas of infection, the propagation of the virus, and the necessity for isolated rooms and healthcare workers throughout this emergency. AI can assist in preventing future virus and illness outbreaks by using earlier mentored data over more recent data. It identifies the traits, underlying causes, and transmission mechanisms of sickness. Hereafter, this method will be essential in the fight against pandemics and other epidemics. It can protect you from harm and treat a variety of illnesses. AI will be essential in the future for strong forecasting and preventive healthcare (Gupta & Misra, 2020).

8.2.3 Role of AI in Cancer

The progress of information analysis and the enhancement of clinical judgment quality are two of the main advantages of applying artificial intelligence to cancer research. By utilizing hitherto unheard-of data quantities, intelligent systems (IS) and translational medicine seek to understand the underlying diverse effects and variables related to individuals' results. Because IS efficiency and functioning are linked to

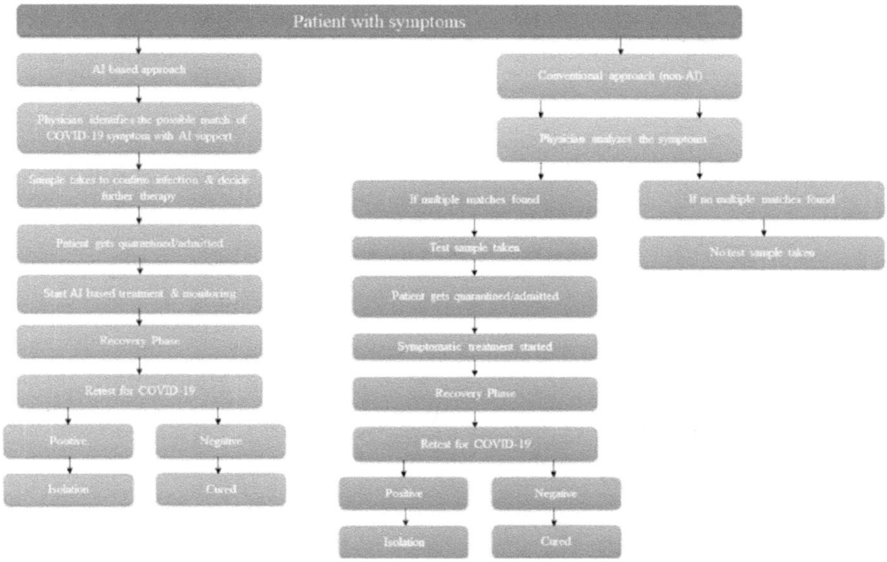

FIGURE 8.4 Impact of AI and non-AI in treatment.

complicated diagnosis and treatment, a wide range of trends and characteristics seen in high-dimensional data may be crucial for making judgments (Capobianco, 2022). Early tumour detection and artificial intelligence (AI) are two fields that are both quickly developing and have significant points of overlap (Dlamini et al., 2020).

Artificial intelligence (AI) is the mimicking of human intelligence by computers. ML is the practice of teaching computer algorithms to generate predictions based on prior performance. It is a branch of AI. It can be broadly divided into supervised and unsupervised learning. Supervised learning occurs when the computer is given access to outcome data. Both techniques search for data patterns to predict outcomes, such as the presence or absence of cancer, survival rates, or risk groups. In oncology and more generally, natural language processing (NLP) is a method that is commonly utilized for evaluating unstructured clinical data. NLP transforms unstructured free text into a computer-analyzable format, allowing labour-intensive tasks to be automated (Bitterman et al., 2021). Cancer in its early diagnosis could be revolutionized using AI in healthcare data, and automation could support worries about capacity, as shown in Figure 8.5. We may be able to interpret complex data from a variety of sources, such as clinical studies, and genomic studies, with the help of AI.

8.3 IDENTIFICATION OF SPECIFIC DRUGS TO TARGET VARIOUS DISEASES USING AI

A crucial part in drug development is played by artificial intelligence (AI), as shown in Figure 8.6. This field is driven particularly by artificial neural networks like deep neural networks or recurrent networks. The robustness of this technique in QSPR or

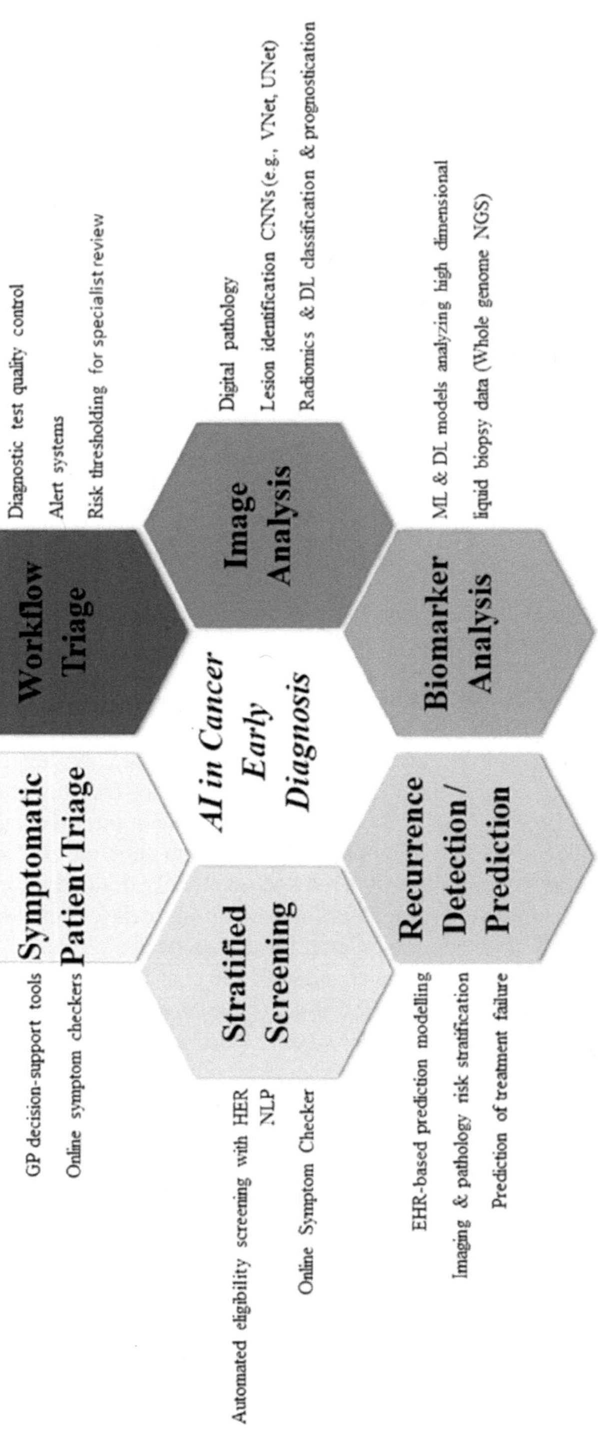

FIGURE 8.5 Utilizing AI in cancer early diagnosis.

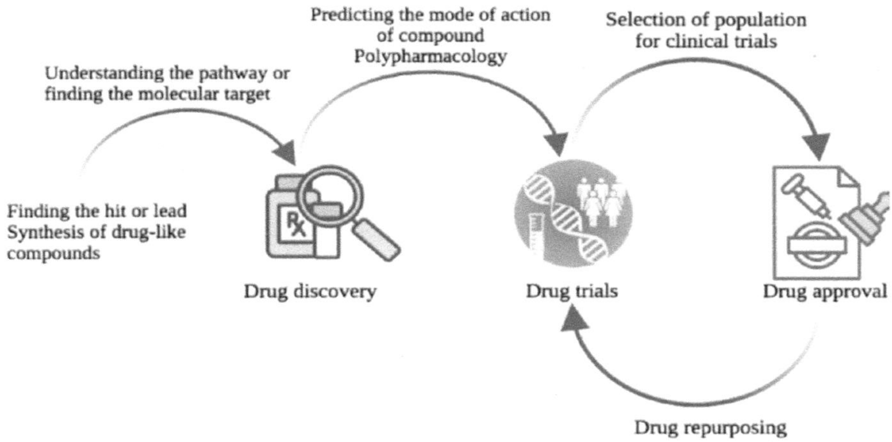

FIGURE 8.6 Drug development roles played by artificial intelligence.

quantitative structure–activity relationships (QSAR) is supported by a large number of applications in properties or activity predictions, such as ADMET and physicochemical characteristics, that have newly emerged. De novo design using artificial intelligence directs the creation of functional new biologically active molecules toward desired qualities. The effectiveness of artificial intelligence in this area is demonstrated in several cases. It is possible to combine drug discovery with synthesis planning and simplicity of synthesis, and shortly, more automated drug discovery by the system is anticipated (Hessler & Baringhaus, 2018a).

8.3.1 Prediction of Targets Using Artificial Intelligence

Clinical potential molecules for drugs must satisfy a variety of requirements. The medication must be reasonably selective against unwanted targets, have good physicochemical and ADMET qualities, and have the right potency for the biological target (absorption, metabolism, distribution, excretion, and toxicity characteristics). Thus, compound escalation is a complex issue. Throughout the optimization process, a range of in silico prediction approaches is employed for efficient compound design. Numerous machine-learning techniques, in particular, include support vector machines (SVM) and random forests (RF) (Teles et al., 2021). Access to huge datasets, a requirement for using AI, is a key factor in the success of machine learning for property identification. Large amounts of data are gathered in the pharmaceutical business during chemical refinement for a variety of features. To drive compound optimization, such sizable datasets are consistently used across numerous chemical series for targets and anti-targets. An example is the prediction of activity against certain kinases. Larger datasets are produced through selectivity profiling in several kinase programs, and these datasets have systematically been used to create models (Sharma & Rani, 2021). Bayesian QSAR models were created for binary profiling QSAR using a sparsely populated data matrix of 130,000 chemicals on 92 distinct kinases. These algorithms are used to novel compounds to build an affinity fingerprint, which is then used to predict metabolic pathways against new kinases using a small number of data points. Models are iteratively refined using new experimental results. As a result, machine learning has been used as an iterative strategy to find new kinase inhibitors. Another example of forecasting kinase activities was merging publicly accessible datasets with internal datasets to successfully construct random forest models for about 200 distinct kinases (Merget et al., 2017). Random forest models outperformed other machine-learning methods in terms of performance. Only a DNN performed similarly, with higher sensitivity but poorer specificity. However, the authors preferred the random forest models since they are simpler to train. Several recent reviews cover a wide range of new machine-learning subjects (Ghasemi et al., 2018; Varnek & Baskin, 2012). Large amounts of data are readily accessible through the public domain and can be utilized to create models using machine learning that forecast cross-target activity (Keiser et al., 2007). These models can be used to find new targets for an existing medicine, a process known as drug repurposing. SEA (similarity ensemble approach) technology has been used successfully to repurpose chemicals (Pushpakom et al., 2019). Ensembles of compounds with each receptor are evaluated using the similarity-based approach known as SEA. To measure the relevance of found similarities in a random distribution, similarities are compared to a distribution formed using random comparisons. The analysis can also be done using a little material searched against an ensemble of ligands for each protein target to reuse a ligand. Deep neural networks have been utilized to handle numerous challenges involving property prediction as a result of the success of the Kaggle competition. Artificial neural networks, which are modelled after the human brain, include deep neural networks. Like the neurons in the brain, several nodes, also known as neurons, are linked together. As seen in Figure 8.7, signals arriving from various

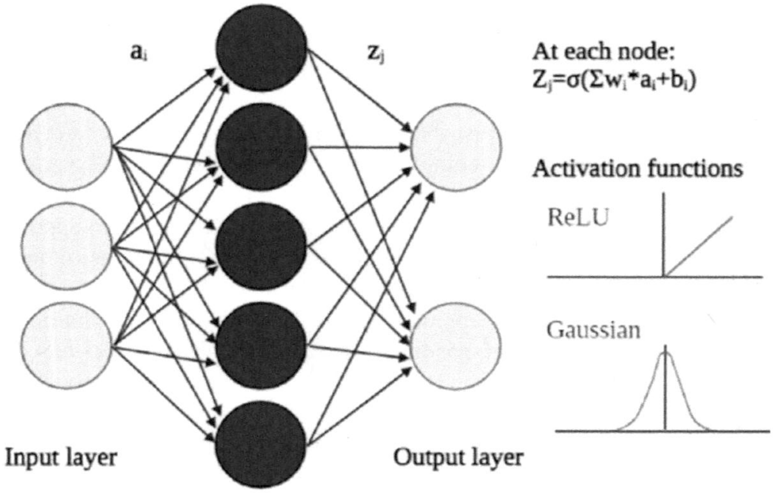

FIGURE 8.7 Activation functions of incoming signals in neurons.

nodes are modified before being cascaded to the neurons of the subsequent layer. Hidden layers are those layers that exist between the input and output layers. Weights and biases at the various nodes are changed during the training process of a neural network. In comparison to shallow architectures, deep neural networks include a substantially higher number of hidden layers and nodes (Srivastava et al., 2014). As a result, a lot of variables need to be fitted when the neural network is being trained. To solve the overfitting problem, it was therefore required to boost computing power and make a variety of algorithmic advancements, like dropout or the use of rectified linear units to solve the vanishing gradient problem (Nair & Hinton, 2010).

8.3.2 Natural Product Drug Discovery

AI in drug discovery is utilized in many areas, as shown in Figure 8.8. The primary use of natural products (NPs) is as favoured structures for interacting with protein pharmacological targets. Even if the pharmaceutical industry has mostly given up, scientists are still in awe of their distinctive qualities and structural variety for inspiring the creation of new medications. Artificial intelligence (AI) is becoming more widely used in various industries and fields of study because of high-performance computer hardware, ample storage, accessible software, and reasonably priced online education (Saldívar-González et al., 2022).

8.3.3 Synthetic Drugs

8.3.3.1 Antimalarial

Chemical property forecasting has been a field where artificial AI, using either structure-based or ligand-based techniques, has been shown to perform extremely well.

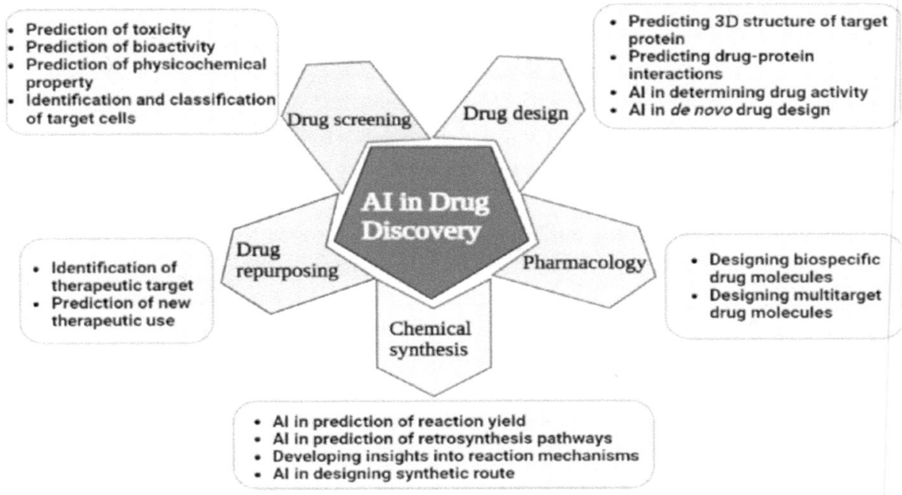

FIGURE 8.8 AI in drug discovery.

Due to extensive medication resistance, the number of available treatment options for malaria is becoming increasingly small. There is an ongoing need for new treatment options because resistance has been observed for all currently available malaria medications, including artemisinin (Keshavarzi Arshadi et al., 2020). Artemisinin-based combined treatment (ACT), the standard treatment for *Plasmodium falciparum* malaria without complications, is progressively losing their efficacy in several Southeast Asian nations (van der Pluijm et al., 2020). We have very limited treatment options in light of reports that the pharmacological combination therapy using dihydroartemisinin and piperaquine failed in Cambodia Laos (Hamilton et al., 2019). This dire circumstance highlights the essential need to create new antimalarial drugs that act on undiscovered targets. There are many lead compounds in preclinical development as a result of the recent increase in novel antimalarial discovery efforts (Ashley & Phyo, 2018). Due to the anticipated loss of new antimalarial medications because of the development of resistance, a learning model was created to predict the inhibition of compounds in *Plasmodium falciparum* using readily available data (van Heerden et al., 2021). Using data from earlier tests, a validation dataset was produced. To aid in hyper-parameter optimization, a comprehensive review has enhanced in this work. Transfer learning was used to create the deep learning model from a vast corpus of unrelated data. To uncover new pharmaceutical choices, the model was evaluated using a separate macrocyclic test dataset. Deep Malaria identified 72.32% of the active compounds in the validation dataset and 87.75% of those in the test dataset, demonstrating reasonable accuracy in an unbalanced situation. Deep learning automatic feature extraction outperforms the classical technique of fingerprint classification by uncovering chemical patterns that can be applied to novel and unstudied datasets. Deep Malaria's increasing accuracy in forecasting more strong chemicals was a vital aspect that made sure that no nanomolar active/non-cytotoxic molecule was overlooked. Additionally, the beneficial chemicals were condensed into a single, quick-acting medication that worked against *P. falciparum* at all stages of growth. As a result of its effect on the apicoplast, DC-9236 also showed suppression of *P. falciparum*'s second developmental cycle, delaying mortality. Compounds having delayed death characteristics may be ideal candidates for combination therapy (Kennedy et al., 2019). By utilizing Deep Malaria, eight medications have possible antimalarial properties. All scaffolds were predicted to be hits for *Plasmodium falciparum*, which are shown in Figure 8.9.

8.3.3.2 COVID-19

Repurposing or repositioning current drugs is one approach to addressing novel and challenging illnesses like COVID-19. Drug repurposing has emerged as a viable strategy due to the promise of shorter research timetables and cheaper total costs. Artificial intelligence (AI) and network medicine provide cutting-edge information science applications to define disease, medicine, therapeutics, and targets with the fewest errors feasible in the big data era. Using AI to accelerate pharmaceutical repositioning or repurposing is a task for which AI tools are not only tenacious but also critical. Using COVID-19 drug repurposing as an example, we examine the applicability of AI models to precision medicine. The rapid evolution, potency, and innovation of network medicine and AI technologies can accelerate the discovery of new treatments. The use of AI aids in the repurposing of drugs to treat human disease, especially during the COVID-19 pandemic (Zhou et al., 2020).

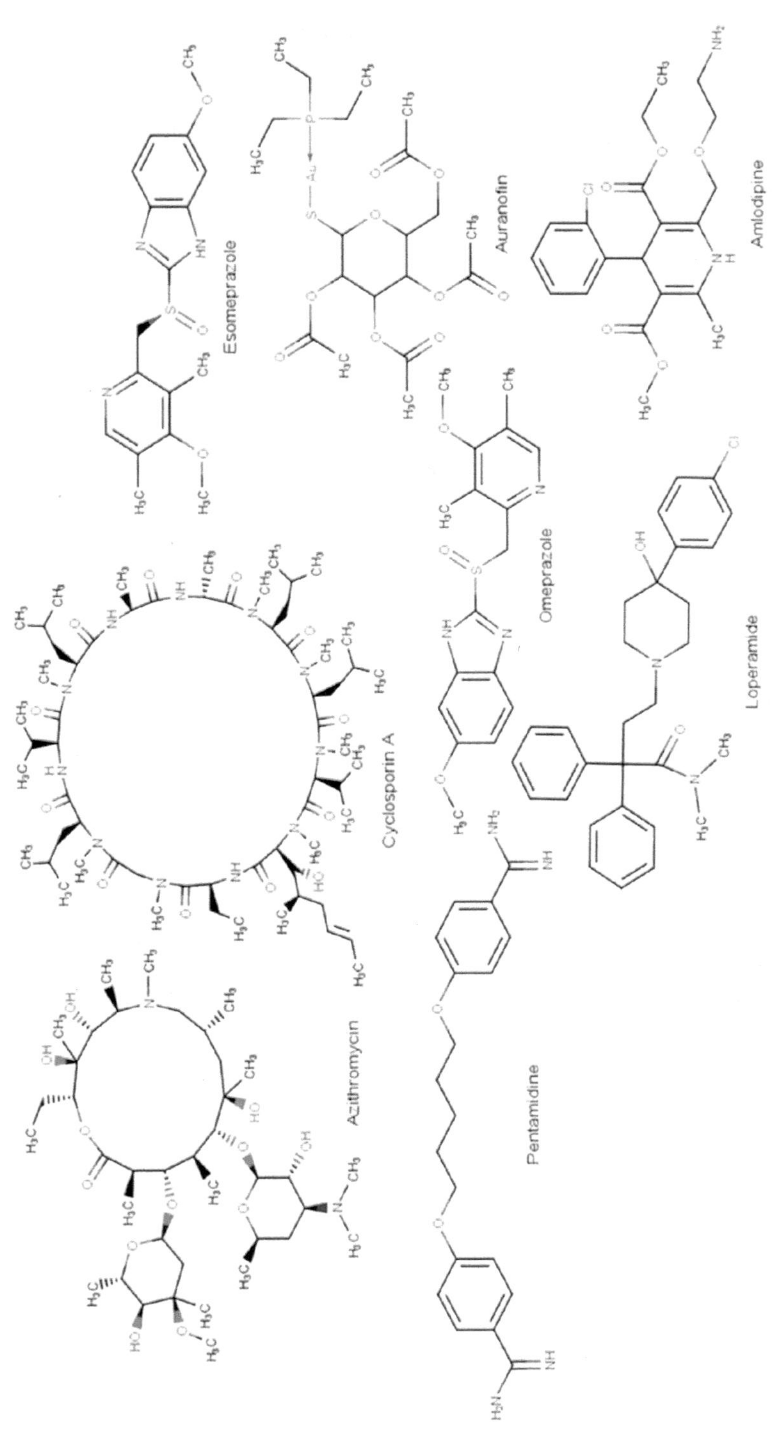

FIGURE 8.9 Eight medications have possible antimalarial properties. All scaffolds were predicted to be hits for *Plasmodium falciparum* by Deep Malaria.

8.3.4 Research on Repurposed Medications for COVID-19

Antiviral medicines and host-targeting treatments are just two examples of repurposed pharmaceuticals that are now being researched or have already been studied in clinical trials for COVID-19. In a study by Sanders and colleagues, repurposed medications for COVID-19 are covered in great depth. It was first thought that remdesivir, a monophosphate prodrug of an active C-adenosine nucleoside triphosphate analogue, would be used to treat the Ebola virus sickness (Sanders et al., 2020). The FDA granted emergency use clearance for remdesivir after it demonstrated potential in the treatment of COVID-19 (shown in Table 8.2), however, the indication is only for severe disease. The FDA reached this conclusion based on preliminary studies suggesting that the medication might hasten recovery for COVID-19 hospital patients. Remdesivir has been demonstrated to block the viral RNA-dependent RNA polymerase in terms of mechanism (Yin et al., 2020). Some of the tools utilized in COVID-19 outbreak are shown in Figure 8.10.

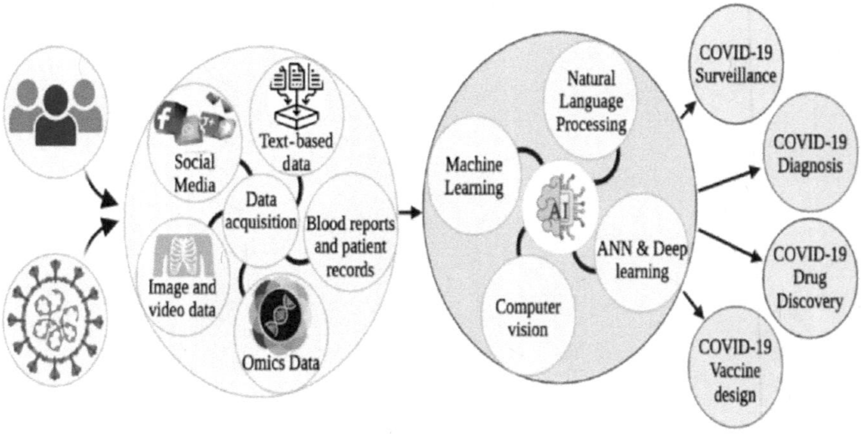

FIGURE 8.10 The COVID-19 pandemic and the involvement of AI tools. The picture shows how ML and other AI methods are applied to handpicked datasets from several perspectives to address the issues brought on by the COVID-19 outbreak.

TABLE 8.1
List of Organizations Using Artificial Intelligence to Create COVID-19 Treatments (Kaushik & Raj, 2020)

Strategy	Name of the Company	Status
Repurposing existing drugs	Benevolent AI	The UK-based company, which is renowned for its work in AI-based drug discovery, identified the six most likely candidates for baricitinib-containing compounds. Because of this company's intriguing findings, Eli Lilly has already contacted them and has begun the clinical validation procedure.

TABLE 8.1 (*Continued*)
List of Organizations Using Artificial Intelligence to Create COVID-19 Treatments (Kaushik & Raj, 2020)

Strategy	Name of the Company	Status
Repurposing existing drugs	Innoplexus	Three combination therapies against COVID-19 were successfully proposed by an Indo-German business, and these combinations are currently going through in vitro and in vivo validation processes: (a) Using tocilizumab and chloroquine together; (b) using remdesivir and chloroquine together; (c) combining hydroxychloroquine with plerixafor or clarithromycin.
Repurposing existing drugs	Deargen	Atazanavir is an antiviral medication with a high level of potency that was developed by a Korean company in partnership with Dankook University. However, it is still undergoing clinical studies.
Repurposing existing drugs	Gero	Using its AI platform, this Singaporean startup has discovered nine medications. The most powerful of these are niclosamide and nitazoxanide.
Repurposing existing drugs	Cyclica	The Canadian business is presently analyzing 6700 chemicals using their AI-based medication repurposing platform MatchMaker, which includes FDA-approved pharmaceuticals and compounds in phase I human trials.
Repurposing existing drugs	Healx	A UK-based company is also working to develop a combination-based therapy using already-approved medications to combat this infection.
Repurposing existing drugs	VantAI	A New York-based company is currently moving toward a systems or network biology approach to investigate how viral and human proteins interact as the infection progresses.
Designing new drugs	Insilico Medicine	The seven potential COVID-19 inhibitors were developed by a Hong Kong-based company, and two of them have already been produced for testing.
Designing new drugs	Exscientia	A UK-based company, in collaboration with the UK's synchrotron facility, Diamond Light Source, screened 15,000 clinically validated compounds from the Scripps Research Institute in California, US, and is also working to understand the mechanism of the SARS-CoV-2 virus's operation through data modelling and artificial intelligence.
Designing new drugs	Iktos and SRI International	Iktos, a French AI-based company, designs new, powerful chemicals. Iktos has partnered with SRI Biosciences, a US-based company, to use its completely automated synthetic chemistry system to synthesize and evaluate new compounds.

8.4 ARTIFICIAL INTELLIGENCE FOR PREDICTION IN DESIGNING AND TARGETING

8.4.1 Physicochemical Property Forecasting

To build the computer-assisted drug discovery program, ML (machine learning) makes use of substantial data sets produced during prior chemical optimization (Yang et al., 2019). Drug design methods use molecule descriptors, like electron density around the molecule, SMILES in the String database, coordinates of atoms in 3D, and potential energy readings, which allows researchers to create structures of compounds using DNN and then predict their properties (Hessler & Baringhaus, 2018b). The lipophilicity and solubility of several components can be predicted at a time using the ADMET predictor and ALGOPS software (Paul et al., 2021). To forecast a substance's acid dissociation constant, kernel ridge-based models, ANN-based models, and graph kernels were created (Chopra et al., 2022).

8.4.2 Analysis of Bioactivity

Web applications like ChemMapper and the similarity ensemble technique (SEA) (Huang et al., 2018) are useful for predicting drug–target interactions. To determine DTBA, a variety of methods integrating ML and DL have been employed, such as SimBoost, PADME, KronRLS, and DeepDTA. Drug target binding affinity (DTBA) is evaluated using ML-based approaches such as Kronecker-regularized least squares (KronRLS), which evaluates the similarity of drug and protein molecules. DTBA was predicted using regression trees, similar to SimBoost, which considers feature-based and similarity-based interactions. Extended connectivity fingerprints, ligand maximal common substructures (LMCS), SMILES drug characteristics, or a mix of these may also be considered (Öztürk et al., 2018).

8.4.3 Predicting the Structure of the Target Protein

To treat patients effectively, choosing the appropriate target during therapeutic molecule development is essential. The progression of the disease is influenced by several overexpressed proteins. As a result, forecasting the structure of the target protein when creating the therapeutic chemical to particularly target disease is critical. AI can aid in structure-based drug development by anticipating the 3D protein structure since the design is in tune with the chemical environment of the target protein region. This makes it easier to predict how a molecule will behave on the target while also considering safety before it is synthesized or made (Wan & Zeng, 2016). The 3D target protein structure can be predicted using the AI tool Alpha Fold, which is based on DNNs, by analyzing the separations between neighbouring amino acids and the corresponding angles of the peptide bonds.

8.4.4 Drug–Protein Interaction Forecasting

Drug–protein interactions are crucial for getting the effectiveness of the desired components. Understanding the efficacy of the component and its effectiveness and predicting how it will interact with a receptor or protein enables drug repurposing and avoids polypharmacology.

8.5 DATABASE AND COMPUTATIONAL TOOLS

Large chemical libraries are screened for potential hits, these hits are converted into leads, and these leads are improved through the optimization of lead molecules for further investigation in the preclinical study and through clinical trials. The process of creating a new medicine, from its inception to its introduction to the market, can take up to 15 to 20 years, and estimated expenses would be more than $1 billion. In the never-ending search for life-saving medications, computational techniques (Table 8.2) have proven indispensable at various phases of drug discovery. The work of evaluating the generated big data has unavoidably become extremely challenging and advancements in the synthesis of massive chemical libraries have. Public databases like Binding DB, PubChem, and ChEMBL provide information about the protein targets and their characters in binding data with another protein or bioactive constituents (Valdés-Jiménez et al., 2021).

In comparison with experimental screening, virtual screening is proven to have a crucial role in the drug development process. Structure-based and ligand-based virtual screenings are the two subcategories of virtual screening. The primary premise of ligand-based virtual screening, which employs ligands for virtual screening, is that compounds with similar chemical structures frequently have related biological roles (Floresta et al., 2018). Fundamentally, the chemical fingerprints of ligands can be used to identify them. For instance, using the Tanimoto coefficient or other distance-based methods, one might extrapolate from the fingerprints of known active compounds to look for new molecules with similar features. Quantitative structure–activity relationship (QSAR) is a ligand-based virtual screening tool which also predicts the bioactivity data by ligand (Nantasenamat et al., 2010; Nantasenamat et al., 2015; Chen et al., 2012). This method involves quantifying the ligands using molecular descriptors like autocorrelations, constitution, and topology, which are then correlated with the corresponding bioactivity using machine-learning techniques. One notable application of QSAR in drug development is the prediction of ADMET features (Li et al., 2014), drug-likeness profiles (Bitew et al., 2021) (Ejeh et al., 2021), and the inhibition of target proteins (Halder & Cordeiro, 2021), cancer cells (Pingaew et al., 2013), and other pathogens (Worachartcheewan et al., 2013).

Incompatibility difficulties may have precluded the broad use of computational tools in the past when they were restricted to a few distinct operating systems. In recent years, tools have moved from desktop-based to cloud-based apps, becoming more and more platform-independent. Reproducible research is a difficulty in the life sciences that affects drug discovery as well.

For instance, Galaxy (Giardine et al., 2005) is a programming language web platform that offers interactive genomic analysis. Furthermore, by integrating all of the cheminformatics toolkits into a single CSB (Mendenhall et al., 2020), Cinfony (Cereto-Massagué et al., 2015) and Biskit (Grünberg et al., 2007), which are in the Python module, promote a platform for toolkits. Python modules are combined with many computational structural biology and structural bioinformatics methods into a single base. A widely used Python framework called BioServices allows programmatic access to the data retrieved from biological databases (such as UniProt, BioModels, KEGG, and ChEMBL) (Sahni et al., 2020). QSAR-ML (Nantasenamat, 2020) embeds the information of structures of desired components and their descriptors with detailed information on the implementations of the software, detailed QSAR datasets, and the values in the format of XML-based file. A revolutionary framework called Chem-Bio-RDF (David et al., 2020) implements interoperability by using semantic web technologies to combine data from various sources and public databases (Table 8.3).

TABLE 8.2
Computational Tools in the Drug Discovery Process

SL No	Computational Tools	Description	References
1.	Swiss target prediction	An online tool for predicting the bioactive small molecule targets in people and other animals. This is useful to forecast off-target effects of known chemicals or to rationalize probable side effects, as well as to explain the molecular processes that result in a certain phenotypic or bioactivity.	www.swisstargetprediction.ch/
2.	ProteomicsDB	A resource for life science research with a wide range of organisms and omics. It includes information on the proteomics, transcriptomics, and phenomics of species including humans, mice, rice, Arabidopsis, and so on. There are several visualization options that, for instance, enable protein- and drug-centric inquiries.	www.proteomicsdb.org/
3.	KEGG (Kyoto Encyclopedia of Genes and Genomes)	A group of databases covering genomes, biological pathways, illnesses, medications, and chemicals, which is considered a knowledge repository that connects genomic data with higher-order functional data for the systematic analysis of gene functions.	www.genome.jp/kegg/
4.	DIAMOnD (DIseAse MOdule Detection)	This provides details about the disease. The fact that related proteins frequently interact with one another has sparked the growth of network-based methods to clarify the molecular causes of human disease. These strategies are predicated on the idea that protein interaction networks can be considered maps where diseases can be located with a localized perturbation in a specific area.	(Ghiassian et al., 2015)
5.	PASS (Prediction of Activity Spectra for Substances)	This can be used to identify new biological targets for particular ligands and, in the opposite direction, to reveal new ones for those targets. PASS uses a substance's structural formula to anticipate more than 300 pharmacological effects and metabolic pathways.	www.way2drug.com/

TABLE 8.3
Databases in the Drug Discovery Process

SL No	Computational Tools	Description	References
1.	DisGeNET	This explains the traits of disease genes, how to create hypotheses about the therapeutic effects and side effects of medications, how to validate disease genes that have been predicted computationally, and how to look into the molecular causes of human diseases and associated comorbidities.	www.disgenet.org/
2.	Disease-Connect	A web server offering full knowledge on mechanism-based connection analysis and visualization among diseases.	https://disease-connect.org/
3.	DrugBank	A resource with extensive annotations that integrates knowledge of pharmaceuticals, drug effects, and drug targets.	www.drugbank.com/
4.	AYUSH Research Portal	Publicizing information on AYUSH systems and recent research updates solely for academic purposes to foster a scientific mindset and improve the calibre of research, teaching, and training in the AYUSH field.	https://ayushportal.nic.in/
5.	Dr. Duke's Phytochemical and Ethnobotanical Database	Enables thorough searches for plants, chemicals, bioactivity, and ethnobotany using scientific or common names. We can download search results as spreadsheets or PDFs. Pharmaceutical, nutritional, and biological research, as well as complementary treatments and herbal items, are all of interest.	https://phytochem.nal.usda.gov/ phytochrome/search
6.	PubChem	Molecular Libraries Roadmap Initiatives of the US National Institutes of Health launched a public repository for data on chemical compounds and their biological effects in 2004.	https://pubchem.ncbi.nlm.nih.gov/
7.	Gene Ontology	This knowledge base is the most comprehensive source of knowledge about the purposes of genes. This information, which can be read by both machines and humans, can be utilized to computationally analyze extensive genetics and molecular biology studies in biomedical research.	http://geneontology.org/
8.	DAVID (The Database for Annotation, Visualization, and Integrated Discovery)	A biological knowledgebase and analytical tool that work together to decipher the biological significance of enormous gene/protein lists produced by various high-throughput genomic research.	https://david.ncifcrf.gov/
9.	SIGNOR (SIGnaling Network Open Resource) 2.0 database	A public database that holds biological entity-to-entity binary causal linkages for signalling information. A signed directed graph is used to visually portray the information that has been collected. Each signalling relationship has an impact (the target entity's up- or down-regulation) and a method (for example, binding, phosphorylation, transcriptional activation, etc.) producing the up- or down-regulation.	https://signor.uniroma2.it/

8.6 FUTURE PROSPECTS AND LIMITATIONS

There is evidence that AI applications are beginning to become ubiquitous in the development of pharmaceuticals. These strategies are slowly exceeding some of the expectations of the community. More clarity should come on these methods and will be effective in assisting the creation and synthesis of "better medication candidates" by researchers (P. Schneider et al., 2020). Methods depending on more "raw" chemical representations (such as graphs for ligand-based property prediction neural networks and recurrent neural networks built on SMILES) can be expected to perform at least average models based on descriptors.

Additionally, deep learning techniques apply to a larger class of chemical substances and more effective use of data for modelling tasks, as in the case of multitasking and online education. However, conformation-aware deep learning, particularly when considering techniques that incorporate 3D symmetries into their basic design, is still in its early stages. Rapid evolution was expected for its use in the discovery of drugs and similar fields like quantum physics and material science, especially as a stand-in for computationally more taxing first principle calculations.

Over the past few years, rule-based and rule-free approaches to de novo drug design have quietly increased in popularity. The latter have constraints, such as a limited ability to be synthesized, but they show promise in exploring hitherto unexplored chemical space. Combining rule-free and rule-based methodologies (sometimes known as "hybrid") may offer a workable solution. Paying close attention will move toward generative methods that can be sources of data for early studies on gene expression (Humbeck et al., 2018), conformational space (Button et al., 2019), and knowledge of ligand binding sites (Miyao et al., 2016).

To forecast reactions and design automated synthesis, the processing of natural language advances will proceed to motivate and encourage innovation. Topics including yield estimation, side-product generation, and other frequently under-researched areas will receive much-needed attention and the forecasting of favourable reaction circumstances.

In the upcoming years, synthesis will be automated. The growing popularity of explainable AI (Jiménez-Luna et al., 2020) using techniques like feature attribution (Riniker & Landrum, 2013) and instance-based uncertainty, a molecular counterfactual explanation (Numeroso & Bacciu, 2020) based on estimates (A. Nguyen et al., 2015), will broaden the appeal of AI-supported drug development.

The creation and approval of these techniques will necessitate additional multidisciplinary research. A relevant focus will also be placed on methods that can take advantage of data in low-data regimes, such as transfer learning multitasking (C. Q. Nguyen et al., 2020), and meta-learning. For interested practitioners, the obstacles to learning and subsequently implementing deep learning approaches have significantly decreased in recent years. As broad high-level research, the formation of software packages (Paszke et al., 2019), and understandable documentation continue to emerge, the present trend indicates that these methodologies will become more widely available shortly.

However, there are still some difficulties. AI has shown tremendous promise in drug discovery. AI must overcome several obstacles, including a dearth of data, a lack of interoperability, and the curse of dimensionality. Every industry using AI must deal with the issue of data scarcity. Five samples are required for biological research to be considered valid. The majority of machine-learning algorithms, however, need to be taught on tens of thousands of data points or samples to be effective. Lack of interpretability is another problem. It can be challenging to describe how a model works and why it makes certain predictions. With deep learning, the likelihood of this happening increases because each layer makes the model more complicated. As the number of layers rises, the explanation of each layer's outputs can get increasingly more complicated.

REFERENCES

Agrebi, S., & Larbi, A. (2020). Use of artificial intelligence in infectious diseases. In *Artificial intelligence in precision health* (pp. 415–438). Elsevier.

Aminian, A., Safari, S., Razeghian-Jahromi, A., Ghorbani, M., & Delaney, C. P. (2020). COVID-19 outbreak and surgical practice: Unexpected fatality in perioperative period. *Annals of Surgery, 272*(1), e27–e29. https://doi.org/10.1097/SLA.0000000000000392

Ashley, E. A., & Phyo, A. P. (2018). Drugs in development for malaria. *Drugs*, *78*(9), 861–879.

Biswas, N., Mustapha, T., Khubchandani, J., & Price, J. H. (2021). The nature and extent of COVID-19 vaccination hesitancy in healthcare workers. *Journal of Community Health*, *46*(6), 1244–1251. https://doi.org/10.1007/s10900-021-00984-3

Bitew, M., Desalegn, T., Demissie, T. B., Belayneh, A., Endale, M., & Eswaramoorthy, R. (2021). Pharmacokinetics and drug-likeness of antidiabetic flavonoids: Molecular docking and DFT study. *PLoS ONE*, *16*(12), e0260853.

Bitterman, D. S., Miller, T. A., Mak, R. H., & Savova, G. K. (2021). Clinical natural language processing for radiation oncology: A review and practical primer. *International Journal of Radiation Oncology* Biology* Physics*, *110*(3), 641–655.

Boon, I. S., Au Yong, T. P., & Boon, C. S. (2018). Assessing the role of artificial intelligence (AI) in clinical oncology: Utility of machine learning in radiotherapy target volume delineation. *Medicines*, *5*(4), 131.

Button, A., Merk, D., Hiss, J. A., & Schneider, G. (2019). Automated de novo molecular design by hybrid machine intelligence and rule-driven chemical synthesis. *Nature Machine Intelligence*, *1*(7), 307–315.

Capobianco, E. (2022). High-dimensional role of AI and machine learning in cancer research. *British Journal of Cancer*, *126*(4), 523–532.

Cereto-Massagué, A., Ojeda, M. J., Valls, C., Mulero, M., Garcia-Vallvé, S., & Pujadas, G. (2015). Molecular fingerprint similarity search in virtual screening. *Methods*, *71*, 58–63.

Chen, J. H., & Asch, S. M. (2017). Machine learning and prediction in medicine—Beyond the peak of inflated expectations. *The New England Journal of Medicine*, *376*(26), 2507.

Chen, L., Li, Y., Yu, H., Zhang, L., & Hou, T. (2012). Computational models for predicting substrates or inhibitors of P-glycoprotein. *Drug Discovery Today*, *17*(7), 343–351. https://doi.org/10.1016/j.drudis.2011.11.003

Chen, S., Yang, J., Yang, W., Wang, C., & Bärnighausen, T. (2020). COVID-19 control in China during mass population movements at New Year. *The Lancet*, *395*(10226), 764–766.

Chopra, H., Baig, A. A., Gautam, R. K., & Kamal, M. A. (2022). Application of artificial intelligence in drug discovery. *Current Pharmaceutical Design*, *28*(33), 2690–2703.

David, L., Thakkar, A., Mercado, R., & Engkvist, O. (2020). Molecular representations in AI-driven drug discovery: A review and practical guide. *Journal of Cheminformatics*, *12*(1), 1–22.

Dlamini, Z., Francies, F. Z., Hull, R., & Marima, R. (2020). Artificial intelligence (AI) and big data in cancer and precision oncology. *Computational and Structural Biotechnology Journal*, *18*, 2300–2311.

Ejeh, S., Uzairu, A., Shallangwa, G. A., & Abechi, S. E. (2021). Computational insight to design new potential hepatitis C virus NS5B polymerase inhibitors with drug-likeness and pharmacokinetic ADMET parameters predictions. *Future Journal of Pharmaceutical Sciences*, *7*, 1–13.

Floresta, G., Amata, E., Barbaraci, C., Gentile, D., Turnaturi, R., Marrazzo, A., & Rescifina, A. (2018). A structure-and ligand-based virtual screening of a database of "Small" marine natural products for the identification of "Blue" Sigma-2 receptor ligands. *Marine Drugs*, *16*(10), 384.

Ghasemi, F., Mehridehnavi, A., Pérez-Garrido, A., & Pérez-Sánchez, H. (2018). Neural network and deep-learning algorithms used in QSAR studies: Merits and drawbacks. *Drug Discovery Today*, *23*(10), 1784–1790.

Ghiassian, S. D., Menche, J., & Barabási, A.-L. (2015). A DIseAse MOdule Detection (DIAMOnD) algorithm derived from a systematic analysis of connectivity patterns of disease proteins in the human interactome. *PLoS Computational Biology*, *11*(4), e1004120. https://doi.org/10.1371/journal.pcbi.1004120

Giardine, B., Riemer, C., Hardison, R. C., Burhans, R., Elnitski, L., Shah, P., Zhang, Y., Blankenberg, D., Albert, I., Taylor, J., Miller, W., Kent, W. J., & Nekrutenko, A. (2005). Galaxy: A platform for interactive large-scale genome analysis. *Genome Research*, *15*(10), 1451–1455. https://doi.org/10.1101/gr.4086505

Gozes, O., Frid-Adar, M., Greenspan, H., Browning, P. D., Zhang, H., Ji, W., Bernheim, A., & Siegel, E. (2020). Rapid AI development cycle for the coronavirus (Covid-19) pandemic: Initial results for automated detection & patient monitoring using deep learning CT image analysis. *ArXiv Preprint ArXiv:2003.05037.*

Grünberg, R., Nilges, M., & Leckner, J. (2007). Biskit—A software platform for structural bioinformatics. *Bioinformatics (Oxford, England)*, *23*(6), 769–770. https://doi.org/10.1093/bioinformatics/btl655

Gupta, R., Ghosh, A., Singh, A. K., & Misra, A. (2020). Clinical considerations for patients with diabetes in times of COVID-19 epidemic. *Diabetes & Metabolic Syndrome*, *14*(3), 211.

Gupta, R., & Misra, A. (2020). Contentious issues and evolving concepts in the clinical presentation and management of patients with COVID-19 infectionwith reference to use of therapeutic and other drugs used in Co-morbid diseases (Hypertension, diabetes etc). *Diabetes & Metabolic Syndrome: Clinical Research & Reviews*, *14*(3), 251–254.

Halder, A. K., & Cordeiro, M. N. D. (2021). Multi-target in silico prediction of inhibitors for mitogen-activated protein kinase-interacting kinases. *Biomolecules*, *11*(11), 1670.

Haleem, A., Javaid, M., & Vaishya, R. (2020). Effects of COVID-19 pandemic in daily life. *Current Medicine Research and Practice*, *10*(2), 78.

Haleem, A., Vaishya, R., Javaid, M., & Khan, I. H. (2020). Artificial Intelligence (AI) applications in orthopaedics: An innovative technology to embrace. *Journal of Clinical Orthopaedics and Trauma*, *11*(Suppl 1), S80.

Hamilton, W. L., Amato, R., van der Pluijm, R. W., Jacob, C. G., Quang, H. H., Thuy-Nhien, N. T., Hien, T. T., Hongvanthong, B., Chindavongsa, K., & Mayxay, M. (2019). Evolution and expansion of multidrug-resistant malaria in southeast Asia: A genomic epidemiology study. *The Lancet Infectious Diseases*, *19*(9), 943–951.

Hessler, G., & Baringhaus, K.-H. (2018a). Artificial intelligence in drug design. *Molecules, 23*(10), 2520.

Hessler, G., & Baringhaus, K.-H. (2018b). Artificial intelligence in drug design. *Molecules, 23*(10), Article 10. https://doi.org/10.3390/molecules23102520

Huang, H., Zhang, G., Zhou, Y., Lin, C., Chen, S., Lin, Y., Mai, S., & Huang, Z. (2018). Reverse screening methods to search for the protein targets of chemopreventive compounds. *Frontiers in Chemistry, 138.*

Humbeck, L., Weigang, S., Schäfer, T., Mutzel, P., & Koch, O. (2018). CHIPMUNK: A virtual synthesizable small-molecule library for medicinal chemistry, exploitable for protein–protein interaction modulators. *ChemMedChem, 13*(6), 532–539.

Im, H., Pathania, D., McFarland, P. J., Sohani, A. R., Degani, I., Allen, M., Coble, B., Kilcoyne, A., Hong, S., & Rohrer, L. (2018). Design and clinical validation of a point-of-care device for the diagnosis of lymphoma via contrast-enhanced microholography and machine learning. *Nature Biomedical Engineering, 2*(9), 666–674.

Jiménez-Luna, J., Grisoni, F., & Schneider, G. (2020). Drug discovery with explainable artificial intelligence. *Nature Machine Intelligence, 2*(10), 573–584.

Kaushik, A. C., & Raj, U. (2020). AI-driven drug discovery: A boon against COVID-19? *AI Open, 1*, 1–4.

Keiser, M. J., Roth, B. L., Armbruster, B. N., Ernsberger, P., Irwin, J. J., & Shoichet, B. K. (2007). Relating protein pharmacology by ligand chemistry. *Nature Biotechnology, 25*(2), 197–206.

Kennedy, K., Cobbold, S. A., Hanssen, E., Birnbaum, J., Spillman, N. J., McHugh, E., Brown, H., Tilley, L., Spielmann, T., & McConville, M. J. (2019). Delayed death in the malaria parasite Plasmodium falciparum is caused by disruption of prenylation-dependent intracellular trafficking. *PLoS Biology, 17*(7), e3000376.

Keshavarzi Arshadi, A., Salem, M., Collins, J., Yuan, J. S., & Chakrabarti, D. (2020). DeepMalaria: Artificial intelligence driven discovery of potent antiplasmodials. *Frontiers in Pharmacology, 10*, 1526.

Krittanawong, C. (2018). The rise of artificial intelligence and the uncertain future for physicians. *European Journal of Internal Medicine, 48*, e13–e14.

Li, D., Chen, L., Li, Y., Tian, S., Sun, H., & Hou, T. (2014). ADMET evaluation in drug discovery. 13. Development of in silico prediction models for P-glycoprotein substrates. *Molecular Pharmaceutics, 11*(3), 716–726. https://doi.org/10.1021/mp400450m

Li, J., Huang, J., Zheng, L., & Li, X. (2020). Application of artificial intelligence in diabetes education and management: Present status and promising prospect. *Frontiers in Public Health, 8*, 173.

Luo, H., Tang, Q., Shang, Y., Liang, S., Yang, M., Robinson, N., & Liu, J. (2020). Can Chinese medicine be used for prevention of corona virus disease 2019 (COVID-19)? A review of historical classics, research evidence and current prevention programs. *Chinese Journal of Integrative Medicine, 26*(4), 243–250.

Mak, K.-K., & Pichika, M. R. (2019). Artificial intelligence in drug development: Present status and future prospects. *Drug Discovery Today, 24*(3), 773–780.

Marlow, M. P., & McLain, B. (2011). Assessing the impacts of experiential learning on teacher classroom practice. *Research in Higher Education Journal, 14.*

Mendenhall, J., Brown, B. P., Kothiwale, S., & Meiler, J. (2020). BCL: Conf: Improved open-source knowledge-based conformation sampling using the crystallography open database. *Journal of Chemical Information and Modeling, 61*(1), 189–201.

Merget, B., Turk, S., Eid, S., Rippmann, F., & Fulle, S. (2017). Profiling prediction of kinase inhibitors: Toward the virtual assay. *Journal of Medicinal Chemistry, 60*(1), 474–485.

Miyao, T., Kaneko, H., & Funatsu, K. (2016). Inverse QSPR/QSAR analysis for chemical structure generation (from y to x). *Journal of Chemical Information and Modeling*, *56*(2), 286–299.

Nair, V., & Hinton, G. E. (2010). Rectified linear units improve restricted boltzmann machines. Proceedings of the 27th International Conference on Machine Learning, Haifa, 21 June 2010, 807–814.

Nantasenamat, C. (2020). Best practices for constructing reproducible QSAR models. *Ecotoxicological QSARs*, 55–75.

Nantasenamat, C., Isarankura-Na-Ayudhya, C., & Prachayasittikul, V. (2010). Advances in computational methods to predict the biological activity of compounds. *Expert Opinion on Drug Discovery*, *5*(7), 633–654. https://doi.org/10.1517/17460441.2010.492827

Nantasenamat, C., Worachartcheewan, A., Jamsak, S., Preeyanon, L., Shoombuatong, W., Simeon, S., Mandi, P., Isarankura-Na-Ayudhya, C., & Prachayasittikul, V. (2015). AutoWeka: Toward an automated data mining software for QSAR and QSPR studies. *Methods in Molecular Biology (Clifton, N.J.)*, *1260*, 119–147. https://doi.org/10.1007/978-1-4939-2239-0_8

Nguyen, A., Yosinski, J., & Clune, J. (2015). Deep neural networks are easily fooled: High confidence predictions for unrecognizable images. 2015 IEEE Conference on Computer Vision and Pattern Recognition (CVPR), 427–436. https://doi.org/10.1109/CVPR.2015.7298640

Nguyen, C. Q., Kreatsoulas, C., & Branson, K. M. (2020). Meta-learning gnn initializations for low-resource molecular property prediction. *ArXiv Preprint ArXiv:2003.05996.*

Nimri, R., Bratina, N., Kordonouri, O., Avbelj Stefanija, M., Fath, M., Biester, T., Muller, I., Atlas, E., Miller, S., & Fogel, A. (2017). MD-Logic overnight type 1 diabetes control in home settings: A multicentre, multinational, single blind randomized trial. *Diabetes, Obesity and Metabolism*, *19*(4), 553–561.

Noble, J. A., & Valdes, A. M. (2011). Genetics of the HLA region in the prediction of type 1 diabetes. *Current Diabetes Reports*, *11*(6), 533–542. https://doi.org/10.1007/s11892-011-0223-x

Numeroso, D., & Bacciu, D. (2020). Explaining deep graph networks with molecular counterfactuals. *ArXiv Preprint ArXiv:2011.05134.*

Öztürk, H., Özgür, A., & Ozkirimli, E. (2018). DeepDTA: Deep drug–target binding affinity prediction. *Bioinformatics*, *34*(17), i821–i829. https://doi.org/10.1093/bioinformatics/bty593

Paszke, A., Gross, S., Massa, F., Lerer, A., Bradbury, J., Chanan, G., Killeen, T., Lin, Z., Gimelshein, N., & Antiga, L. (2019). Pytorch: An imperative style, high-performance deep learning library. *Advances in Neural Information Processing Systems*, *32*.

Paul, D., Sanap, G., Shenoy, S., Kalyane, D., Kalia, K., & Tekade, R. K. (2021). Artificial intelligence in drug discovery and development. *Drug Discovery Today*, *26*(1), 80.

Pingaew, R., Worachartcheewan, A., Nantasenamat, C., Prachayasittikul, S., Ruchirawat, S., & Prachayasittikul, V. (2013). Synthesis, cytotoxicity and QSAR study of N-tosyl-1,2,3,4-tetrahydroisoquinoline derivatives. *Archives of Pharmacal Research*, *36*(9), 1066–1077. https://doi.org/10.1007/s12272-013-0111-9

Pushpakom, S., Iorio, F., Eyers, P. A., Escott, K. J., Hopper, S., Wells, A., Doig, A., Guilliams, T., Latimer, J., & McNamee, C. (2019). Drug repurposing: Progress, challenges and recommendations. *Nature Reviews Drug Discovery*, *18*(1), 41–58.

Quinn, C. C., Shardell, M. D., Terrin, M. L., Barr, E. A., Ballew, S. H., & Gruber-Baldini, A. L. (2011). Cluster-randomized trial of a mobile phone personalized behavioral intervention for blood glucose control. *Diabetes Care*, *34*(9), 1934–1942.

Riniker, S., & Landrum, G. A. (2013). Similarity maps-a visualization strategy for molecular fingerprints and machine-learning methods. *Journal of Cheminformatics*, *5*(1), 1–7.

Sahni, S., Khanna, A., & Rodrigues, J. J. (2020). Analysis of biological information using statistical techniques in cloud computing. In *Applications of cloud computing* (pp. 1–24). Chapman and Hall/CRC.

Saldívar-González, F. I., Aldas-Bulos, V. D., Medina-Franco, J. L., & Plisson, F. (2022). Natural product drug discovery in the artificial intelligence era. *Chemical Science, 13*(6), 1526–1546.

Sanders, J. M., Monogue, M. L., Jodlowski, T. Z., & Cutrell, J. B. (2020). Pharmacologic treatments for coronavirus disease 2019 (COVID-19): A review. *Jama, 323*(18), 1824–1836.

Schneider, G. (2019). Mind and machine in drug design. *Nature Machine Intelligence, 1*(3), 128–130.

Schneider, P., Walters, W. P., Plowright, A. T., Sieroka, N., Listgarten, J., Goodnow, R. A., Fisher, J., Jansen, J. M., Duca, J. S., & Rush, T. S. (2020). Rethinking drug design in the artificial intelligence era. *Nature Reviews Drug Discovery, 19*(5), 353–364.

Sharma, A., & Rani, R. (2021). A systematic review of applications of machine learning in cancer prediction and diagnosis. *Archives of Computational Methods in Engineering, 28*(7), 4875–4896.

Silver, D., Schrittwieser, J., Simonyan, K., Antonoglou, I., Huang, A., Guez, A., Hubert, T., Baker, L., Lai, M., & Bolton, A. (2017). Mastering the game of go without human knowledge. *Nature, 550*(7676), 354–359.

Sohrabi, C., Alsafi, Z., O'Neill, N., Khan, M., Kerwan, A., Al-Jabir, A., Iosifidis, C., & Agha, R. (2020). World Health Organization declares global emergency: A review of the 2019 novel coronavirus (COVID-19). *International Journal of Surgery, 76*, 71–76.

Srivastava, N., Hinton, G., Krizhevsky, A., Sutskever, I., & Salakhutdinov, R. (2014). Dropout: A simple way to prevent neural networks from overfitting. *The Journal of Machine Learning Research, 15*(1), 1929–1958.

Teles, G., Rodrigues, J. J., Rabêlo, R. A., & Kozlov, S. A. (2021). Comparative study of support vector machines and random forests machine learning algorithms on credit operation. *Software: Practice and Experience, 51*(12), 2492–2500.

Valdés-Jiménez, A., Peña-Varas, C., Borrego-Muñoz, P., Arrue, L., Alegría-Arcos, M., Nour-Eldin, H., Dreyer, I., Nuñez-Vivanco, G., & Ramírez, D. (2021). Psc-db: A structured and searchable 3d-database for plant secondary compounds. *Molecules, 26*(4), 1124.

Vamathevan, J., Clark, D., Czodrowski, P., Dunham, I., Ferran, E., Lee, G., Li, B., Madabhushi, A., Shah, P., Spitzer, M., & Zhao, S. (2019). Applications of machine learning in drug discovery and development. *Nature Reviews Drug Discovery, 18*(6), Article 6. https://doi.org/10.1038/s41573-019-0024-5

van der Pluijm, R. W., Tripura, R., Hoglund, R. M., Phyo, A. P., Lek, D., Ul Islam, A., Anvikar, A. R., Satpathi, P., Satpathi, S., & Behera, P. K. (2020). Triple artemisinin-based combination therapies versus artemisinin-based combination therapies for uncomplicated Plasmodium falciparum malaria: A multicentre, open-label, randomised clinical trial. *The Lancet, 395*(10233), 1345–1360.

van Heerden, A., van Wyk, R., & Birkholtz, L. M. (2021). Machine learning uses chemo-transcriptomic profiles to stratify antimalarial compounds with similar mode of action. *Frontiers in Cellular and Infection Microbiology, 11*, 688256. https://doi.org/10.3389/fcimb.2021.688256

Varnek, A., & Baskin, I. (2012). Machine learning methods for property prediction in chemoinformatics: Quo Vadis? *Journal of Chemical Information and Modeling, 52*(6), 1413–1437.

Walsh, J., Roberts, R., Weber, D., Faber-Heinemann, G., & Heinemann, L. (2015). Insulin pump and CGM usage in the United States and Germany: Results of a real-world survey with 985 subjects. *Journal of Diabetes Science and Technology, 9*(5), 1103–1110.

Walters, W. P., & Barzilay, R. (2020). Applications of deep learning in molecule generation and molecular property prediction. *Accounts of Chemical Research*, *54*(2), 263–270.

Wan, F., & Zeng, J. (Michael). (2016). Deep learning with feature embedding for compound-protein interaction prediction. *bioRxiv*, 086033. https://doi.org/10.1101/086033

Worachartcheewan, A., Nantasenamat, C., Isarankura-Na-Ayudhya, C., & Prachayasittikul, V. (2013). Predicting antimicrobial activities of benzimidazole derivatives. *Medicinal Chemistry Research*, *22*(11), 5418–5430. https://doi.org/10.1007/s00044-013-0539-y

Wu, Z., Ramsundar, B., Feinberg, E. N., Gomes, J., Geniesse, C., Pappu, A. S., Leswing, K., & Pande, V. (2018). MoleculeNet: A benchmark for molecular machine learning. *Chemical Science*, *9*(2), 513–530.

Yang, X., Wang, Y., Byrne, R., Schneider, G., & Yang, S. (2019). Concepts of artificial intelligence for computer-assisted drug discovery. *Chemical Reviews*, *119*(18), 10520–10594. https://doi.org/10.1021/acs.chemrev.8b00728

Yin, W., Mao, C., Luan, X., Shen, D.-D., Shen, Q., Su, H., Wang, X., Zhou, F., Zhao, W., & Gao, M. (2020). Structural basis for inhibition of the RNA-dependent RNA polymerase from SARS-CoV-2 by remdesivir. *Science*, *368*(6498), 1499–1504.

Zhou, Y., Wang, F., Tang, J., Nussinov, R., & Cheng, F. (2020). Artificial intelligence in COVID-19 drug repurposing. *The Lancet Digital Health*, *2*(12), e667–e676.

9 Significance of Artificial Intelligence in the Recognition, Characterization, and Prediction of Hepatocellular Carcinoma

Smriti Parashar and Rupesh K. Gautam**,†*
*Vedic Institute of Pharmaceutical Education and Research, Sagar, India; **Department of Pharmacology, Indore Institute of Pharmacy, Rau-Indore, India
†Corresponding Author: drrupeshgautam@gmail.com

ABBREVIATIONS

AI	Artificial intelligence
ANN	Artificial neural network
ART	Assessment for retreatment with TACE
BCLC	Barcelona clinical liver cancer
CCA	Cholangiocarcinoma
CEUS	Contrast-enhanced ultrasound
CNN	Convolutional neural network
CT	Computed tomography
C-US	Contrast-enhanced ultrasound
DI	Deep learning
EASL	European Association for the Study of the Liver
EHR	Electronic health record
FDG	Fluorine 18 fluorodeoxyglucose
FNH	Focal nodular hyperplasia
HCC	Hepatocellular carcinoma
MI	Machine learning
MRI	Magnetic resonance imaging

DOI: 10.1201/9781032699882-9

NAFLD	Non-alcoholic fatty liver disease
NASH	Non-alcoholic liver steatohepatitis
NLP	Natural language processing
PET	Positron emission tomography
R-BMode	Radiomics-based B-Mode images model
R-DLCEUS	Radiomic deep learning contrast-enhanced ultrasound
R-TIC	Radiomics-based time-intensity curve
SVM	Support vector machines
TACE	Transcatheter arterial chemoembolization
TERT	Telomerase reverse transcriptase

9.1 INTRODUCTION

The fourth most common adult liver malignancy is hepatocellular carcinoma (HCC), which is considered the third leading cause of mortality and morbidity in the world. Over time, significant progress has been seen in HCC diagnosis, surveillance, and understanding of its pathogenesis, improving its prevention management. But HCC is still a challenge for physicians globally (McGlynn et al. 2021). Its characterization, recognition, and diagnostic challenges are still to be explored. HCC is a challenge because of its heterogeneity, malignant progression range, and imitators such as i-CCA (i-cholangiocarcinoma) or c-CCA (c-cholangiocarcinoma). HCC is complicated due to its heterogenous pathogenesis and multiple recognized risk factors, which create inconsistencies in staging systems and prediction. Even after preventive measures with surgical resection and liver transplantation, it has a high recurrence rate (Kumar et al. 2020).

Artificial intelligence (AI) technology uniquely emerged as a tool to cover all spectrums and challenges of pharmacology. AI, with its subsections like machine learning (ML), deep learning (DL), natural language processing (NLP), and algorithms, can overcome such challenges and detect detailed information about HCC. To increase accuracy and precision in the diagnosis of HCC, various DL models, large datasets, biomarkers, image sense modality, and electronic health records (EHRs) are recommended (Nakamura et al. 2021). AI-based methods help in the early diagnosis of HCC and can define its range by predicting disease progression and consequences (Martinino et al. 2022). The recognition, characterization, and prediction of hepatocellular carcinoma can be technically resolved by the development of AI as a unique novel tool. Although AI is almost an old concept that prevailed in the 50s, recently, a breakthrough was seen in this technique that can effectively manage complex information from big data available in the field of pharmacology. It is a technology that is an alternative to human intellect or manpower (Pérez et al. 2020). ML creates algorithms to analyze data and recognize the pattern of symptoms which helps in characterization and prediction. An innovative ML with a new subtype, DL, helps in creating multi-layered neural network algorithms, making it more effective with convolutional neural networks, artificial neural networks, and support vector machines (Sato et al. 2021). Here in this chapter, AI-based concoctions will be discussed in three dimensions, which are the recognition, characterization, and prediction of HCC. In this context, AI-based recognition with imaging and clinical datasets highlights the liver abnormality. Then, AI-based characterization of

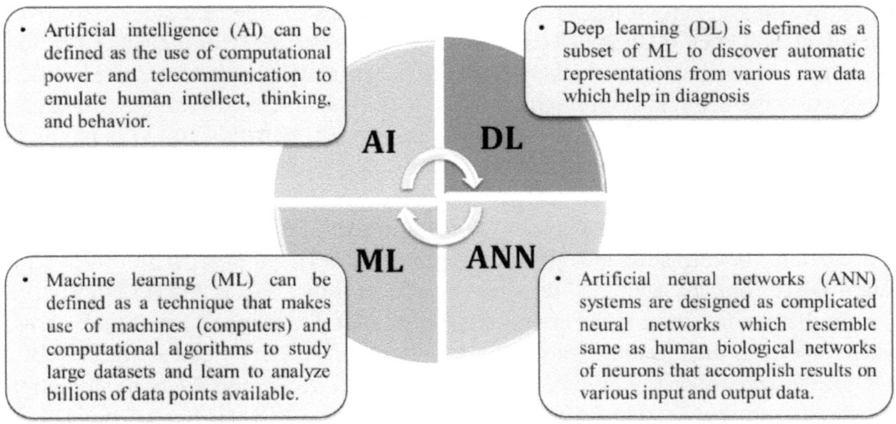

FIGURE 9.1 A simple explanation of the terms: artificial intelligence (AI), machine learning (MI), deep learning (DI), and artificial neural network (ANN).

HCC differentiates previously diagnosed hepatic abnormalities in detail with their malignant range and progression (Martinino et al. 2022). The AI-based prediction of HCC evaluates tumor succession, long-term outcomes, assessment of treatment response, and overall survival. Artificial intelligence (AI) can be defined as the use of computational power and telecommunication to emulate human intellect, thinking, and behavior (Szolovits 2019). Machine learning (ML) can be defined as a technique that makes use of machines (computers) and computational algorithms to study large datasets and learns to analyze billions of data points available. Deep learning (DL) is defined as a subset of ML used to discover automatic representations from various raw data which help in diagnosis (Álvarez-Machancoses and Fernández-Martínez 2019). There are two types of ML: first, supervised learning, and second, unsupervised learning. Supervised learning experts supervise various available inputs to predict consequences, whereas unsupervised learning works without a supervisor to find rationally occurring patterns without a pre-delineated outcome (Becker 2019). Artificial neural network (ANN) systems are designed as complicated neural networks which resemble human biological networks of neurons that accomplish results on various input and output data. A convolutional neural network (CNN) is defined as a multilayer ANN that uses pooling and convolution multilayers for processing grid patterns of available images to produce the required outcome (He et al. 2019). Discussed terms related to artificial intelligence in Figure 9.1 will be useful to understand the further chapter.

9.2 HEPATOCELLULAR CARCINOMA (HCC) PATHOPHYSIOLOGY

Hepatocellular carcinoma (HCC), or liver cancer, occurs when a tumor develops in the liver, predominantly in patients with chronic hepatitis B and C. Symptoms of HCC comprise weight loss, pain in the abdomen, or yellow skin (jaundice). HCC preventive measures require surgery, freezing up or heating the cancerous cells, liver transplant, and chemotherapy (Kumar et al. 2020). About 90 % of patients suffering from liver cirrhosis are more likely to develop a primary tumor of the liver, which is termed hepatocellular carcinoma (HCC). HCC is considered the second leading cause of death due to cancer. As shown in Figure 9.2, hepatitis B and hepatitis C viruses, liver damage due to alcohol, and liver steatohepatitis increase the chance or danger of developing HCC. Viral hepatitis (hepatitis B virus and hepatitis C virus) is responsible for 85% of HCC cases (Martinino et al. 2022). The hepatitis B virus is a partially double-stranded virus belonging to the *Hepadnavirus* family with a round DNA complex genome. Telomerase reverse transcriptase (TERT) developer sites of the genome in humans are targeted by the viral genome of hepatitis B virus, which results in various mutations including alterations in beta-1 catenin (CTNNBI), ARID2 (chromatin proliferation), TP53 (affecting cell cycle), and AT-rich interaction domain-containing protein 1A (ARID1A). The hepatitis C virus is a partially double-stranded RNA virus belonging to the family *Flaviviridae*. It contains genotypes of 11 types and 15 subtypes. The hepatitis C virus 1b genotype is mainly responsible for causing HCC. Liver damage by drinking alcohol is another factor that contributes to the pathogenesis of HCC. An alcoholic person is more likely to develop liver cirrhosis, which can lead to HCC. Excessive alcohol increases liver inflammation and increases reactive oxidative stress. Another liver pathologic condition termed NASH, which means non-alcoholic liver steatohepatitis, is where the accumulation of fat in the liver occurs in a non-alcoholic person. Patients with a history of metabolic syndrome develop NAFLD, which means non-alcoholic fatty liver disease.

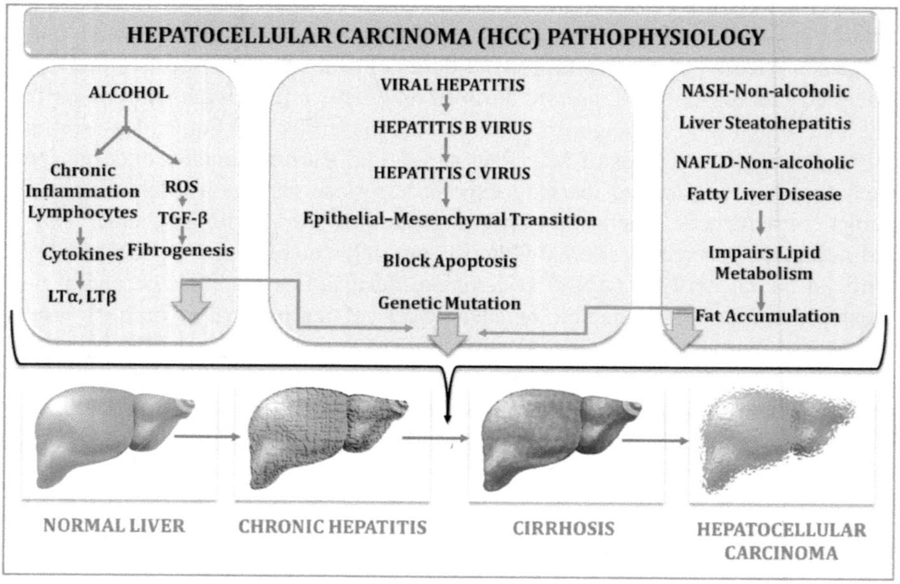

FIGURE 9.2 Pathophysiology of hepatocellular carcinoma.

Patients with abdominal obesity, hypertension, and hypertriglyceridemia are more prone to NAFLD (Mokrane et al. 2020; Kumar et al. 2020).

9.3 RECOGNITION OF HCC

To recognize HCC, traditional diagnostic methods are improved with the use of AI-driven techniques such as machine learning (ML), deep learning (DL), natural language processing (NLP), artificial neural network (ANN) systems, convolutional neural networks (CNNs), and algorithms (Sato et al. 2019). Diagnostic output produced by ultrasound, magnetic resonance imaging (MRI), abdomen tomography, positron emission tomography (PET), and liver section histopathology is made accurately precise when CNN and ANN multilayer networks study all types of input data to recognize the biological pattern (Mokrane et al. 2020; Martinino et al. 2022). Table 9.1 shows some examples of AI-based recognition of HCC. All the obtained patterns and output are processed by an AI technique-based HCC diagnostic system to produce the exact detailed result (Azer 2019; Martinino et al. 2022). Figure 9.3 explains the innovative concept of artificial intelligence in the recognition of HCC. The following reports some AI-based HCC diagnostic kits:

9.3.1 AI-Based Abdominal Ultrasound Kit

Patients with HCC or hepatic cirrhosis are subjected to abdominal ultrasound conditions frequently. Ultrasound is one of the most efficient tools to evaluate HCC and to check new space-occupying lesions in the liver with cirrhosis (Lai et al. 2020). But ultrasound images are not always easy to process and recognize the variability, so to make abdominal ultrasound more effective, it is blended with AI (Pérez et al. 2020; Martinino et al. 2022). With an AI-based algorithm and ultrasound blend, it is possible to conclude or recognize hepatic cirrhosis in its early stage, which was not possible with only ultrasound imaging. Liver capsule morphology images were classified by an AI-based algorithm and were able to verify the early-stage presence or absence of hepatic cirrhosis (Liu et al. 2017). An AI-based method was used where an ANN model combined with an ultrasound technique to clarify various stages of hepatic disease, including normal liver condition, chronic liver condition, cirrhosis condition, and HCC. In this model, accuracy was detected to be 97% (Bharti et al. 2018). Table 9.1 shows some examples of AI-based recognition of HCC. A blending kit with an AI-based DL system and ultrasound imaging was used to identify hepatic space-lodging lesions. A radiological report with a database containing 367 images of hepatic cells was studied and recognized by the algorithm. It differentiated between benign and malignant hepatic cells with their stage of progression (Schmauch et al. 2019). In a new way, contrast-enhanced ultrasound (C-US) was also combined with DL (a subset of AI), which refined its ability to identify hepatic cancer in three phases, including the normal liver condition, chronic liver condition, and cirrhosis condition, which increases the accurateness, sensitivity, and feature of the study (Guo et al. 2018).

TABLE 9.1
Artificial Intelligence-Based Recognition, Characterization, and Prediction of Hepatocellular Carcinoma

HCC case category	Number of cases (N)	Artificial intelligence	Validation	Precision/ Specificity/AUC	Remark	Reference
1. Cirrhosis (HBV) on entecavir HCC case	T:86/424 V: 316	Deep learning CNN/ ANN neural network	Validated externally	C-stats 0.719 (T); 0.782 (V)	Cirrhosis (HBV) patients results which are on entecavir were outpaced under several conventional algorithms	Nam *et al.* 2020
2. HCC recognition using AI based analysis of Transcriptome biomarker	HCC: 2,316 non-tumorous tissue:1,665	AI based Multiple methods combined	Validated externally	0.91–0.96	Pre-HCC/ HCC were diagnosed and characterized by transcriptome biomarker which are analysed by AI based Multiple methods; Due to group analysis heterogeneity is seen in data	Kaur *et al.* 2020
3. HCC characterisation using digitised histopathology study	T: 194 V: 328	AI based Artificial neural network ANN	Validated externally	C-stats: 0.78	After resection it is predicted for survival.	Saillard *et al.* 2020
4. HCC prediction using AI based CT imaging method	T: 562 V: 227	AI based convolutional neural network (CNN)	Validated externally	AUC: >0.95	Transcatheter arterial chemoembolization treatment was predicted using CNN (AI based) with complete and partial response with accuracy	Peng *et al.* 2020

5. HCC prognostication using contrast-enhanced ultrasound imaging method	36	Distance weighted discrimination	Internal and cross validation (leave-one-out)	Accuracy: 85% Specificity: 82% Sensitivity: 88.9%	Prediction of Transcatheter arterial chemoembolization response with AI based contrast-enhanced ultrasound imaging method	Oezdemir *et al.* 2020
6. HCC prognostication by MRI imaging method and analysing clinical big data	36	Regression analysis, logistic regression random forest	Internal and cross validation (leave-one-out)	Accuracy: 79% Specificity: 82% Sensitivity: 63%	Prediction of Transcatheter arterial chemoembolization response with AI based MRI imaging method and analysing clinical big data	Abajian *et al.* 2018
7. HCC recognition and characterisation by CT images and clinical data	T: 210 V: 107	RSF/MRMR	Validated externally	C-statistic: 0.73	HCC reocurrence is predicted after resection.	Ji *et al.* 2019
8. Serum as biomarkers for HCC prognostication	1,582	Multiple techniques combined	No validation only development	0.844–0.940	Single centre, internally validated studies with small sample size	Sato *et al.* 2019
9. AI based system used to study the chronic HCV to detect HCC	T: 10,741	AI based Artificial neural network ANN	Validated internally by randomly splitting sample	0.89	Study to find out the range of progression of chronic Hepatitis B/C infection into HCC. There was a limitation in the study that no external validation was done.	Ioannou *et al.* 2019

(*Continued*)

TABLE 9.1 (*Continued*)
Artificial Intelligence-Based Recognition, Characterization, and Prediction of Hepatocellular Carcinoma

HCC case category	Number of cases (N)	Artificial intelligence	Validation	Precision/ Specificity/AUC	Remark	Reference
10. Cirrhosis/ fibrosis/ hepatitis B/ hepatitis C based HCC cases	165	Support vector machine	Internal and cross validation	0.88	Viral status and clinical data are used to develop anlysis. There was a limitation in the study that only small sample size were taken and studied.	Książek *et al.* 2019
11. Pre-HCC disease models Population screening for NAFLD	500 cases: 146 controls: 354	Regression analysis, logistic regression	Internal and cross validation	0.87 (0.83–0.90)	They used Retrosceptive study design There was a limitation in the study that no external validation was done.	Yip *et al.* 2017
12. Gene co-expression as biomarkers for HCC prognostication	57	*Principal Component Analysis*	No validation only development	N/A	They used retrospective gene databases which was studied under neural network and no clinical applicability	Zhang *et al.* 2017
13. Cirrhosis/ fibrosis/ hepatitis B/ hepatitis C based HCC cases	T:165/6,092	AI based Artificial neural network ANN	N/A	AUROC:0.96	Study to find out the range of progression of chronic hepatitis infection into hepatic cirrhosis.	Reddy *et al.* 2017
14. Biomarker identification for HCC prognostication	N/A	Data mining	Internal and cross validation	F-score 0.89	Impact factor used as scoring tool and systematic bias was introduced into the results.	Chang *et al.* 2017

15. Urine as biomarkers for HCC prognostication	15	*Principal ComponentAnalysis*, Random forest	Validated internally	AUC: 0.903	There was a limitation in the study that only small sample size were taken and studied.	Liang *et al*. 2016
16. Pre-HCC disease models NAFLD/NASH	15	Random forest machine learning algorithm	No validation only development	N/A	Only animal (murine) model were used which do not replicated on humans	Chiappini *et al*. 2016
17. HCC detection on multi-phase CT scans in pre-HCC disease models	25	CT Temporal subtraction, 3D global matching	No validation only development	N/A	There was a limitation in the study that only small sample were taken and studied.	Lee *et al*. 2015
18. Cirrhosis/ fibrosis/ hepatitis B/ hepatitis C based HCC cases	533 (184 fibrosis cases)	Random forest machine learning algorithm	Validated internally	0.84 (0.82–0.86)	Study to find out the range of progression of chronic Hepatitis C infection into fibrosis.	Konerman *et al*. 2015
19. Genes Biomarkers for HCC prognostication	95	AI based Artificial neural network ANN	Internal and cross validation	N/A	They used retrospective gene databases which was studied under neural network.	Gui *et al*. 2015
20. miRNA Biomarkers are used for HCC prognostication	N/A	Deep Belief Networks (DBNs)	Internal and cross validation	F1-score 75%	There was a limitation in the study that no external validation was done.	Ibrahim *et al*. 2014

(Continued)

TABLE 9.1 (*Continued*)

Artificial Intelligence-Based Recognition, Characterization, and Prediction of Hepatocellular Carcinoma

HCC case category	Number of cases (N)	Artificial intelligence	Validation	Precision/ Specificity/AUC	Remark	Reference
21. Cirrhosis cases are studied and analysed using AI based system.	T: 41/442 V: 88/1,050	Random forest	Validated externally (HALT-C trial)	C-statistic 0.64 Accuracy: 80.5%	Outpaced HALT-C model for predicting HCC (IDI = 0.01, $p = 0.04$; NRI = 0.39, $p < 0.001$)	Singal *et al.* 2013
22. MRI imaging results for HCC cases studied using AI based algorithm.	MRI images: 40	AI based Artificial neural network ANN	No validation only development	accuracy 92%	SPIO-MRI used to study liver tissue nodule (HCC) in rat models Animal models used; there was no test-retest replicability.	Guo *et al.* 2009

(HCC: hepatocellular carcinoma, AUC: area under the curve, T: training, V: validation)

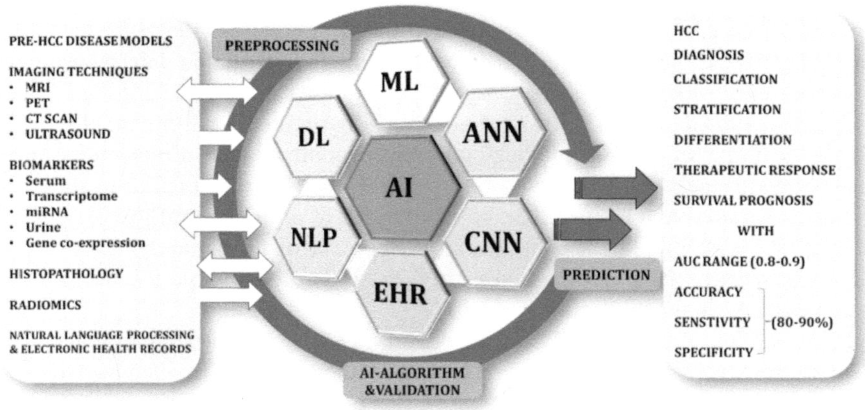

FIGURE 9.3 Innovative concept of artificial intelligence in the recognition, characterization, and prediction of hepatocellular carcinoma: Different input data are pre-processed under an AI-based algorithm and validated to classify and differentiate HCC. These neural networks help to record accurate therapeutic responses and survival prognosis. (HCC: hepatocellular carcinoma, MRI: magnetic resonance imaging, PET: positron emission tomography, CT: computed tomography, AI: artificial intelligence, DL: deep learning, ML: machine learning, ANN: artificial neural network, CNN: convolutional neural network, NLP: natural language processing, EHR: electronic health record, AUC: area under the curve).

9.3.2 AI-Based Magnetic Resonance Imaging (MRI)

A blend of the system was prepared in which MRI liver lesions images were studied by DL-based CNN. The concluded outcome showed 92% accuracy and sensitivity, and 98% of the images were classified specifically (Hamm et al. 2019). AI-based MRI systems were further enhanced by including clinical data and risk factor data. Then, MRI liver lesion images were classified into five types, including adenoma, cyst, hemangioma, HCC, and metastasis (Jansen et al. 2019). In another study, a deep neural network with a multi-phase training framework was used to study MRI results in 20 patients and promisingly classified liver tissue for a better outcome (Zhang et al. 2018; Martinino et al. 2022).

9.3.3 AI-Based Computed Tomography (CT) Scan and Positron Emission Tomography (PET)

To recognize HCC accurately after ultrasound imaging, abdominal computed tomography (CT) or intravenous (IV) contrast-enhanced computed tomography is preferred (Heimbach et al. 2018; Nakamura et al. 2021). In a traditional study, 178 patients suffering from liver cirrhosis were studied for HCC via biopsy followed by CT scan according to European Association for the Study of the Liver (EASL) guidelines. Then, using the ML technique blended with CT scan imaging, liver nodules were studied under the trained unit, calibrated unit, and validated unit to differentiate liver nodules as cancerous or not. The area under the curve was 0.70 (95%CI: 0.61–0.80) and 0.66 (95%CI: 0.64–0.84) for the discovery unit and validation unit, respectively (Mokrane et al. 2020; Martinino et al. 2022). Another systematic combination of CT images with CNN multilayer ANN successfully segmented liver cancerous cells with an accuracy of 82.67% and helped in the recommendation of preventive treatment (Li 2015). The segmentation of infected liver cells is very crucial to study the presence of lesions and to conclude the stage or range of infection. Liver lesions are heterogenic, which makes it complicated to segment them manually, so AI-based diagnosis helps in accurate segmenting (Pérez et al. 2020). Table 9.1 shows some examples of AI-based recognition of HCC.

In one study, an ANN-based contrast-enhanced CT system was used to recognize HCC where ANN showed three layers. Obtained images were classified into five categories: a) basic HCC; b) cancer other than HCC; c) unspecified masses, nodules, and early-stage HCC; d) hemangiomas; and e) cysts (Yasaka et al. 2018). With the help of AI plus CT studies, HCC relapses or recurrence can also be recognized (Vivanti et al. 2017).

A study was performed where the ANN technique was evaluated for liver uptake of fluorine 18 fluorodeoxyglucose (FDG) with positron emission tomography (PET). About 98 patients were studied with FDG positron emission tomography (18F-FDG PET) and MRI liver lesion imaging (Preis et al. 2011). Liver malignancies were detected with high accuracy and sensitivity. ANN with 18F-FDG PET had greater applicability to identifying metastatic liver disease. From the result, it was very clear that PET used in conjunction with ANN improves accuracy. Results obtained by ANN incorporating lesion data showed in area under the curve of 0.905 (standard error, 0.0370), whereas ANN independent of lesion data showed an area under the curve of 0.896 (standard error, 0.0386) (Pérez et al. 2020; Martinino et al. 2022).

9.3.4 AI-Based Histopathology

Histopathology is a crucial step in identifying and classifying the HCC. To take preventive measures for liver cirrhosis and to determine the treatment regimen for HCC, its recognition is important. To enhance histopathology, AI-based techniques are used to add computational and telecommunication power. ANN and CNN neural networks further help in the classification of various stages of liver tumors (Martinino et al. 2022). ML and DL, which are subsets of AI, help in analyzing various available big data to produce an output with accuracy, specificity, and sensitivity.

9.3.5 AI-Based Pre-HCC Recognition

HCC generally develops due to viral infections of hepatitis B and C, but there are also some non-virus reasons to study such as non-alcoholic fatty liver disease and non-alcoholic steatohepatitis, which can cause HCC. So, an AI-based pre-HCC model can be a perfect blend to identify high-risk individuals who can develop HCC in the future (Kawka et al. 2022). Research was conducted where serum, lipid levels, and 23 other clinical parameters were studied in non-alcoholic fatty liver disease and non-alcoholic steatohepatitis murine cancer models. This study was supervised by ML algorithm-based randosm forest analysis, where the area under the curve was obtained to be 0.88 (95%CI: 0.84–0.91) (Chiappini et al. 2016; Martinino et al. 2022). In another study, an area under the curve was obtained as high as 0.962 with a sophisticated ANN-based ML model for diagnosing HCC development from viral infection hepatitis B or C (Reddy et al. 2017; Ioannou et al. 2019). In recent research, an ANN-based ML model was used to study various reports of patients, including 23 quantitative and 26 qualitative features, viral infection data, laboratory results data, and histopathology data. This study has shown 88% accuracy (Książek et al. 2019; Kawka et al. 2022).

9.3.6 AI-Based Recognition with Biomarkers

Biomarkers are widely studied as a way to accurately recognize HCC. Nowadays, AI-based technology and bioinformatics can perfectly blend with these biomarkers data to generate 'big biological data' and help in the amalgamation of multiple datasets. To accurately recognize the stage, progression, and range of HCC, many types of 'omics' datasets (genome, proteome, transcriptome) can be used (Manzoni et al. 2018). 'Omics' can be combined with DL, CNN-based ANN systems, and AI-based algorithms with suitable biomarkers to analyze available 'big biological data' and conclude the best possible therapy after correct diagnosis (Chen et al. 2020). In a study where a traditional method for HCC diagnosis using the serological marker alpha-fetoprotein, integration with CNN and ANN neural networks produced diagnostic results with a sensitivity of 88% (Poon et al. 2001; Kaur et al. 2020).

Previous classical methods' results when compared with the new ones obtained from AI-based systems increase in sensitivity from 65% to 80%. A large-scale study was also conducted where about 2,000 HCC cancerous tissue samples and about 1,000 non-cancerous tissue samples from healthy patients were taken (Kaur et al. 2020). Specifically, blood samples from both HCC and healthy patients were taken to analyze mononuclear cells with the help of ML as subsets of the AI system, and transcriptomic profiling was done (Ibrahim et al. 2014; Gui et al. 2015). The outcome included three-gene initials, first, FCN3; second, CLEC1B; and third, PRC1, with an area under curve of 0.92–0.95 (Kaur et al. 2020). Many HCC biomarkers such as miRNA, genes, serum, gene expression prototypes, and urine biomarkers are used with the combination of AI-based systems (ML, CNN, ANN) to improve a potential HCC recognition system (Zhang et al. 2017). When studied with various urine biomarkers, about 37 samples with 25 HCC samples and 12 controls showed effective outcomes with a sensitivity of 95% and specificity of 85% (Liang et al. 2016; Kaur et al. 2020). You can refer to Table 9.1 for examples of AI-based recognition of HCC.

9.4 CHARACTERIZATION OF HCC

AI-based systems to diagnose HCC can further be equipped with more computational technology to characterize HCC clearly and specifically (Laino et al. 2022). AI-based biomarker diagnostic techniques have shown accurate results to detect pre-HCC or HCC conditions. As discussed earlier, biomarkers are used to diagnose HCC. When it comes to the characterization of HCC, ML-based AI techniques can be used to differentiate or classify its different stages, its range, or its progression. So, using the ML technique to study biomarker profiles obtained in HCC recognition can create a clear picture of HCC by its stratification. Based on these classifications, a better treatment therapy can be developed (Martinino et al. 2022). Figure 9.3 explains the innovative concept of artificial intelligence in the characterization of HCC. In a study, ML-based AI analysis was used to study DNA methylation patterns in epigenomics as well as in genomics. Results obtained were very accurate about the various stages of HCC and specifically characterized early- or late-stage HCC (Kalapala et al. 2023). In another study, AI-based analysis was conducted on biomarker profile and cytokine profile data from serum samples to characterize HCC into viral hepatitis B-caused HCC, hepatitis C-caused HCC, or non-viral HCC (Kalapala et al. 2023). Secondly, various imaging methods are used to diagnose HCC like magnetic resonance imaging (MRI), computed tomography (CT) scanning, positron emission tomography (PET), and ultrasound (UT) (Lupsor-Platon et al. 2021). These imaging methods are enhanced with AI based on computer-aided characterization of HCC. To characterize and differentiate liver pathology, AI focuses on studying the region of interest and examining characteristics (lesion edges or texture) that help in identifying benign and malignant tumors and HCC (Kalapala et al. 2023). This AI-based characterization is very accurate in differentiating the stage, range, and progression of HCC. A study using CNN-based ANN with ultrasound scanning technique characterized HCC with 95% accuracy and differentiated between liver cirrhosis and HCC (Maruyama et al. 2021). AI-based neural networks help in creating a network that resembles a human biological network, which helps in concluding the clear image of atypical HCC and focal nodular hyperplasia (FNH) (Cao et al. 2021; Tiyarattanachai et al. 2022).

Another research work was performed with contrast-enhanced ultrasound (CEUS), which characterizes HCC imaging profile grades. Characterization of HCC into well-distinguished, moderately distinguished, and poorly distinguished HCC using CEUS showed an area under the curve of 0.86–0.87 (Tiyarattanachai et al. 2022). Tumor dissection algorithms with contrast-enhanced CT scans and positron emission tomography (PET) characterize HCC to a higher extent. They produce 3D projections and conclude the stage, range, progression, and reoccurrence of HCC. These algorithms help to create clinical management planning for effective treatment.

Recently a new approach is used to create an innovative blend of magnetic resonance imaging (MRI), computed tomography (CT), positron emission tomography (PET), and ultrasound (UT) imaging methods (Urhut et al. 2022) with radiomics for the characterization of HCC (Tiyarattanachai et al. 2021). Now, what is radiomics? Radiomics is a technique that employs data-characterization algorithms to extract a large number of characteristics from different pathological images (Castaldo et al. 2021). This type of characterization can uncover different HCC tumoral patterns. The computational technique of radiomics drives big data from radiological characteristics using image assets, subdivision, feature mining, and automatic analysis of tumor patterns. As discussed earlier, AI-driven characterization with a blend of biomarkers and imaging methods creates an innovative future perspective to develop a technology that can characterize HCC with a perfect picture (Dana et al. 2022). This technology can differentiate all stages of liver tumors and can tell the types (viral or non-viral HCC), stages, ranges, progression, and chances of recurrence of hepatic cancer (Laino et al. 2022).

Thirdly, liver pathology is another way to characterize HCC. An AI-based liver pathology is now a new approach to stratifying HCC successfully and accurately. Liver pathology results from biopsy and sectioning of liver tumors are analyzed by an AI-based system (Laino et al. 2022). In a study of hematoxylin and eosin-stained liver tissue sections, slides were analyzed by AI, which showed 85% differentiation accuracy. These AI-based models show high recognition and characterization accuracy of approximately 88% in classifying liver healthy tissue and HCC (Lin et al. 2022). These models have future potential to prognosticate HCC and can also predict treatment response in patients. Studies also proved that by analyzing (AI-based models) nuclei and the texture of liver tissue section slides, HCC can be differentiated into low-grade HCC or high-grade HCC (Calderaro and Kather 2021; Laino et al. 2022). A traditional gold-standard method of using frozen sections of liver tissue, which is both time-consuming and needs skilled personnel, now has an alternative method of an AI-based deep learning model (88.1% accuracy) (Laino et al. 2022). Table 9.1 shows some examples of AI-based characterization of HCC. Finally, an AI-based solution offers a perfect kit that is laboratory free and provides accurate real-time diagnoses and characterization (Eisenbrey et al. 2021; Chapiro 2022).

9.5 AI-BASED TREATMENT AND PREDICTION OF HCC

All patients with HCC differ from one another due to different clinical conditions and therapeutic responses (Craig et al. 2020). So, this creates a hindrance in the clinical assessment of treatment regimens for every individual accordingly (Villanueva and Llovet 2011). That is why potential AI-based stratification and characterization systems are needed to prepare treatment plans and predict treatment outcomes. AI-based systems can play a significant role in the therapeutic approach to HCC. AI-based treatment and prediction of HCC involve the use and analysis of genetic features, histopathological data, radiological images, and radiomic reports along with clinical data (Gillies et al. 2016; Castaldo et al. 2021; Chapiro 2022).

A new technique of AI-based software in combination with radiomics is not exclusively used in medical practice (Castaldo et al. 2021). But it is an upcoming area of interest for predicting medication outcomes for HCC because it extracts large, computable objective data which is analyzed to produce accurate diagnostic and prognostic reports (Lambin et al. 2017; Castaldo et al. 2021). Surgical resections are analyzed with the help of a computer model to identify the risk of tumor recurrence to avoid redundant treatment. Vascular micro-invasion is a recommended independent variable to predict tumor recurrence (Erstad and Tanabe 2019; Xu et al. 2019). Much research is based on predicting pre-operational vascular micro-invasion status with the help of radiomic monograms (Ma et al. 2019; Erstad and Tanabe 2019; Dong et al. 2020). In one study, a radiomic blended surgical resection model was studied for predicting the recurrence of liver tumors, and results showed a C-index of 0.63–0.69.

When this model was augmented with clinical data, it could identify the stratification of the liver tissue section, which gives a clear picture to develop a treatment profile for any individual (Ji et al. 2019). In the management regimen of HCC, transcatheter arterial chemoembolization (TACE) is considered the treatment of choice in Barcelona clinical liver cancer (BCLC). Some adverse secondary effects were reported under this treatment, so AI-based techniques need to be used to diagnose radiological images, radiomics data, and genomic profiles (Peng et al. 2020). AI-based techniques can identify the stage of HCC, which helps in predicting the required medication and outcome. In one study, researchers evaluated the therapeutic response to TACE treatment for HCC. For this, they developed an automated ML algorithm that uses CT images of liver tissue and also the available pre-treatment clinical data of patients. The results showed 75% accuracy and specificity (Morshid et al. 2019).

In another study, a DL algorithm was used to predict TACE therapeutic response using CT images, and it estimated the response with 85% of accuracy and a value of 0.9 for the area under the curve (Peng et al. 2020; Chapiro 2022). An AI-based DL radiomics–C-US model was used for predicting treatment outcome from TACE; it was highly precise, specific, and sensitive. It showed an area under the curve for R-DLCEUS (radiomic deep learning contrast-enhanced ultrasound), R-TIC (radiomics-based time-intensity curve), and R-BMode (radiomics-based B-Mode images model) of 0.93 (95%CI: 0.80–0.98), 0.80 (95%CI: 0.64–0.90), and 0.81 (95%CI: 0.67–0.95), respectively (Liu et al. 2020; Saillard et al. 2020). In a trial, 36 patients were treated with TACE and underwent MRI before the treatment. MRI images were analyzed by an AI-based ML algorithm and predicted responses with accuracy, sensitivity, and specificity of 78%, 62%, and 82%, respectively (Abajian et al. 2018; Turco et al. 2022). Another way to predict the TACE outcome is to find out the survival status of patients. A prediction neural network model was prepared using an ANN that included all ART (assessment for retreatment with TACE) (Sieghart et al. 2013), ABCR (Adhoute et al. 2015), and SNACOR (Kim et al. 2016) parameters for predicting scores (Mähringer-Kunz et al. 2020). Survival status was observed for one year, and prediction showed an area under curve, specificity, and sensitivity of 0.7%, 80%, and 78%, respectively (Mähringer-Kunz et al. 2020; Schoenberg et al. 2020). TACE therapeutic response can also be studied with genetic analysis. So, to predict response, a support vector machine (SVM), which is an influential ordering and regression tool in various ML-based techniques, was used to study the genetic mutation (Ziv et al. 2017; Ahsan 2022). Table 9.1 shows some more examples of AI-based prediction of therapeutic response to the treatment of HCC.

9.6 FUTURE PROSPECTS AND LIMITATIONS

Recent advancement in AI-based technologies in HCC management is quickly taking place in the pharma world. In the future, AI will be one of the most relevant and progressive fields to add to the diagnosis and recognition of HCC to build up curative management for HCC. AI can help to process and analyze a large amount of data to quickly resolve the different types of diagnostic and characterization data for HCC cases.

Now let us talk about limitations because every type of technology has some restrictions. Firstly, the requirement of trained personnel for AI technology is a must because, without the presence of trained healthcare professionals, this technology cannot be explored at its fullest. This technology is a supportive system to support human intelligence, which makes it versatile. The second limitation is the use of such a high-quality AI-based predictive model by the researcher at a small level by demonstrating small-size samples because it needs to be used at a wider perspective level for big data. The researcher should validate such technology with large and multicenter studies. The third limitation of the AI model is the inadequate reproducibility of various purposes in therapeutic practice. The predictive model has a limited area of work according to its design, and there is a special requirement of various software programs for algorithm AI calculations. Fourth is the high cost of developing such a vast AI system with high-tech software and to train the required professional to make it work at a large level for various studies (Pérez et al. 2020; Cao et al. 2021).

However, by accounting for the limitations of AI technology, we can further validate and study the problems. This can resolve the problems of trained health care professionals, reproducibility in heterogeneity of imaging possession, and non-existence of multicenter validation. So, AI technology can be prepared to develop accurate and reproducible predictive models for diagnosis, recognition, and characterization of HCC, empowering its application to treat HCC patients.

9.7 CONCLUSION

In this chapter, we explored what AI-based HCC management looks like. So, here we compiled all the AI-based technology with HCC diagnosis, classification, and prediction methods. This combination is a wide-ranging field that encourages scientists and clinicians to overcome the various challenges which are faced in HCC management. Traditional methods for HCC diagnosis or recognition like ultrasound, magnetic resonance imaging (MRI), abdomen tomography, positron emission tomography (PET), biomarkers, and liver section histopathology have their limitations. These methods are costly, tedious, time-consuming, and lack precision when compared with automated AI techniques. When all these methods are combined with AI-based technology like ML, DL, ANN, CNN, EHR, and algorithms, they recognize and characterize HCC with full accuracy, specificity, and sensitivity. This increases the chance of develop a future perspective with AI-based techniques in HCC for its treatment management and response outcome prediction.

REFERENCES

Abajian, Aaron, Nikitha Murali, Lynn Jeanette Savic, Fabian Max Laage-Gaupp, Nariman Nezami, James S. Duncan, Todd Schlachter, MingDe Lin, Jean-François Geschwind, and Julius Chapiro. "Predicting treatment response to intra-arterial therapies for hepatocellular carcinoma with the use of supervised machine learning—an artificial intelligence concept." *Journal of Vascular and Interventional Radiology* 29, no. 6 (2018): 850–857.

Adhoute, Xavier, Guillaume Penaranda, Sebastien Naude, Jean Luc Raoul, Herve Perrier, Olivier Bayle, Olivier Monnet, et al. "Retreatment with TACE: The ABCR SCORE, an aid to the decision-making process." *Journal of Hepatology* 62, no. 4 (2015): 855–862.

Ahsan, Zarish. "Artificial intelligence used for the diagnosis, treatment and surveillance of hepatocellular carcinoma: A systematic review." *Undergraduate Research in Natural and Clinical Science and Technology Journal* (2022): 1–13.

Álvarez-Machancoses, Óscar, and Juan Luis Fernández-Martínez. "Using artificial intelligence methods to speed up drug discovery." *Expert Opinion on Drug Discovery* 14, no. 8 (2019): 769–777.

Azer, Samy A. "Deep learning with convolutional neural networks for identification of liver masses and hepatocellular carcinoma: A systematic review." *World Journal of Gastrointestinal Oncology* 11, no. 12 (2019): 1218.

Becker, Aliza. "Artificial intelligence in medicine: What is it doing for us today?." *Health Policy and Technology* 8, no. 2 (2019): 198–205.

Bharti, Puja, Deepti Mittal, and Rupa Ananthasivan. "Preliminary study of chronic liver classification on ultrasound images using an ensemble model." *Ultrasonic Imaging* 40, no. 6 (2018): 357–379.

Calderaro, Julien, and Jakob Nikolas Kather. "Artificial intelligence-based pathology for gastrointestinal and hepatobiliary cancers." *Gut* 70, no. 6 (2021): 1183–1193.

Cao, J.S., Z.Y. Lu, M.Y. Chen, B. Zhang, S. Juengpanich, J.H. Hu, S.J. Li, W. Topatana, X.Y. Zhou, X. Feng, and J.L. Shen. "Artificial intelligence in gastroenterology and hepatology: Status and challenges." *World Journal of Gastroenterology* 27, no. 16 (2021): 1664.

Castaldo, Anna, Davide Raffaele De Lucia, Giuseppe Pontillo, Marco Gatti, Sirio Cocozza, Lorenzo Ugga, and Renato Cuocolo. "State of the art in artificial intelligence and radiomics in hepatocellular carcinoma." *Diagnostics* 11, no. 7 (2021): 1194.

Chang, Nai-Wen, Hong-Jie Dai, Yung-Yu Shih, Chi-Yang Wu, Mira Anne C. Dela Rosa, Rofeamor P. Obena, Yu-Ju Chen, Wen-Lian Hsu, and Yen-Jen Oyang. "Biomarker identification of hepatocellular carcinoma using a methodical literature mining strategy." *Database* 2017 (2017).

Chapiro, Julius. "Translating artificial intelligence from code to bedside: The road towards AI-driven predictive biomarkers for immunotherapy of hepatocellular carcinoma." *Journal of Hepatology* 77, no. 1 (2022): 6–8.

Chen, Bin, Lana Garmire, Diego F. Calvisi, Mei-Sze Chua, Robin K. Kelley, and Xin Chen. "Harnessing big 'omics' data and AI for drug discovery in hepatocellular carcinoma." *Nature Reviews Gastroenterology & Hepatology* 17, no. 4 (2020): 238–251.

Chiappini, Franck, Christophe Desterke, Justine Bertrand-Michel, Catherine Guettier, and François Le Naour. "Hepatic and serum lipid signatures specific to nonalcoholic steatohepatitis in murine models." *Scientific Reports* 6, no. 1 (2016): 1–9.

Craig, Amanda J., Johann Von Felden, Teresa Garcia-Lezana, Samantha Sarcognato, and Augusto Villanueva. "Tumour evolution in hepatocellular carcinoma." *Nature Reviews Gastroenterology & Hepatology* 17, no. 3 (2020): 139–152.

Dana, Jérémy, Aïna Venkatasamy, Antonio Saviano, Joachim Lupberger, Yujin Hoshida, Valérie Vilgrain, Pierre Nahon, Caroline Reinhold, Benoit Gallix, and Thomas F. Baumert. "Conventional and artificial intelligence-based imaging for biomarker discovery in chronic liver disease." *Hepatology International* (2022): 1–14.

Dong, Yi, Liu Zhou, Wei Xia, Xing-Yu Zhao, Qi Zhang, Jun-Ming Jian, Xin Gao, and Wen-Ping Wang. "Preoperative prediction of microvascular invasion in hepatocellular carcinoma: Initial application of a radiomic algorithm based on grayscale ultrasound images." *Frontiers in Oncology* 10 (2020): 353.

Eisenbrey, John R., Helena Gabriel, Esika Savsani, and Andrej Lyshchik. "Contrast-enhanced ultrasound (CEUS) in HCC diagnosis and assessment of tumor response to locoregional therapies." *Abdominal Radiology* 46, no. 8 (2021): 3579–3595.

Erstad, Derek J., and Kenneth K. Tanabe. "Prognostic and therapeutic implications of microvascular invasion in hepatocellular carcinoma." *Annals of Surgical Oncology* 26, no. 5 (2019): 1474–1493.

Gillies, Robert J., Paul E. Kinahan, and Hedvig Hricak. "Radiomics: Images are more than pictures, they are data." *Radiology* 278, no. 2 (2016): 563.

Gui, Tuantuan, Xiao Dong, Rudong Li, Yixue Li, and Zhen Wang. "Identification of hepatocellular carcinoma–related genes with a machine learning and network analysis." *Journal of Computational Biology* 22, no. 1 (2015): 63–71.

Guo, Dongmei, Tianshuang Qiu, Jie Bian, Wei Kang, and Li Zhang. "A computer-aided diagnostic system to discriminate SPIO-enhanced magnetic resonance hepatocellular carcinoma by a neural network classifier." *Computerized Medical Imaging and Graphics* 33, no. 8 (2009): 588–592.

Guo, Le-Hang, Dan Wang, Yi-Yi Qian, Xiao Zheng, Chong-Ke Zhao, Xiao-Long Li, Xiao-Wan Bo, et al. "A two-stage multi-view learning framework based computer-aided diagnosis of liver tumors with contrast enhanced ultrasound images." *Clinical Hemorheology and Microcirculation* 69, no. 3 (2018): 343–354.

Hamm, Charlie A., Clinton J. Wang, Lynn J. Savic, Marc Ferrante, Isabel Schobert, Todd Schlachter, MingDe Lin, et al. "Deep learning for liver tumor diagnosis part I: development of a convolutional neural network classifier for multi-phasic MRI." *European Radiology* 29, no. 7 (2019): 3338–3347.

He, Jianxing, Sally L. Baxter, Jie Xu, Jiming Xu, Xingtao Zhou, and Kang Zhang. "The practical implementation of artificial intelligence technologies in medicine." *Nature Medicine* 25, no. 1 (2019): 30–36.

Heimbach, Julie K., Laura M. Kulik, Richard S. Finn, Claude B. Sirlin, Michael M. Abecassis, Lewis R. Roberts, Andrew X. Zhu, M. Hassan Murad, and Jorge A. Marrero. "AASLD guidelines for the treatment of hepatocellular carcinoma." *Hepatology* 67, no. 1 (2018): 358–380.

Ibrahim, Rania, Noha A. Yousri, Mohamed A. Ismail, and Nagwa M. El-Makky. "Multi-level gene/MiRNA feature selection using deep belief nets and active learning." In *2014 36th Annual International Conference of the IEEE Engineering in Medicine and Biology Society*, pp. 3957–3960. IEEE, 2014.

Ioannou, George N., Weijing Tang, Lauren A. Beste, Monica A. Konerman, Grace L. Su, Tony Van, Elliot B. Tapper, Amit G. Singal, Ji Zhu, and Akbar K. Waljee. "498–deep learning models accurately predict development of HCC in 146,218 patients with Chronic Hepatitis C." *Gastroenterology* 156, no. 6 (2019): S-1201.

Ioannou, George N., Weijing Tang, Lauren A. Beste, Monica A. Tincopa, Grace L. Su, Tony Van, Elliot B. Tapper, Amit G. Singal, Ji Zhu, and Akbar K. Waljee. "Assessment of a deep learning model to predict hepatocellular carcinoma in patients with hepatitis C cirrhosis." *JAMA Network Open* 3, no. 9 (2020): e2015626–e2015626.

Jansen, Mariëlle J.A., Hugo J. Kuijf, Wouter B. Veldhuis, Frank J. Wessels, Max A. Viergever, and Josien P.W. Pluim. "Automatic classification of focal liver lesions based on MRI and risk factors." *PLoS ONE* 14, no. 5 (2019): e0217053.

Ji, Gu-Wei, Fei-Peng Zhu, Qing Xu, Ke Wang, Ming-Yu Wu, Wei-Wei Tang, Xiang-Cheng Li, and Xue-Hao Wang. "Machine-learning analysis of contrast-enhanced CT radiomics predicts recurrence of hepatocellular carcinoma after resection: A multi-institutional study." *EBioMedicine* 50 (2019): 156–165.

Kalapala, Rakesh, Hardik Rughwani, and D. Nageshwar Reddy. "Artificial intelligence in hepatology-ready for the primetime." *Journal of Clinical and Experimental Hepatology* 13, no. 1 (2023): 149–161.

Kaur, Harpreet, Anjali Dhall, Rajesh Kumar, and Gajendra P.S. Raghava. "Identification of platform-independent diagnostic biomarker panel for hepatocellular carcinoma using large-scale transcriptomics data." *Frontiers in Genetics* 10 (2020): 1306.

Kawka, Michal, Aleksander Dawidziuk, Long R. Jiao, and Tamara M.H. Gall. "Artificial intelligence in the detection, characterisation and prediction of hepatocellular carcinoma: A narrative review." *Translational Gastroenterology and Hepatology* 7 (2022): 41.

Kim, Beom Kyung, Ju Hyun Shim, Seung Up Kim, Jun Yong Park, Do Young Kim, Sang Hoon Ahn, Kang Mo Kim, Young-Suk Lim, Kwang-Hyub Han, and Han Chu Lee. "Risk prediction for patients with hepatocellular carcinoma undergoing chemoembolization: Development of a prediction model." *Liver International* 36, no. 1 (2016): 92–99.

Konerman, Monica A., Yiwei Zhang, Ji Zhu, Peter D.R. Higgins, Anna S.F. Lok, and Akbar K. Waljee. "Improvement of predictive models of risk of disease progression in chronic hepatitis C by incorporating longitudinal data." *Hepatology* 61, no. 6 (2015): 1832–1841.

Książek, Wojciech, Moloud Abdar, U. Rajendra Acharya, and Paweł Pławiak. "A novel machine learning approach for early detection of hepatocellular carcinoma patients." *Cognitive Systems Research* 54 (2019): 116–127.

Kumar, Ashish, Subrat K. Acharya, Shivaram P. Singh, Anil Arora, Radha K. Dhiman, Rakesh Aggarwal, Anil C. Anand, et al. "2019 update of Indian national association for study of the liver consensus on prevention, diagnosis, and management of hepatocellular carcinoma in India: The puri II recommendations." *Journal of Clinical and Experimental Hepatology* 10, no. 1 (2020): 43–80.

Lai, Quirino, Gabriele Spoletini, Gianluca Mennini, Zoe Larghi Laureiro, Diamantis I. Tsilimigras, Timothy Michael Pawlik, and Massimo Rossi. "Prognostic role of artificial intelligence among patients with hepatocellular cancer: A systematic review." *World Journal of Gastroenterology* 26, no. 42 (2020): 6679.

Laino, Maria Elena, Luca Viganò, Angela Ammirabile, Ludovica Lofino, Elena Generali, Marco Francone, Ana Lleo, Luca Saba, and Victor Savevski. "The added value of artificial intelligence to LI-RADS categorization: A systematic review." *European Journal of Radiology* (2022): 110251.

Lambin, Philippe, Ralph T.H. Leijenaar, Timo M. Deist, Jurgen Peerlings, Evelyn E.C. De Jong, Janita Van Timmeren, Sebastian Sanduleanu, et al. "Radiomics: The bridge between medical imaging and personalized medicine." *Nature Reviews Clinical Oncology* 14, no. 12 (2017): 749–762.

Lee, Jeongjin, Kyoung Won Kim, So Yeon Kim, Juneseuk Shin, Kyung Jun Park, Hyung Jin Won, and Yong Moon Shin. "Automatic detection method of hepatocellular carcinomas using the non-rigid registration method of multi-phase liver CT images." *Journal of X-Ray Science and Technology* 23, no. 3 (2015): 275–288.

Li, Wen. "Automatic segmentation of liver tumor in CT images with deep convolutional neural networks." *Journal of Computer and Communications* 3, no. 11 (2015): 146.

Liang, Qun, Han Liu, Cong Wang, and Binbing Li. "Phenotypic characterization analysis of human hepatocarcinoma by urine metabolomics approach." *Scientific Reports* 6, no. 1 (2016): 1–8.

Lin, Biaoyang, Yingying Ma, and ShengJun Wu. "Multi-omics and artificial intelligence-guided data integration in chronic liver disease: Prospects and challenges for precision medicine." *OMICS: A Journal of Integrative Biology* 26, no. 8 (2022): 415–421.

Liu, Dan, Fei Liu, Xiaoyan Xie, Liya Su, Ming Liu, Xiaohua Xie, Ming Kuang, et al. "Accurate prediction of responses to transarterial chemoembolization for patients with hepatocellular carcinoma by using artificial intelligence in contrast-enhanced ultrasound." *European Radiology* 30, no. 4 (2020): 2365–2376.

Liu, Xiang, Jia Lin Song, Shuo Hong Wang, Jing Wen Zhao, and Yan Qiu Chen. "Learning to diagnose cirrhosis with liver capsule guided ultrasound image classification." *Sensors* 17, no. 1 (2017): 149.

Lupsor-Platon, Monica, Teodora Serban, Alexandra Iulia Silion, George Razvan Tirpe, Alexandru Tirpe, and Mira Florea. "Performance of ultrasound techniques and the potential of artificial intelligence in the evaluation of hepatocellular carcinoma and non-alcoholic fatty liver disease." *Cancers* 13, no. 4 (2021): 790.

Ma, Xiaohong, Jingwei Wei, Dongsheng Gu, Yongjian Zhu, Bing Feng, Meng Liang, Shuang Wang, Xinming Zhao, and Jie Tian. "Preoperative radiomics nomogram for microvascular invasion prediction in hepatocellular carcinoma using contrast-enhanced CT." *European Radiology* 29, no. 7 (2019): 3595–3605.

Mähringer-Kunz, Aline, Franziska Wagner, Felix Hahn, Arndt Weinmann, Sebastian Brodehl, Sebastian Schotten, Jan B. Hinrichs, et al. "Predicting survival after transarterial chemoembolization for hepatocellular carcinoma using a neural network: A pilot study." *Liver International* 40, no. 3 (2020): 694–703.

Manzoni, Claudia, Demis A. Kia, Jana Vandrovcova, John Hardy, Nicholas W. Wood, Patrick A. Lewis, and Raffaele Ferrari. "Genome, transcriptome and proteome: The rise of omics data and their integration in biomedical sciences." *Briefings in bioinformatics* 19, no. 2 (2018): 286–302.

Martinino, Alessandro, Mohammad Aloulou, Surobhi Chatterjee, Juan Pablo Scarano Pereira, Saurabh Singhal, Tapan Patel, Thomas Paul-Emile Kirchgesner, et al. "Artificial intelligence in the diagnosis of hepatocellular carcinoma: A systematic review." *Journal of Clinical Medicine* 11, no. 21 (2022): 6368.

Maruyama, Hitoshi, Tadashi Yamaguchi, Hiroaki Nagamatsu, and Shuichiro Shiina. "AI-based radiological imaging for HCC: Current status and future of ultrasound." *Diagnostics* 11, no. 2 (2021): 292.

McGlynn, Katherine A., Jessica L. Petrick, and Hashem B. El-Serag. "Epidemiology of hepatocellular carcinoma." *Hepatology* 73 (2021): 4–13.

Mokrane, Fatima-Zohra, Lin Lu, Adrien Vavasseur, Philippe Otal, Jean-Marie Peron, Lyndon Luk, Hao Yang, et al. "Radiomics machine-learning signature for diagnosis of hepatocellular carcinoma in cirrhotic patients with indeterminate liver nodules." *European Radiology* 30, no. 1 (2020): 558–570.

Morshid, Ali, Khaled M. Elsayes, Ahmed M. Khalaf, Mohab M. Elmohr, Justin Yu, Ahmed O. Kaseb, Manal Hassan, et al. "A machine learning model to predict hepatocellular carcinoma response to transcatheter arterial chemoembolization." *Radiology. Artificial Intelligence* 1, no. 5 (2019).

Nakamura, Yuko, Toru Higaki, Yukiko Honda, Fuminari Tatsugami, Chihiro Tani, Wataru Fukumoto, Keigo Narita, Shota Kondo, Motonori Akagi, and Kazuo Awai. "Advanced CT techniques for assessing hepatocellular carcinoma." *La radiologia medica* 126, no. 7 (2021): 925–935.

Nam, Joon Yeul, Jeong-Hoon Lee, Junho Bae, Young Chang, Yuri Cho, Dong Hyun Sinn, Bo Hyun Kim, et al. "Novel model to predict HCC recurrence after liver transplantation obtained using deep learning: A multicenter study." *Cancers* 12, no. 10 (2020): 2791.

Oezdemir, Ipek, Corrine E. Wessner, Colette Shaw, John R. Eisenbrey, and Kenneth Hoyt. "Tumor vascular networks depicted in contrast-enhanced ultrasound images as a predictor for transarterial chemoembolization treatment response." *Ultrasound in Medicine & Biology* 46, no. 9 (2020): 2276–2286.

Peng, Jie, Shuai Kang, Zhengyuan Ning, Hangxia Deng, Jingxian Shen, Yikai Xu, Jing Zhang, et al. "Residual convolutional neural network for predicting response of transarterial chemoembolization in hepatocellular carcinoma from CT imaging." *European Radiology* 30, no. 1 (2020): 413–424.

Pérez, Miguel Jiménez, and Rocío González Grande. "Application of artificial intelligence in the diagnosis and treatment of hepatocellular carcinoma: A review." *World Journal of Gastroenterology* 26, no. 37 (2020): 5617.

Poon, Terence Chuen-Wai, Anthony Tak-Cheung Chan, Benny Zee, Stephen King-Wah Ho, Tony Shu-Kam Mok, Thomas Wai-Tong Leung, and Philip James Johnson. "Application of classification tree and neural network algorithms to the identification of serological liver marker profiles for the diagnosis of hepatocellular carcinoma." *Oncology* 61, no. 4 (2001): 275–283.

Preis, Ori, Michael A. Blake, and James A. Scott. "Neural network evaluation of PET scans of the liver: A potentially useful adjunct in clinical interpretation." *Radiology* 258, no. 3 (2011): 714–721.

Reddy, Raja, and Timothy D. Imler. "Artificial neural networks are highly predictive for hepatocellular carcinoma in patients with cirrhosis." *Gastroenterology* 152, no. 5 (2017): S1193.

Saillard, Charlie, Benoit Schmauch, Oumeima Laifa, Matahi Moarii, Sylvain Toldo, Mikhail Zaslavskiy, Elodie Pronier, et al. "Predicting survival after hepatocellular carcinoma resection using deep learning on histological slides." *Hepatology* 72, no. 6 (2020): 2000–2013.

Sato, Masaya, Kentaro Morimoto, Shigeki Kajihara, Ryosuke Tateishi, Shuichiro Shiina, Kazuhiko Koike, and Yutaka Yatomi. "Machine-learning approach for the development of a novel predictive model for the diagnosis of hepatocellular carcinoma." *Scientific Reports* 9, no. 1 (2019): 1–7.

Sato, Masaya, Ryosuke Tateishi, Yutaka Yatomi, and Kazuhiko Koike. "Artificial intelligence in the diagnosis and management of hepatocellular carcinoma." *Journal of Gastroenterology and Hepatology* 36, no. 3 (2021): 551–560.

Schmauch, B., P. Herent, P. Jehanno, O. Dehaene, C. Saillard, Christophe Aubé, Alain Luciani, N. Lassau, and S. Jégou. "Diagnosis of focal liver lesions from ultrasound using deep learning." *Diagnostic and Interventional Imaging* 100, no. 4 (2019): 227–233.

Schoenberg, Markus Bo, Julian Nikolaus Bucher, Dominik Koch, Nikolaus Börner, Sebastian Hesse, Enrico Narciso De Toni, Max Seidensticker, et al. "A novel machine learning algorithm to predict disease free survival after resection of hepatocellular carcinoma." *Annals of Translational Medicine* 8, no. 7 (2020).

Sieghart, Wolfgang, Florian Hucke, Matthias Pinter, Ivo Graziadei, Wolfgang Vogel, Christian Mueller, Harald Heinzl, Michael Trauner, and Markus Peck-Radosavljevic. "The ART of decision making: Retreatment with transarterial chemoembolization in patients with hepatocellular carcinoma." *Hepatology* 57, no. 6 (2013): 2261–2273.

Singal, Amit G., Ashin Mukherjee, B. Joseph Elmunzer, Peter D.R. Higgins, Anna S. Lok, Ji Zhu, Jorge A. Marrero, and Akbar K. Waljee. "Machine learning algorithms outperform conventional regression models in predicting development of hepatocellular carcinoma." *The American Journal of Gastroenterology* 108, no. 11 (2013): 1723.

Szolovits, Peter. "Artificial intelligence and medicine." In *Artificial Intelligence in Medicine*, pp. 1–19. Routledge, 2019.

Tiyarattanachai, Thodsawit, Terapap Apiparakoon, Sanparith Marukatat, Sasima Sukcharoen, Nopavut Geratikornsupuk, Nopporn Anukulkarnkusol, Parit Mekaroonkamol, et al. "Development and validation of artificial intelligence to detect and diagnose liver lesions from ultrasound images." *PLoS ONE* 16, no. 6 (2021): e0252882.

Tiyarattanachai, Thodsawit, Terapap Apiparakoon, Sanparith Marukatat, Sasima Sukcharoen, Sirinda Yimsawad, Oracha Chaichuen, Siwat Bhumiwat, et al. "The feasibility to use artificial intelligence to aid detecting focal liver lesions in real-time ultrasound: A preliminary study based on videos." *Scientific Reports* 12, no. 1 (2022): 1–12.

Turco, Simona, Thodsawit Tiyarattanachai, Kambez Ebrahimkheil, John Eisenbrey, Aya Kamaya, Massimo Mischi, Andrej Lyshchik, and Ahmed El Kaffas. "Interpretable machine learning for characterization of focal liver lesions by contrast-enhanced ultrasound." *IEEE Transactions on Ultrasonics, Ferroelectrics, and Frequency Control* 69, no. 5 (2022): 1670–1681.

Urhut, Cristiana Marinela, Costin Theodor Streaba, Ion Rogoveanu, Madalin Mamuleanu, Suzana Danoiu, and Daniela Larisa Sandulescu. "Evaluation of liver tumors by using artificial intelligence in contrast-enhanced ultrasound." *Ultrasound in Medicine & Biology* 48 (2022): S21.

Villanueva, Augusto, and Josep M. Llovet. "Targeted therapies for hepatocellular carcinoma." *Gastroenterology* 140, no. 5 (2011): 1410–1426.

Vivanti, Refael, Adi Szeskin, Naama Lev-Cohain, Jacob Sosna, and Leo Joskowicz. "Automatic detection of new tumors and tumor burden evaluation in longitudinal liver CT scan studies." *International Journal of Computer Assisted Radiology and Surgery* 12, no. 11 (2017): 1945–1957.

Xu, Xun, Hai-Long Zhang, Qiu-Ping Liu, Shu-Wen Sun, Jing Zhang, Fei-Peng Zhu, Guang Yang, Xu Yan, Yu-Dong Zhang, and Xi-Sheng Liu. "Radiomic analysis of contrast-enhanced CT predicts microvascular invasion and outcome in hepatocellular carcinoma." *Journal of Hepatology* 70, no. 6 (2019): 1133–1144.

Yasaka, Koichiro, Hiroyuki Akai, Osamu Abe, and Shigeru Kiryu. "Deep learning with convolutional neural network for differentiation of liver masses at dynamic contrast-enhanced CT: A preliminary study." *Radiology* 286, no. 3 (2018): 887–896.

Zhang, Chaoyang, Li Peng, Yaqin Zhang, Zhaoyang Liu, Wenling Li, Shilian Chen, and Guancheng Li. "The identification of key genes and pathways in hepatocellular carcinoma by bioinformatics analysis of high-throughput data." *Medical Oncology* 34, no. 6 (2017): 1–13.

Zhang, Fan, Junlin Yang, Nariman Nezami, Fabian Laage-Gaupp, Julius Chapiro, Ming De Lin, and James Duncan. "Liver tissue classification using an auto-context-based deep neural network with a multi-phase training framework." In *International Workshop on Patch-based Techniques in Medical Imaging*, pp. 59–66. Springer, 2018.

Ziv, Etay, Hooman Yarmohammadi, F. Edward Boas, Elena Nadia Petre, Karen T. Brown, Stephen B. Solomon, David Solit, Diane Reidy, and Joseph P. Erinjeri. "Gene signature associated with upregulation of the Wnt/β-catenin signaling pathway predicts tumor response to transarterial embolization." *Journal of Vascular and Interventional Radiology* 28, no. 3 (2017): 349–355.

10 Artificial Intelligence Applied to Neuromotor Rehabilitation Engineering

Advances and Challenges

Cristian David Guerrero-Mendez,*
Cristian Felipe Blanco-Díaz,†,*
*Sebastián Jaramillo-Isaza**,*
Teodiano Freire Bastos-Filho, and*
*Andrés Felipe Ruiz-Olaya***
*Federal University of Espírito Santo, Postgraduate Program in Electrical Engineering, Vitoria, Brazil; **Antonio Nariño University, Faculty of Mechanical, Electronic and Biomedical Engineering, Bogotá, Colombia
†Corresponding Author: cristian.diaz@edu.ufes.br

ABBREVIATIONS

ADLs	Activities of daily living
AI	Artificial intelligence
ALS	Amyotrophic lateral sclerosis
ALSFRS	ALS functional rating scale
ANN	Artificial neural network
BCI	Brain–computer interface
BMI	Brain–machine interface
BPNN	Backpropagation neural network
CC	Coefficient of correlation
CNN	Convolutional neural network
CNS	Central nervous system
Conv-LSTM	Stacked convolutional and long short-term memory network
DBN	Dynamic Bayesian network
DL	Deep learning
DOF	Degrees of freedom
DT	Decision tree

DOI: 10.1201/9781032699882-10

EC	Ensemble classifier
EcoG	Electrocorticography
EEG	Electroencephalography
EOG	Electrooculography
ERP	Event-related potential
FFNN	Feed-forward neural network
Het-TCN	Heterogeneous kernel-based temporal convolutional network
hHMI	Hybrid human–machine interface
HMI	Human–machine interface
HRI	Human–robot interaction
IMU	Inertial measurement units
IoT	Internet of Things
ITR	Information transfer rate
KNN	k-nearest neighbors
LDA	Linear discriminant analysis
LR	Linear regression
LRCN	Long-term recurrent convolution network
LR-LSTM	Linear regression and LSTM-integrated method
LSTM	Long short-term memory
MEG	Magnetoencephalography
MI	Motor imagery
ML	Machine learning
MLP	Multi-layer perceptron
mLR	Multiple linear regression
MRI	Magnetic resonance imaging
MS	Multiple sclerosis
NB	Naïve Bayes
OCT	Optical coherence tomography
PBP	Progressive bulbar palsy
PD	Parkinson's disease
PET	Positron emission tomography
PMA	Progressive muscular atrophy
PNS	Peripheral nervous systems
QDA	Quadratic discriminant analysis
R^2	Coefficient of determination
RMSE	Root mean square error
RNN	Recurrent neural network
SAE-DNN	Stacked autoencoder-based deep neural network
sEMG	Surface electromyography
SMA	Spinal muscular atrophy
SNR	Signal-to-noise ratio
soft-DTW	Smoothed version of the dynamic time warping neural network
SSVEP	Steady-state visually evoked potentials
SVM	Support vector machine
SVR	Support vector regression
UKF	Unscented Kalman filter decoder
VS	Vital sign

10.1 INTRODUCTION

Motor impairment is the partial or total loss of function of a body part, usually a limb or limbs. This may result in muscle weakness, poor stamina, lack of muscle control, or total paralysis. Motor impairment is often evident in neurological conditions such as cerebral palsy, Parkinson's disease, stroke, and multiple sclerosis (Gilja et al. 2015). Such conditions typically affect movement, gross motor ability, gait, posture, fine motor ability, muscle weakness and fatigue, impaired sensation and poor balance, and muscle contracture and spasticity, all of which are required to carry out most of the daily activities. Thus, motor impairment is a major cause of physical disability. The World Health Organization (WHO) defines rehabilitation as "a set of interventions designed to optimize functioning and reduce disability in individuals with health conditions in interaction with their environment" (World Health Organization (WHO) 2013). It is estimated that between 76% and 85% of people with disabilities in developing countries have not accessed diagnostic, treatment, or follow-up programs (World Health Organization (WHO) 2013). The 2030 Agenda for Sustainable Development promotes health and well-being for people requiring rehabilitation. It emphasizes universal health coverage (UHC) to ensure a sustainable development for everybody.

Rehabilitation engineering is the use of engineering principles to 1) develop technological solutions and devices to assist individuals with disabilities and 2) aid in the recovery of physical and cognitive functions lost because of disease or injury (National Institute of Biomedical Imaging and Bioengineering (NIBIB) 2013). Thus, rehabilitation engineering has recently emerged with the aim of applying various technologies (sensing, actuation, control, signal processing, etc.) to help in the rehabilitation and assistance processes of disabled people.

Artificial intelligence (AI) is an area of computer science born in the middle of the 1950s that can solve problems and perform several tasks that typically require human intelligence by using algorithms, computing frameworks, probability, and other kinds of uncertainties (Ertel 2017; Stuart J. Russell and Peter Norvig 2003). Nowadays, AI is changing almost every industry and every field of human everyday life. Its applications in medical practice and biomedical engineering are expanding into areas that were previously thought to be only the province of human experts, such as disease detection, diagnosis, risk predictions, treatment selection, data processing, and the design of devices (Bhardwaj, Banyal, and Sharma 2019; K.-H. Yu, Beam, and Kohane 2018).

In rehabilitation engineering, technologies, including artificial intelligence, have provided systems that improve the quality of life in people with some neuromotor disabilities. Emerging technological developments in machine learning (supervised and unsupervised learning), deep learning, neural networks, fuzzy logic, and artificial intelligence play an important role in rehabilitation engineering to meet the specific needs of motor-disabled people during their rehabilitation process.

The integration of artificial intelligence and rehabilitation devices is becoming a potential tool to enhance physical therapy traditional. These devices offer a follow-up of measurable parameters during supervision and intervention by the therapist; furthermore, they provide feedback with quantitative information about the rehabilitation process. Thus, the integration of artificial intelligence and rehabilitation engineering aids reach goals from the 2030 Agenda for Sustainable Development. Considering this, the use of AI proposes different advances and challenges related to rehabilitation systems for neuromotor disabilities that will be discussed in this chapter.

10.2 ADVANCES IN REHABILITATION ENGINEERING

10.2.1 Classification Techniques for Device Control

As aforementioned, supervised learning allows the finding of patterns that come from historic data by linking the input features with a marked output, known as class. This type of problem is called classification, and has been widely used for the development of rehabilitation techniques because, considering the information source, it is possible to decode the user's intention and, in a discrete form, associate it with a task to be executed, e.g., device control (Nizamis et al. 2021). Figure 10.1 summarizes the classification process considering the input and output variables. In the field of neurorehabilitation, it is of great importance to consider the individual's range of movement, as well as the source information that allows an adequate recognition of the intention, as well as the individual's comfortability with the sensors. For this reason, AI classification techniques have been combined with different kinds of sensors for rehabilitation device control, as shown in Figure 10.1. Among them, it is possible to highlight in the last years' sensors based on biomechanics and bioelectric information. The most used sensors in rehabilitation sciences are those that can be placed in a non-invasive way on the individual, allowing enough relevant information to be measured with the highest possible SNR. Thus, this section focuses on classification techniques applied to sEMG, EEG, biomechanical, and hybrid sensors.

10.2.1.1 Surface Electromyography (sEMG)

Surface electromyography consists of a measurement technique of muscular electrical activity with electrodes located on the skin. This technique has been widely implemented in assistance technology and rehabilitation for the control of prostheses and orthoses, among others. However, these signals have problems related to SNR, added to the fact

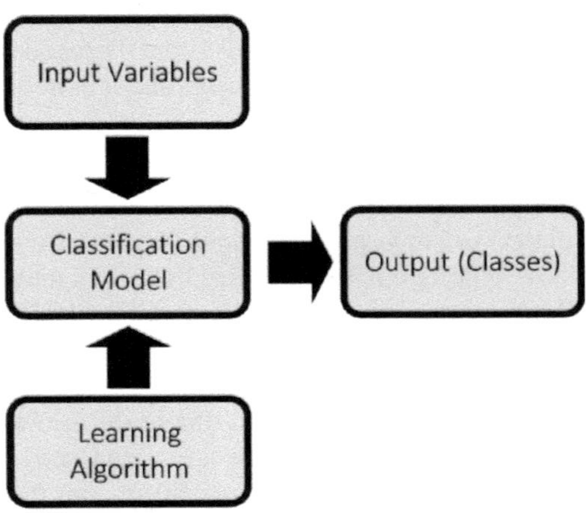

FIGURE 10.1 Classification methodology using AI techniques.

TABLE 10.1
Accuracy of Some Existing sEMG Classification Methods

Authors	Classifiers	Number of Classes (Movements)	Accuracy (%)
(Sui, Wan, and Zhang 2019)	SVM	6	90.66
(Williams et al. 2022)	CNN	5	92
(Azlan Abu et al. 2020)	MLP	5	80
(Gao et al. 2020)	SVM	3	90
(S. Lee, Sung, and Choi 2020)	CNN	8	91.3
(Too et al. 2019)	KNN	17	93
(Hu et al. 2018)	CNN	4	94
(Morbidoni et al. 2019)	MLP	2 (gait cycle)	95
(Too et al. 2018)	SVM	10	95
(Yang et al. 2018)	LDA, MLP, SVM	9	96, 97 and 99
(Ishii, Murooka, and Tajima 2016)	SVM	7	89.7

that the activation of motor units is required for recognition, which generates limitations in people whose PNS is at a critical level of disability. Thus, information transfer in the nerve–muscle link is practically impossible. In addition, one of the challenges in sEMG acquisition is the correct placement of the electrodes to allow high movement decoding using as few sources as possible with enough accuracy (Fang et al. 2020). For this reason, sEMG has been combined with AI classification techniques to identify the patient's intention with information from a group of resting muscles with high accuracy. Different classification methods have been used, such as deep, incremental, and machine learning methods. Among the methods that are highlighted are SVM, CNN, and MPL, among others, which can be used to identify different movements in multiclass problems. Some of these methods used in the last years are available in Table 10.1.

As shown in Table 10.1, these classification algorithms provide accuracy suitable to decode movements through sEMG signals by using ML techniques. The most used features are in the time domain, which have been used toward the construction of neuromotor rehabilitation devices related to myoelectric prostheses and orthoses (Fang et al. 2020).

10.2.1.2 Electroencephalography (EEG)

EEG is a technique in which it is possible to get brain information through non-invasive electrodes placed on the scalp. This method is used in the design of rehabilitation systems whose objective is to recognize the user's intention by generating patterns in the cerebral cortex related to the execution of different tasks. These systems are known as BCI or BMI. Such systems are very useful for neuromotor rehabilitation because they work as a bridge between the user and the environment without using the PNS but using the CNS data (the brain). However, in the field of neuroengineering, pattern recognition is challenging, considering the low SNR of EEG signals (order of μV), the inter-subject variability, and the involved artifacts due to physiological conditions, among others (Padfield et al. 2019; Cristian Felipe

Blanco-Díaz, Guerrero-Méndez, Bastos-Filho et al. 2022). For this reason, classification techniques are very useful for the identification of brain patterns and the control of neuromotor rehabilitation systems, such as prostheses, exoskeletons, and wheelchairs, among others. The most decoded patterns are related to the paradigms of MI, ERP-P300, and SSVEP (Cristian David Guerrero-Mendez, Blanco-Diaz, and Ruiz-Olaya 2021a; C.F. Blanco-Díaz, Guerrero-Méndez, and Ruiz-Olaya 2023). Following are the details of each paradigm:

- MI is a technique where the user must imagine their own movement (upper or lower limb), which is associated with a desynchronization in the parieto-central cortex in the frequency band between 8 and 30 Hz (Gert Pfurtscheller and Neuper 2003).
- ERP-P300 is a potential that appears in the parieto-central cortex of the brain approximately 300 ms after the presentation of a stimulus of interest (Picton 1992).
- SSVEPs are a form of brain response that is described by a frequency pattern at the visual stimulus frequency (or its harmonics) in the occipital cortex (Becedas 2012).

Table 10.2 shows different classification algorithms for pattern recognition using EEG signals using different paradigms. It should be highlighted that the three aforementioned paradigms are very different respecting the phenomena in the brain. For this reason, the application changes, and the classification problem can be binary or multiclass.

The BCI community has been working on the construction of new algorithms from traditional ML strategies to DL architectures due to the currently available computing resources. The classification of EEG is currently possible thanks to the

TABLE 10.2
Accuracy of Some Existing EEG Classification Methods by Paradigm

Authors	Classifiers	Paradigm	Accuracy (%)
(Blanco-Diaz, Antelis, and Ruiz-Olaya 2022)	LDA	MI	74
(Hashmi et al. 2022)	SVM	P300	98.53
(Zhu et al. 2021)	CNN	SSVEP	81.74
(Blanco-Diaz and Ruiz Olaya 2020)	LDA	P300	83.5
(Kundu and Ari 2020)	CNN	P300	96
(M.-H. Lee et al. 2019)	LDA	P300	96
(Amin et al. 2019)	CNN	MI	75.7
(Acevedo et al. 2019)	LDA	P300	78
(H. K. Lee and Choi 2018)	CNN	MI	78.93
(Kong et al. 2018)	ANN	P300	72
(Cristian David Guerrero-Mendez, Blanco-Diaz, and Ruiz-Olaya 2021b)	CCA	SSVEP	95

use of such cutting-edge techniques, making possible the reduction of calibration times and allowing the implementation in real-time scenarios as control of rehabilitation devices.

10.2.1.3 Biomechanical Sensors

Biomechanical sensing can be considered the use of mechanical sensors adapted to the body. The most used, due to their advantages in real-time acquisition and costs, are inertial sensors (IMUs) and force-based sensors. Force-based sensors allow recording of the muscle activity in the force domain, which can be measured from the local pressure change at the sensor location (Jiang et al. 2022). This kind of sensor has been used in hand gesture recognition to control prosthetic devices, making use of ML algorithms to identify different movements of the subjects and to discretize the user's intention. In this context, Belyea *et al.* reported in their research the use of SVM for the classification of five different hand movements by using sensors of force, with an accuracy of approximately 90% (Belyea, Englehart, and Scheme 2019). IMU is a combination of accelerometers and gyroscopes (and sometimes magnetometers as well) that allows measuring inertial variables based on movement, which is useful for the control of rehabilitation devices. Different classification methods have been used to recognize hand gestures. For instance, Liu *et al.* used ANN to classify eight different hand movements, whereas Ommeren *et al.* used SVM to identify four grasp tasks of post-stroke patients. On the other hand, Hwang *et al.* used SVM to classify different hand tasks and performed a comparison of performance between healthy users and post-stroke patients using an ML algorithm (Liu et al. 2022; van Ommeren et al. 2019; Hwang, Lu, and Lin 2022). Classification techniques have also been combined with IMU for the identification of lower-limb movements toward exoskeleton control. For instance, Tanna *et al.* reported an accuracy of 90% for the classification of eight foot moves of healthy users by using SVM (Tanna and Vithalani 2022), and Brand *et al.* used CNN and a combination of ANN to classify pathological gait between healthy users and Parkinson patients, obtaining 99% accuracy (Brand et al. 2022). Other types of sensors used for motion analysis involved in biomechanics studies can be found in high-speed camera-based devices, which have been widely used in the literature for motion analysis (Guerrero-Méndez et al. 2021; Cristian David Guerrero-Méndez, Moreno-Arévalo et al. 2021).

10.2.1.4 Hybrid HMI (hHMI)

When an AI cannot classify the problem with the appropriate metrics, it is necessary to improve the information source. In this context, hHMI proposes a combination strategy among different channels on different interaction levels, generating systems with more physiological compression (implying more robust systems) through data fusion implementation. For example, an hHMI would allow the BCIs the option of increasing both the number of commands and the ITR by implementing techniques of the combination of sEMG signals (Cristian D. Guerrero-Mendez and Ruiz-Olaya 2022). For instance, Tortora *et al.* in their study reported an increase in accuracy of approximately 20% by combining EEG and sEMG features (Tortora et al. 2020). On the other hand, Hooda *et al.* reached an accuracy close to 94% by using an

EEG–sEMG fusion (Hooda, Das, and Kumar 2020). Also, biomechanical sensors have been combined with sEMG to make more robust the decoding of a user's intention in grasp movements. For instance, Belyea *et al.* obtained a 90% classification rate by using force-based sensors and sEMG (Belyea, Englehart, and Scheme 2019). Yuk *et al.* reached an accuracy close to 98% with an ANN for the classification of four hand movements by using the information of sEMG and IMUs (Yuk and Sohn 2022). For lower limbs, Li *et al.* implemented a CNN for the classification of four different daily movement patterns using information from sEMG and IMUs located on an individual's legs, reaching 97% of accuracy in the recognition (Li et al. 2022).

10.2.2 Regression Models of Rehabilitation Techniques

According to the regression models in the scientific literature, different approaches have been found to predict values related to linear and nonlinear regression models (Fahrmeir et al. 2021). The simplest regression model is presented in Equation 1, which is the linear model with a single independent variable. Another type of model is found in multivariate linear regression with multiple independent inputs. On the other hand, nonlinear regression describes the nonlinear relationship in experimental data that can be modeled using polynomial regression. According to this, AI techniques typically use non-parametric and nonlinear regression models due to the experimental data in a real application, which are not ideal and regularly do not exhibit Gaussian distributions (Fahrmeir et al. 2021).

$$V_{out} = \delta_0 + \delta_1 V_{int} + \in, \tag{1}$$

where V_{out} is the output variable, i.e., the dependent estimate variable; V_{int} is the input variable, i.e., the independent variable that acts as a predictor; δ_0 is the y-intercept; δ_1 is the regression coefficient; and $\in$ is the error term.

For rehabilitation engineering, regression models have been used to estimate and predict kinematics and kinetics in the upper- and lower-limb movements to be applied to the motor rehabilitation of ADLs, such as reach-to-grasp tasks and walking (C. Chen et al. 2021; Meattini et al. 2022; Pei et al. 2022; Sosnik and Zheng 2021). Another application in motor rehabilitation is related to the prediction of the user intention to generate more controllability, usability, and reliability in robotics devices (Bi, Feleke, and Guan 2019). Different sources of information related to non-biological signals have been applied to predict user intention, such as head pose, hand position and orientation, and kinematic parameters, among others (Blanco-Diaz et al. 2021; Bi, Feleke, and Guan 2019; Giarmatzis, Zacharaki, and Moustakas 2020). However, biological signals are the most interesting information source to the scientific community due to the ability to obtain more natural and fluent movements in robotics applications. The main techniques for recording biological information are sEMG and EEG signals, as they are non-invasive techniques. However, other biological signals such as EOG (Usakli et al. 2010), ECoG (Schalk and Leuthardt 2011; Jang et al. 2022), and MEG (Yeom, Kim, and Chung 2013) have been applied in the estimation and prediction of kinematic and kinetic parameters.

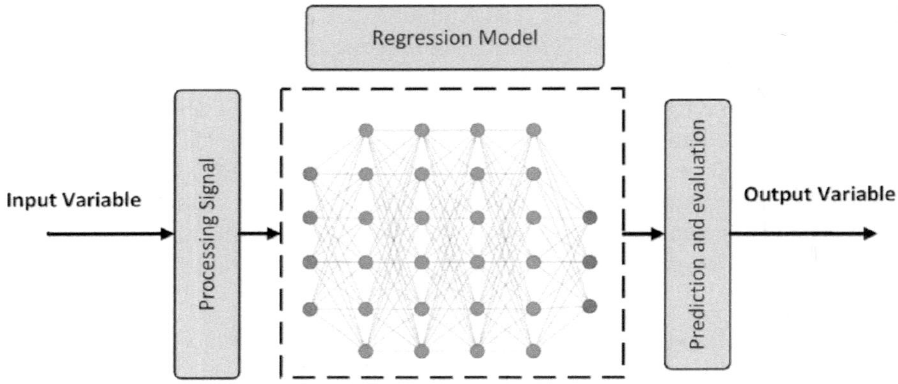

FIGURE 10.2 Block diagram for regression applications.

The methodology for regression application is presented in Figure 10.2. For the input variable, it is usually necessary to perform signal processing to eliminate outliers by means of filters or to extract temporal, frequency, or spatial features. These approaches depend on the objective of the research question. Subsequently, regression models are applied according to the variation of hyperparameter settings of the AI methods. The predicted or estimated values are then obtained and compared with the actual values to validate the models and be used for future applications. Considering that for neuromotor rehabilitation, the main techniques applied are sEMG and EEG, in this section, only these techniques are considered.

10.2.2.1 sEMG Approaches

Recently, the sEMG recording technique has been used to predict and estimate different postures, forces, and torques in the limb movements for motor rehabilitation. Some applications of sEMG signals using different regression models are presented in Table 10.3. Some authors define two different approaches to sEMG-based motion prediction. In this, the model-based approach estimates the relationship between the input and the output variables, that is, the relationship between the sEMG signals and the kinematic, dynamic, and musculoskeletal models using different parameters such as position, orientation, velocity, acceleration, and force, among others (Bi, Feleke, and Guan 2019). The other approach is that of free models that use numerical functions to estimate the values of the input variable to the desired target variable. In this case, sEMG is used as an input variable to estimate kinematic parameters (Bi, Feleke, and Guan 2019).

Several AI approaches have been proposed to estimate kinematic and kinetic parameters from sEMG signals in different applications related to upper- and lower-limb motor rehabilitation. The main approach is related to the implementation of different DL methods from the simplest to the most robust and complex neural networks. The applications in motor rehabilitation are found in the estimation of upper- and lower-limb angles, forces on the grasp objects, and assembly torques in upper limbs tasks, among others presented in Table 10.3. These estimates can be applied in robotic devices

TABLE 10.3
Some AI Approaches using sEMG Signals in Regression Models for Motor Rehabilitation

No	Parameter/Action (Estimation or Prediction)	Approach	Performance	Reference
1	Hip, knee, and ankle joint angles	Conv-LSTM	R^2—0.9334	(Y. Lu et al. 2022)
2	Force in press gesture	LR-LSTM	R^2—0.9604	(Hua, Wang, and Wu 2022)
3	Torque in upper limb tasks	Het-TCN/CNN/LSTM	RMSE—0.09 R^2—0.72	(C. Chen et al. 2021)
4	Grasping postures	soft-DTW	R^2—0.7878 RMSE—0.133	(Meattini et al. 2022)
5	Multiple degrees of freedom (DoFs) kinetics of wrist	SAE-DNN/SVR/LR	R^2—0.82	(Y. Yu et al. 2020)
6	Angular motion of shoulder abduction, forward flexion, spin, and elbow flexion	MLP/LSTM	R^2—0.9171 RMSE—5.53	(Yan Chen et al. 2019)
7	Knee joint angle	LRCN	MAE—0.081	(Gautam et al. 2020)
8	Force intention	CNN/RNN	RMSE—1.435	(Yuyang Chen, Dai, and Chen 2020)
9	Upper limb joint torque	BPNN	RMSE—0.7383 R^2—0.9886	(N. Yang et al. 2022)

to perform rehabilitation of more natural and complex movements related to ADLs. In addition, this improves controllability, usability, and reliability in the use of neuromotor rehabilitation devices such as neuroprostheses, considering the reported high performance. However, more AI applications are found in the literature using sEMG as an input variable to estimate continuous variables such as kinematic and kinetic parameters. Xiong *et al.* present the role of DL approaches in sEMG-based HMIs (Xiong et al. 2021). And Bi *et al.* presented a review of sEMG-based prediction of continuous upper limb movements using different AI approaches (Bi, Feleke, and Guan 2019).

10.2.2.2 EEG Approaches

Recently, there has been a trend to use brain patterns recorded mainly by EEG signals to estimate kinematic variables of upper- and lower-limb movements due to the great application in motor rehabilitation of people with stroke. Stroke is the main cause of disability related to motor limitation of limb movements due to the generated loss of muscle control and coordination (Robinson et al. 2021). However, decoding brain patterns can be a difficult task due to the limitation of the EEG signals related to the low SNR, non-stationary condition, and inter- and intra-subject variability. In addition, predicting values from EEG signals turns out to be more complicated than classification approaches, since regression must approximate fit lines according to the data, and classification determines a discrete decision from the data (Giuseppe Bonaccorso 2017; Fahrmeir et al. 2021). Considering this, to reduce the limitations of EEG and improve the performance of BCI systems, several authors have proposed as a solution the use of more robust and complex AI methods to decode brain patterns, such as the application of DL neural networks (Xiong et al. 2021; R. Zhang et al. 2020).

Currently, in motor rehabilitation, the most interesting application of EEG signals is to predict different kinematic and kinetic parameters in gait movement (Nakagome et al. 2020; Juan et al. 2022; He et al. 2018). Through gait analysis, physicians and therapists can detect and evaluate motor pathologies. For this reason, the prediction of kinematic parameters related to lower-limb movements in gait can be an important tool to facilitate the evaluation of motor pathologies. In addition, the application of AI methods may allow better acquisition and better monitoring of the evolution of patients with motor disabilities (Cristian Felipe Blanco-Díaz, Guerrero-Méndez, Duarte-González et al. 2022). Table 10.4 presents different works related to the estimation of gait kinematic parameters.

Another interesting and recent application of EEG signals to estimate kinematic parameters is based on the MI paradigm. As aforementioned, in the MI paradigm, people must generate patterns related to the imagination of a movement without performing a voluntary muscle contraction. In this new approach, for instance, people must imagine a direct kinematic trajectory of their upper limb movements in a reach-to-grasp task (Sosnik and Zheng 2021; Jang et al. 2022). This can lead to motor rehabilitation of more natural and complex movements such as those involved in ADLs to control robotic devices with various degrees of freedom. Furthermore, with this trajectory estimation, more realistic environments can be developed, and BCI systems can increase control in continuous approaches with high usability and controllability to command these devices. Some works related to trajectory estimation are presented in Table 10.4.

TABLE 10.4
Some AI Approaches Using EEG Signals in Regression Models for Motor Rehabilitation

No	Parameter/Action (Estimation or Prediction)	Approach	Performance	Reference
1	Kinematics of lower-limb movements during walking	Different DL and ML methods	R^2—0.4	(Nakagome et al. 2020)
2	Torque of lower-limb joints in pre-gait movements	MLP	CC—0.86	(Mercado et al. 2021)
3	Hip joint angle in treadmill walking	UKF	R^2—0.64	(He et al. 2018)
4	Lower-limb angles	UKF	CC—0.71	(Luu et al. 2019)
5	Decode lower-limb kinematics	mLR	CC—0.42	(Juan et al. 2022)
6	Kinematic parameters in imagined 3D trajectories	mLR	CC—0.28	(Sosnik and Zheng 2021)
7	The imagined 3D trajectory of the hand joint	mLR	CC—0.60	(Korik et al. 2018)
8	Synergy-based hand kinematics	mLR	CC—0.70	(Pei et al. 2022)
9	Muscle activity and kinematics of hand movements	DL	CC—0.85	(Kumarasinghe, Kasabov, and Taylor 2021)

10.2.2.3 Performance Measurement

To validate the regression models, different performance metrics related to correlation or percentage error have been implemented by several authors. This validation is performed using gold standard measurements (target data) and input data used to estimate or predict the continuous values. According to the application of regression models in motor rehabilitation related to the estimation of kinematic and kinetic variables, the gold standard measurements are related to the use of devices that allow recording these types of variables. To mention a few, these can be IMUs, cameras, force sensors, and pressure platforms. Nevertheless, the main metrics used are presented in Equations 2–4.

$$RMSE = \sqrt{\sum_{i=1}^{N} \frac{(\gamma_i - \beta_i)^2}{N}}, \tag{2}$$

$$CC = \frac{\sum_{i=1}^{N} (\gamma_i - \overline{\gamma})(\beta_i - \overline{\beta})}{\sqrt{\sum_{i=1}^{N} (\gamma_i - \overline{\gamma})^2 \sum_{i=1}^{N} (\beta_i - \overline{\beta})^2}}, \tag{3}$$

$$R^2 = 1 - \frac{\sum_{i=1}^{N} (\beta_i - \gamma_i)^2}{\sum_{i=1}^{N} (\beta_i - \overline{\beta})^2}, \tag{4}$$

where γ is the estimated value; β is the real value; $\overline{\gamma}$ and $\overline{\beta}$ are the means of the estimated and real value, respectively; N is the length of the data point vector; and i is the index of the position in the data point vector. Other performance metrics applied in the regression models for offline and online implementations are described in (Bi, Feleke, and Guan 2019).

10.2.3 Neuromotor Disease Estimation

According to the latest World Health Organization (WHO) report on disability, approximately 2.2% of the global population has limitations in motor functions derived from a disability (World Health Organization (WHO) 2011). There are several causes that generate loss of motor functions; these include spinal cord injury, amputations, stroke, amyotrophic lateral sclerosis, and paralysis, among others (Kandel et al. 2000). Accordingly, AI methods have been implemented to predict and prognosticate neuromotor disabilities, as well as to determine the neurological effects that can be triggered (Myszczynska et al. 2020; Fernandes et al. 2021; Ahlrichs and Lawo 2013). These AI approaches generate great benefits for the public health system due to the reduction of costs for motor rehabilitation processes in this population. In addition, they improve the quality of life of people with motor problems, considering that motor activities are of special importance in the development of essential tasks in the support of daily life. A summary of the application of AI methods for disease estimation is presented in Figure 10.3.

The increased use of regression-based AI methods is because they can learn specific patterns from the input data in the training phase to generate a prediction in

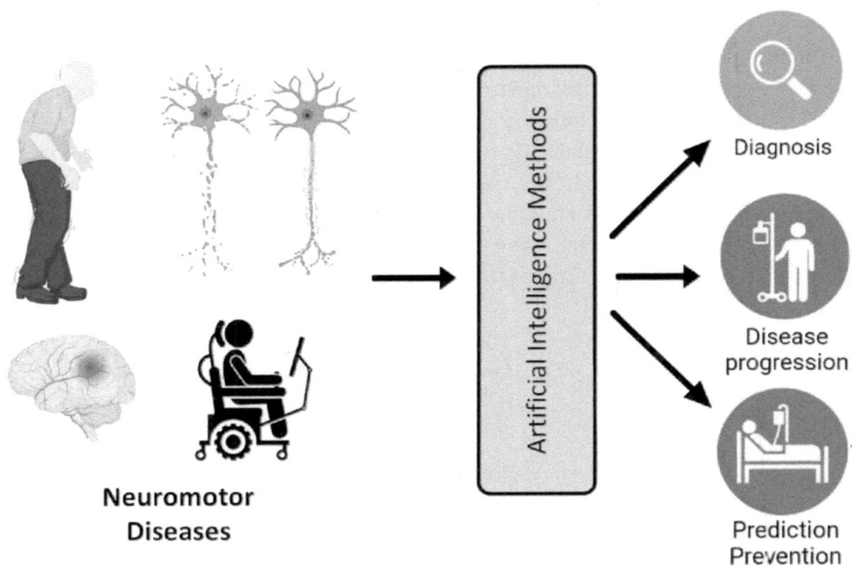

FIGURE 10.3 Summary of the use of AI in the estimation of neuromotor diseases.

the evaluation of the new data. This interest is also due to the recent increase in the amount of clinical data available that can be used in the exploration and creation of new tools based on predictive data to be applied for the benefit of the healthcare system in the early detection of pathologies affecting motor functions (Campagnini et al. 2022). However, ML methods currently perform poorly in reliably predicting data that generate automatic responses to neurological effects of pathologies, which affect monitoring in health prevention (Christodoulou et al. 2019). This may be due to the complexity of data prediction in these types of applications, and because model setup and training methodologies lack more robust and deep validity. Consequently, DL-based methods have been implemented because their configuration allows for more robust processing that provides the ability to decode data in more complex applications, such as those found in the prediction of neurological effects in pathologies that generate neuromotor losses (Myszczynska et al. 2020; Pancotti et al. 2022).

In the literature, different techniques for the acquisition of biological information have been used for the prediction of different chronic pathologies, as well as for diagnosis, including sEMG, MRI, and PET, among others (Nusinovici et al. 2020; Choi et al. 2019; Myszczynska et al. 2020; Campagnini et al. 2022). Through sEMG signals, the electrical muscle activation is recorded, which allows for determining when the person has the intention to perform a movement. In addition, through this information, it is possible to determine patterns associated with a voluntary or involuntary execution of a movement (Fang et al. 2020). Therefore, these signals are of special importance in applications related to the prediction of the evolution of pathologies such as ALS, Parkinson's disease, or stroke (Campagnini et al. 2022; Fernandes et al. 2021; Ahlrichs and Lawo 2013). However, considering that Parkinson's disease generates repetitive and involuntary movements, other potential information acquisition techniques are found in IMUs and EEG signals (Ahlrichs and Lawo 2013; Maitin, Romero Muñoz, and García-Tejedor 2022). On the other hand, in pathologies such as ALS, other types of biological information related to VS such as blood pressure, pulse, respiratory rate, and ALSFRS, among others, have been used (Pancotti et al. 2022).

Several AI approaches, presented in Table 10.5, have been used for the prediction, progression, and diagnosis of pathologies that generate motor limitations. Accordingly, the prediction of pathologies can benefit people with disabilities as well as the clinical sector in the detection of risks, to know in advance when a negative neuromotor effect will occur in the development of ADLs. The use of AI in the prediction of the progression of pathologies is of great interest in the scientific community, as it generates an early understanding of the progression of a pathology, for example, neurodegenerative, to choose the best treatment for the benefit of the patient. On the other hand, in diagnosis, AI methods help in the classification to know exactly when a pathology is occurring. Thus, the accurate detection of a pathology benefits patients and the clinical sector for the selection of an appropriate treatment. Accordingly, a recent article developed by Bede *et al.* presented a classification of different diseases affecting neuromotor functioning, among them ALS, with a percentage higher than 93% using ML approaches (Bede et al. 2022). Additionally, other types of DL applications focus on telerehabilitation for the rehabilitation and treatment of neuromotor speech disorders (Mulfari et al. 2022).

10.2.4 Robotics Applications

HRIs are technologies that acquire, process, identify, and communicate the intention of an individual to a device via control commands. Figure 10.4 shows examples of HRIs.

TABLE 10.5
AI Methods Applied to the Prediction, Progression, and Diagnosis of Neuromotor Diseases

No	Disease	Signal	Method	Goal	Reference
1	ALS	VS, ALSFRS, FVC	FFNN CNN RNN	Predict disease progression	(Pancotti et al. 2022)
2	ALS	iPSCs	CNN	Prediction	(Imamura et al. 2021)
3	ALS	VS ALSFRS	DBN	Progression	(Zandonà et al. 2019)
4	PD	Motor performance tests	LSTM	Diagnosis	(Zhao et al. 2018)
5	MS	OCT	mLR, SVM, DT, KNN, NB, EC, LSTM	Diagnosis and disability prediction	(Montolío et al. 2021)
6	ALS	sEMG	SVM	Diagnosis	(Chatterjee et al. 2019)
7	PD	MR	CNN	Diagnosis	(Sivaranjini and Sujatha 2020)
8	PD	IMU	TCN	Event detection	(Romijnders et al. 2022)

HRI is a complex field that involves AI, robotics, and the social sciences for the purpose of interaction between the user and environment through robots. Robotics devices have been used in the rehabilitation of diseases such as the explained in section 10.2.3.

For instance, robotic gloves have been implemented for the rehabilitation of diseases such as stroke in mirror therapy (Xiaoshi Chen et al. 2020) or Parkinson's detection and damping (Hwang, Lu, and Lin 2022). ML techniques, such as SVM and KNN, have been implemented to classify different hand gestures using features from sEMG (Xiaoshi Chen et al. 2020) and inertial sensors (Hwang, Lu, and Lin 2022; van Ommeren et al. 2019). Robotic hands are useful in mirror therapy and for prosthesis control for objects manipulations tasks, such as done by Blana *et al.*, who used sEMG (Blana et al. 2020), and by Chen *et al.*, who used an information hybrid of sEMG channels and inertial sensors (Xiaoshi Chen et al. 2020). For the case of amputations, robotic prostheses have been used and researched, especially in limbs with complex movements, such as the arms. Robotic arms have been combined with AI techniques for control, with EEG being used to identify the subject's intention. Studies reported by (Padfield et al. 2019) and (Xiaogang Chen et al. 2019) show different types of hand prostheses controlled by EEG signal decoding in MI and SSVEP paradigms, respectively. In addition, Yuk *et al.* show a robotic arm that is controlled by ANN based on information from inertial sensors and sEMG (Yuk and Sohn 2022).

Other approaches of ML for robotic control correspond to exoskeletons, such as those done by (Brambilla et al. 2021), where exoskeletons of the upper and lower limb are used as a robotic device for the rehabilitation of diseases related to hemiparesis, using sEMG and EEG signals for decoding the user's intention. In addition, Azam *et al.* also reported in their study the design of a lower-limb neurorobotic system controlled by EEG signals, using classifiers such as KNN, LDA, and QDA for the rehabilitation of spinal cord injury (Khan et al. 2018). Also, Xu *et al.* reported an upper limb exoskeleton controlled by SSVEP obtained from EEG signals by using linear classifiers (Xu et al. 2022).

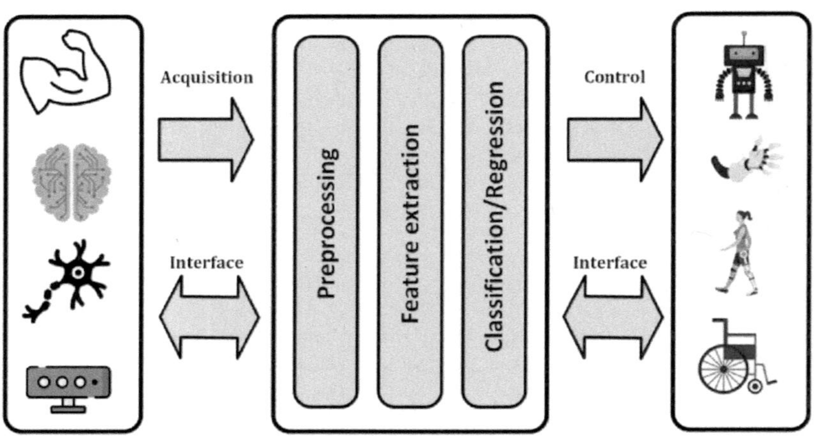

FIGURE 10.4 HRIs are involved in the human intention (EEG, sEMG, kinematics, force-based) and include processing, feature extraction, classification/regression, and finally the control commands for various assistive, rehabilitation, or prosthetic devices.

Previously speaking about lower-limb rehabilitation and assistance techniques, it is also important to highlight the use of assistive treadmills, such as in the study by Hammida *et al.*, who report the use of DL on treadmills for patient monitoring during a walking process with video projections for feedback (Hamidah et al. 2019), or the study reported by Herbert and Munz implementing LSTM-based techniques for the detection of ERPs during gait performance (Herbert and Munz 2020).

Among other AI techniques combined with robotic devices, the use of rehabilitation devices based on cycling or wheelchair tasks can be highlighted, such as the work of Romero-Laiseca *et al.*, who reported the implementation of an MI-controlled robotic unicycle for the rehabilitation of post-stroke patients using linear classifiers (Romero-Laiseca et al. 2020). On the other hand, the work published by Callejas-Cuervo *et al.* reports the use of different acquisition techniques, such as EEG, sEMG, and inertial sensors signals, combined with AI techniques as LDA, SVM, and ANN, for wheelchair navigation control (Callejas-Cuervo, González-Cely, and Bastos-Filho 2020). In addition, Chen *et al.* reported the implementation of a BCI with a wheelchair controlled by P300 and SVM (J.-W. Chen et al. 2020). Some examples of robotic applications using AI techniques are presented in Figure 10.5.

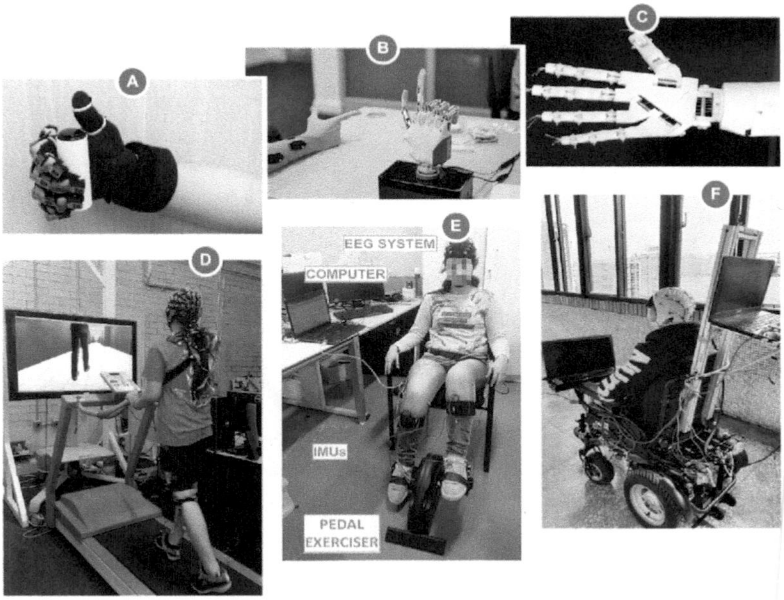

FIGURE 10.5 HRIs based on AI. (a) Glove implemented to decode hand gestures (Hwang, Lu, and Lin 2022); (b) robotic hand controlled by sEMG signals (Fang et al. 2020); (c) prosthetic hand controlled by BCI (Padfield et al. 2019); (d) HMI system based on assistive treadmill with visual feedback (He et al. 2018); (e) system based on MI and pedaling tasks (Rodríguez-Ugarte et al. 2017); (f) wheelchair controlled by SSVEP (W. Chen et al. 2022). The red square represents devices related to inertial sensors; the cyan square shows devices related to sEMG signals; the green square shows devices related to BCI; the purple square represents hybrids HMI, e.g., inertial sensors and EEG. All images presented in this figure are available under the terms of the Creative Commons Attribution 4.0 International License (https://creativecommons.org/licenses/by/4.0/).

10.3 CHALLENGES IN REHABILITATION ENGINEERING

Although technological advances have allowed an evolution in the design of rehabilitation technologies such as HRI, as well as better AI techniques that have been implemented for device control, such as those shown in section 10.2, there are still many challenges for the scientific community that limit the adequate accomplishment of the objectives in the motor rehabilitation of users. Figure 10.6 presents a summary and existing relationship of AI-related challenges in neural signal recognition and estimation, control of rehabilitation systems, and disease and pathology estimation.

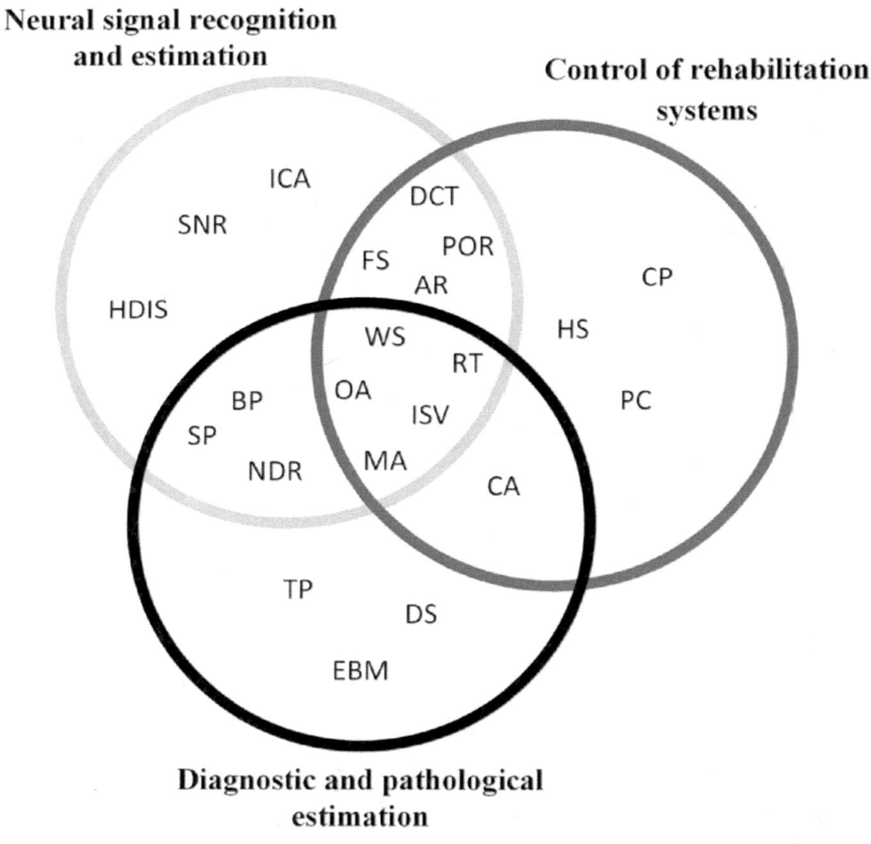

FIGURE 10.6 Coverage challenges in various areas. Wearable sensors (WS), robustness of IA techniques (RT), inter- and intra-subject variability (ISV), multimodal applications (MA), online applications (OA), cloud assistance (CA), biomechanical parameters (BP), new data repository (NDR), signal processing (SP), artifact reduction (AR), feedback to subjects (FS), portability (POR), decoding of complex tasks (DCT), physical challenges (PC), calibration personality (CP), hardware and software (HS), data security (DS), telemonitoring (TP), exploration of benchmark methods (EBM), interpretability of learning algorithms (ICA), signal-to-noise ratio (SNR), high dimensionality of information sources (HDIS).

10.3.1 Neural Signal Recognition and Estimation

Great advances have been evidenced in the field of neurorehabilitation, according to the implementation of intelligent technologies that allow the assistance and rehabilitation of motor functionalities in disabled subjects. Advances related to the use of AI are focused on the identification, estimation, or prediction of commands, as well as risks associated with diseases, in addition to the robotic applications discussed in the previous sections. Accordingly, different challenges can be identified, which are of interest to the scientific community, related to the implementation of computational methods that allow adequate pattern recognition or estimation using neural signals.

Subjects in a condition of disability related to limitations in their neuromotor functionality need methodological strategies that generate reliability in rehabilitation processes making use of technologies such as BCI or HMI systems to control robotic devices such as exoskeletons, prostheses, walkers, and wheelchairs, among others, using neural signals. Accordingly, and considering that neural signals are contaminated by artifacts, biological and non-biological, which makes decoding difficult, it is necessary to deepen processing methods that generate suitable features to be identified or estimated by AI-based algorithms with adequate performance. In this line, the exploration of robust AI-based methodologies for decoding patterns associated with the intention to perform a movement is required. This considers that paradigms immersed in BCI systems such as the MI-based one present several challenges related to the exploration of more natural and complex movement strategies. These include reach-to-grasp movements, moving objects, eating, walking, explosive jumping, running, and balancing, among others. Computationally, these paradigms can be complex to decode due to the number of neural patterns presented in the muscles or in the brain. These patterns can be associated with muscle synergies, i.e., the coordinated activation and coactivation of each muscle to execute complex movements, because each muscle is involved in a specific function in a movement (Cristian D. Guerrero-Mendez and Ruiz-Olaya 2022). Additionally, regarding brain patterns, when dealing with complex movements, more zones and sources of neuronal connection can be activated, as well as deeper phenomena in the cerebral cortex that can be found in the execution of these movements (G. Pfurtscheller and Lopes da Silva 1999; Cristian D. Guerrero-Mendez and Ruiz-Olaya 2022). Considering this, decoding can be a difficult process, so the exploration of AI-based methodologies, more specifically DL, can generate solutions in these approaches.

On the other hand, the identification of patterns in neural signals can be affected by several factors related to substance or medication consumption, subject motivation, concentration in command generation, muscle or eye fatigue, and also previous experience in the use of rehabilitation technologies, among others (Cristian Felipe Blanco-Díaz, Guerrero-Méndez, Bastos-Filho et al. 2022). However, in the literature, it has been reported that rehabilitation systems are often limited according to illiteracy in the use of technologies, generating specific inclusion criteria for their use (Allison and Neuper 2010; Wang, Du, and Dong 2021). This limits their application because the subjects are categorized as inefficient for the use of these technologies. Accordingly, it is considered that the specific use of DL could help mitigate these phenomena due to its capacity to process data with high efficiency and reliability.

Another important point in the application of technologies for rehabilitation lies in the capacity of the systems to generate an instantaneous response to stimuli, i.e., functionality in real time (online). This is important considering that feedback in the subjects generates an increase in the effectiveness of rehabilitation, in addition to generating motivation in the execution of movements or tasks in neurorehabilitation. On the other hand, feedback increases neuroplasticity in subjects who have suffered brain damage due to cerebrovascular accidents (Ang et al. 2014). Considering this, the exploration of new methodological strategies based on AI is important; however, a fundamental point in this trend is to test and ensure that these algorithms can be implemented in real time for task execution. Therefore, an open challenge for the scientific community is to develop algorithms with high efficiency and low computational cost so that they can be applied in real time and can be incorporated into low-cost technologies for neuromotor rehabilitation.

In another aspect, there are currently several technologies based on motion analysis and acquisition, such as high-speed cameras, Kinect, inertial sensors, and fiber optics, among others (Guerrero-Mendez Cristian David et al. 2021; Jiang et al. 2022). However, these technologies can be expensive if high-speed cameras are implemented; unreliable and unusable if Kinect is used; in need of constant calibrations if inertial sensors are used; and subject to information of kinematic variables without having the representation in space, that is, information without a position in cartesian planes, if fiber optics are used. Accordingly, the incorporation of AI-based methods can benefit experiments based on biomechanical analysis, as well as explore and increase the understanding of the CNS through the decoding of kinematic parameters generated by brain patterns. In this sense, it is considered that the use of AI for motion analysis incorporating neural signals can generate greater reliability in the estimation of movements, as well as reduce costs and expand applications of rehabilitation systems for the execution of more complex movements.

Finally, even rehabilitation systems present several limitations related to the number of commands that can be identified or estimated. On the other hand, the use of a single modality may not generate high performance. In addition, the public health system presents a great need to reduce costs and improve rehabilitation processes for people with motor disabilities to increase their quality of life. Considering this, a challenge that is still open is the use of more than one modality, that is, the use of more than one source of biological information or external stimuli for the control and interaction with the environment. In this sense, the exploration of methodologies that incorporate data fusion or connectivity between different signals can increase the performance of rehabilitation systems. For example, the use of EEG and sEMG has generated important results in this area (Brambilla et al. 2021). And, with the incorporation of neural networks focused on data fusion, performance can be increased when the information from both sensors is combined with methods based on adaptive strategies according to parameters related to the signals of each subject. This considering that the feature extraction phases in signal processing can be eliminated if DL methods are implemented because they implement the extraction and classification phase within the same phase (R. Zhang et al. 2020). With this, systems can be incorporated into rehabilitation with a high degree of controllability, usability, and reliability, so that people can interact with the environment in a more natural way.

10.3.2 Control of Rehabilitation Systems

Some of the problems that occur in the control of devices such as prostheses or orthoses that are related to the therapy and rehabilitation of hemiparesis or limb amputations consist of the variability of movements. In the case of hand prostheses, tasks related to grasping recognized by ML have been implemented through biomechanical signals and sEMG; however, grasping can be classified as a binary identification problem, which is a limiting factor in the usability of a prosthesis, considering the degrees of freedom of the user's hand (Yuk and Sohn 2022). The design of new prostheses with more degrees of freedom can be assumed as a solution to this problem; however, with it appears the challenge of the association of different movements that allow this type of control, using fewer information channels (Fang et al. 2020). Different ML algorithms allow decoding movements and, with them, the control of devices. However, as is shown in Table 10.1, although with sEMG signals it is possible to recognize different limb movements with adequate precision and generate movements for a prosthesis, this type of control is imprecise due to the recognition discretization.

In rehabilitation and assistive technologies, an important factor corresponds to the physical characteristics of the sensors and the fact that actuators may not be able to affect the task to be performed. For this reason, in recent years, the scientific community has focused on the design of smaller and lightweight actuators with wearable and comfortable sensors for the prosthesis user. However, this generates a new problem related to the fact that by modifying the physical characteristics of the sensor, its nature can be modified, and thus, information with noise can be obtained, altering the detection of intentionality. At this point, AI appears as a support for information loss, where regression techniques have been used to estimate kinematic phenomena of movements in people, which has applications in rehabilitation devices controlled by models of this magnitude, such as exoskeletons (He et al. 2018; Blanco-Diaz et al. 2021). Additionally, ML techniques have been used for the recognition of actions through biosignals for the application of robotic assistive devices; however, it is necessary to deepen this in computational techniques that allow the elimination of artifacts and the creation of ideal extraction methods.

Additionally, a challenge in the implementation of AI-controlled systems corresponds to the application of high computational cost techniques, which can reduce the data transfer rate. For this reason, it is necessary to explore ideal recognition techniques, as well as the use of classifiers/regressors that allow real-time implementations. To correct this, calibration sessions or stages are usually implemented a priori to the therapy, with the objective of training the AI models. However, this implies extra time in the development of the experimental session (Aggarwal and Chugh 2022). It is worth commenting that the intention recognition applied to robotic device control is limited by the conditions with which the model was trained, so that, at the time of performing an unknown intention, the device could execute an erroneous task. As mentioned earlier, AI techniques have enabled significant progress in rehabilitation engineering; however, a major concern when implementing complex methods is the need for processors and machines with enough resources, such as memory, energy, and portability, that enable real-time compilation and execution.

For this reason, the omnipotent presence of internet resources as well as emerging telecommunications-based technologies have enabled collaborations between cloud computing and service robotics (cloud robotics). In fact, cloud computing empowers robots by offering them faster and more powerful computing capabilities thanks to the ease of data storage and massively parallel computing (Saha and Dasgupta 2018). However, new challenges arise in this modality, which are related to data security and privacy, dynamic data behavior depending on the network topology, considerable delays associated with cloud-to-cloud communication, and the conversion processes for the correct reading and writing of data between local systems and the cloud.

10.3.3 Diagnostic and Pathological Estimation

Considering the large stroke survivor population, which experiences limitations in basic motor functionalities and, with these, limitations in their ADLs and decreased quality of life, different AI-based methodologies have emerged for the prediction and estimation of neurological effects present in this type of users, as discussed in previous sections. Additionally, AI has been implemented for the estimation and prediction of relevant diseases that cause limitations in motor functioning such as MS, PD, and ALS, among others.

According to the reported findings, the main current challenges that can be discussed are in the exploration of new configurations of AI algorithms, which are aimed at the prediction of other types of diseases that cause motor limitations such as PBP, SMA, or PMA. So far, the advances are important; however, the incorporation of these techniques and methodologies for applications in wearable technologies, as well as remote monitoring of the progression of the effects of diseases, is among the open challenges. Due to the importance of neuromotor rehabilitation in these types of diseases, it has been demonstrated that the combination of AI together with wearable sensors allows the measurement of physiological and mechanical variables during therapies and, with it, an improvement in the diagnosis of the evolution of the patient's pathology (L. Lu et al. 2020). Additionally, these sensors combined with other emerging technologies, such as the IoT and cloud storage, open the door for the construction of databases for the design of complete medical systems. This would enable the wider use of these techniques in fields such as telemedicine, preventive medicine, and epidemiology (L. Lu et al. 2020). This could benefit both the people with disability and the treatment clinics, as AI may be used for the prediction of the health condition of these people, generating a rapid response of health personnel and the prevention of negative effects in their care.

Several variations of AI methods have been reported in the literature, where standard methods have been created for case-specific applications for command or pattern detection, such as AlexNet architectures (Krizhevsky, Sutskever, and Hinton 2017). This generates advances in the field of computing because, under gold standard methods, various approaches can be explored and compared with these standard architectures. However, in the field of diagnosis, prediction, or estimation of neuromotor pathologies, there is still no standard technique that allows reliable estimation of pathologies. Therefore, an open challenge lies in the exploration, optimization, and regularization of methodologies in the search for standardized techniques in this area. With this, the creation of data repositories is also required for the validation of models in various pathologies and subjects, considering that each subject reacts differently to pathologies.

Finally, as attributed to the philosopher Desiderius Erasmus, "prevention is better than cure"; AI techniques have been used in the prediction of neurological diseases, with the aim of preventing the user from suffering a disease that leads to a disability. This has been extensively studied in children, where different sensors and databases have been used to estimate conditions such as cerebral palsy (Irshad et al. 2020; Zhang 2017) or to classify typical versus abnormal movements, which may be associated with a neurodegenerative disease (Fitter et al. 2020). This is a challenge for the medical community, considering that empirical detection of such diseases is highly complex and inaccurate for medical staff and must be done at a precise time for the correct intervention by the health system. Thus, AI methods shed light on methodologies that in the future will be of great help for the correct prediction of diseases, offering adequate accuracy in the detection of neuromotor pathologies. This can allow better prevention of diseases, improving the overall health of people, as proposed in the Sustainable Development Goals 2030 proposed by the United Nations (UN) in the category of health and well-being.

10.4 FUTURE PROSPECTS AND LIMITATIONS

Methodological and technological advances, particularly in AI, are revolutionizing neuromotor rehabilitation research, capabilities, and practice. However, AI applications in rehabilitation engineering are still technologically underdeveloped. A lot must be done to validate, adapt, regulate, and implement AI methods used to automate data analysis, assessment, and evaluation.

Due to the medical nature of the data used in AI applications for rehabilitation engineering, patient safety and privacy trump everything; therefore, transparency and patient approval is ethically required and mandatory for data access.

These days, many companies are developing computational algorithms and business models based on them for applications in healthcare and biomedical and rehabilitation engineering. For proprietary reasons, they do not have to reveal the core of their algorithms. This fact highlights the need for new and responsible governance mechanisms, regulations, and standards that can be applied to AI technology internationally in the future.

The intention of using AI is to improve the quality of health care services given and the technological resources available for patients during their neuromotor rehabilitation processes. Thus, it is extremely important that patients can be involved in decision making, aiming to reduce errors/problems/concerns in the laboratory/clinic.

Several reports have shown that the algorithms and technology do not always work well; therefore, AI does not replace medical specialists or engineers but can provide good support for decision making that could improve the patient's rehabilitation process.

Finally, as future perspectives, we believe that there is an open challenge for the scientific community in developing AI algorithms with high efficiency and low computational cost so that they can be applied in real time and can be incorporated into low-cost technologies for neuromotor rehabilitation.

10.5 CONCLUSIONS

This chapter has shown the importance of AI to allow adequate rehabilitation and a significant improvement in the quality of life of people with motor problems. AI techniques can learn specific patterns from input data and generate a prediction on the evaluation of the new data. Thus, AI provides the ability to decode data in more complex applications, such as those found in the prediction of neurological problems in pathologies that generate neuromotor losses.

Several AI approaches have been shown in different applications related to upper- and lower-limb motor rehabilitation. Also, different AI methods have been shown to predict and prognosticate neuromotor disabilities as well as to determine the neurological effects that can be triggered by these disabilities. Such AI approaches have been used not only for prediction but also to foresee the progression and diagnosis of pathologies that generate motor limitations. The special importance of using AI was shown in applications related to the evolution of pathologies such as ALS, Parkinson's disease, and stroke. It is important to emphasize that the prediction of pathologies can benefit people in general as well as the clinical sector in the detection of risks, allowing clinicians know in advance when a negative neuromotor effect may occur.

Regarding neurorehabilitation, this chapter has shown the use of AI to reduce the limitations of EEG and improve the performance of BCI systems using more robust and complex methods to decode brain patterns, such as the application of deep learning neural networks. It is worth mentioning that the importance of this chapter falls into the fact of AI can generate great benefits to the public health system due to the reduction of costs in motor rehabilitation therapies and the improvement in the quality of life of affected people, considering that motor activities are of special importance to the development of essential tasks in the support of their daily life. The use of AI in the prediction of the progression of pathologies is also of great interest in the scientific community, as it generates an early understanding of the progression of pathologies, for example, neurodegenerative pathologies, to choose the best treatment for the benefit of the patient. On the other hand, in diagnosis, AI methods help identify when pathology is occurring.

This chapter shows also that robotics can be combined with AI techniques for motor rehabilitation, showing that the combination of AI with wearable sensors allows the measurement of physiological and mechanical variables during rehabilitation therapies and, with it, an improvement in the diagnosis of the evolution of the patient's pathology.

In fact, AI has been used to estimate kinematic phenomena of movements in people, which has applications in rehabilitation devices, such as exoskeletons and other robotic assistive devices. On the other hand, it is a fact that AI techniques have enabled significant progress in rehabilitation engineering, and that the use of AI for motion analysis incorporating neural signals can generate greater reliability in the estimation of movements, as well as reduce costs and expand applications of rehabilitation systems for the execution of more complex movements.

However, the difficulty in producing neurorehabilitation is because brain signals are contaminated by artifacts (biological and non-biological), which makes decoding difficult. Thus, it is necessary to deepen processing methods that generate suitable features to be identified or estimated by AI-based algorithms with adequate performance. In this line, the exploration of robust AI-based methodologies for decoding patterns associated with the motor intention to perform a movement is required. It is worth noting that the identification of patterns in neural signals can be also affected by several factors related to substance or medication consumption, subject motivation, concentration in command generation, muscle or eye fatigue, and even previous experience in the use of rehabilitation technologies, among others. Thus, it is considered that the specific use of deep learning could help mitigate these phenomena due to its capacity to process data with high efficiency and reliability.

REFERENCES

Acevedo, R., Y. Atum, I. Gareis, J. Biurrun Manresa, V. Medina Bañuelos, and L. Rufiner. 2019. "A Comparison of Feature Extraction Strategies Using Wavelet Dictionaries and Feature Selection Methods for Single Trial P300-Based BCI." *Medical & Biological Engineering & Computing* 57 (3): 589–600. https://doi.org/10.1007/s11517-018-1898-9.

Aggarwal, Swati, and Nupur Chugh. 2022. "Review of Machine Learning Techniques for EEG Based Brain Computer Interface." *Archives of Computational Methods in Engineering* 29 (5): 3001–3020. https://doi.org/10.1007/s11831-021-09684-6.

Ahlrichs, Claas, and Michael Lawo. 2013. "Parkinson's Disease Motor Symptoms in Machine Learning: A Review." *Health Informatics—An International Journal* 2 (4): 1–18. https://doi.org/10.5121/hiij.2013.2401.

Allison, Brendan Z., and Christa Neuper. 2010. "Could Anyone Use a BCI?" In *Brain-Computer Interfaces*, 35–54. https://doi.org/10.1007/978-1-84996-272-8_3.

Amin, Syed Umar, Mansour Alsulaiman, Ghulam Muhammad, Mohamed Amine Mekhtiche, and M. Shamim Hossain. 2019. "Deep Learning for EEG Motor Imagery Classification Based on Multi-Layer CNNs Feature Fusion." *Future Generation Computer Systems* 101 (December): 542–554. https://doi.org/10.1016/j.future.2019.06.027.

Ang, Kai Keng, Cuntai Guan, Kok Soon Phua, Chuanchu Wang, Longjiang Zhou, Ka Yin Tang, Gopal J. Ephraim Joseph, Christopher Wee Keong Kuah, and Karen Sui Geok Chua. 2014. "Brain-Computer Interface-Based Robotic End Effector System for Wrist and Hand Rehabilitation: Results of a Three-Armed Randomized Controlled Trial for Chronic Stroke." *Frontiers in Neuroengineering* 7 (July). https://doi.org/10.3389/fneng.2014.00030.

Azlan Abu, Mohd, Syazwani Rosleesham, Mohd Zubir Suboh, Mohd Syazwan Md Yid, Zainudin Kornain, and Nurul Fauzani Jamaluddin. 2020. "Classification of EMG Signal for Multiple Hand Gestures Based on Neural Network." *Indonesian Journal of Electrical Engineering and Computer Science* 17 (1): 256–263. https://doi.org/10.11591/ijeecs.v17.i1.

Becedas, J. 2012. "Brain–Machine Interfaces: Basis and Advances." *IEEE Transactions on Systems, Man, and Cybernetics, Part C (Applications and Reviews)* 42 (6): 825–836. https://doi.org/10.1109/TSMCC.2012.2203301.

Bede, Peter, Aizuri Murad, Jasmin Lope, Stacey Li Hi Shing, Eoin Finegan, Rangariroyashe H. Chipika, Orla Hardiman, and Kai Ming Chang. 2022. "Phenotypic Categorisation of Individual Subjects with Motor Neuron Disease Based on Radiological Disease Burden Patterns: A Machine-Learning Approach." *Journal of the Neurological Sciences* 432 (January): 120079. https://doi.org/10.1016/j.jns.2021.120079.

Belyea, Alex, Kevin Englehart, and Erik Scheme. 2019. "FMG Versus EMG: A Comparison of Usability for Real-Time Pattern Recognition Based Control." *IEEE Transactions on Biomedical Engineering* 66 (11): 3098–3104. https://doi.org/10.1109/TBME.2019.2900415.

Bhardwaj, Kartik Krishna, Siddhant Banyal, and Deepak Kumar Sharma. 2019. "Artificial Intelligence Based Diagnostics, Therapeutics and Applications in Biomedical Engineering and Bioinformatics." In *Internet of Things in Biomedical Engineering*, 161–187. Elsevier. https://doi.org/10.1016/B978-0-12-817356-5.00009-7.

Bi, Luzheng, Aberham -->Genetu Feleke, and Cuntai Guan. 2019. "A Review on EMG-Based Motor Intention Prediction of Continuous Human Upper Limb Motion for Human-Robot Collaboration." *Biomedical Signal Processing and Control* 51 (May): 113–127. https://doi.org/10.1016/j.bspc.2019.02.011.

Blana, Dimitra, Antonie J. van den Bogert, Wendy M. Murray, Amartya Ganguly, Agamemnon Krasoulis, Kianoush Nazarpour, and Edward K. Chadwick. 2020. "Model-Based Control of Individual Finger Movements for Prosthetic Hand Function." *IEEE Transactions on Neural Systems and Rehabilitation Engineering* 28 (3): 612–620. https://doi.org/10.1109/TNSRE.2020.2967901.

Blanco-Diaz, Cristian Felipe, Javier M. Antelis, and Andrés Felipe Ruiz-Olaya. 2022. "Comparative Analysis of Spectral and Temporal Combinations in CSP-Based Methods for Decoding Hand Motor Imagery Tasks." *Journal of Neuroscience Methods* 371 (April): 109495. https://doi.org/10.1016/j.jneumeth.2022.109495.

Blanco-Díaz, Cristian Felipe, Cristian David Guerrero-Méndez, Teodiano Bastos-Filho, Sebastián Jaramillo-Isaza, and Andrés Felipe Ruiz-Olaya. 2022. "Effects of the Concentration Level, Eye Fatigue and Coffee Consumption on the Performance of a BCI System Based on Visual ERP-P300." *Journal of Neuroscience Methods* 382 (December): 109722. https://doi.org/10.1016/j.jneumeth.2022.109722.

Blanco-Diaz, Cristian Felipe, Cristian David Guerrero-Mendez, Mario Enrique Duarte-González, and Sebastián Jaramillo-Isaza. 2021. "Estimation of Limbs Angles Amplitudes During the Use of the Five Minute Shaper Device Using Artificial Neural Networks." In *Applied Computer Sciences in Engineering*, 213–224. https://doi.org/10.1007/978-3-030-86702-7_19.

Blanco-Díaz, Cristian Felipe, Cristian David Guerrero-Méndez, Mario Enrique Duarte-González, and Sebastián Jaramillo-Isaza. 2022. "Implementación de Métodos Computacionales Para Estimar Las Amplitudes Angulares de Los Miembros Inferiores Durante El Squat." *TecnoLógicas* 25 (53): e2164. https://doi.org/10.22430/22565337.2164.

Blanco-Díaz, C.F., C.D. Guerrero-Méndez, and A.F. Ruiz-Olaya. 2023. "Enhancing P300 Detection Using a Band-Selective Filter Bank for a Visual P300 Speller." *IRBM* 44 (3): 100751. https://doi.org/10.1016/j.irbm.2022.100751.

Blanco-Diaz, Cristian Felipe, and Andres Felipe Ruiz Olaya. 2020. "A Novel Method Based on Regularized Logistic Regression and CCA for P300 Detection Using a Reduced Number of EEG Trials." *IEEE Latin America Transactions* 18 (12): 2147–2154. https://doi.org/10.1109/TLA.2020.9400443.

Bonaccorso, Giuseppe. 2017. *Machine Learning Algorithms: A reference guide to popular algorithms for data science and machine learning.* Birmingham: Packt Publishing Ltd.

Brambilla, Cristina, Ileana Pirovano, Robert Mihai Mira, Giovanna Rizzo, Alessandro Scano, and Alfonso Mastropietro. 2021. "Combined Use of EMG and EEG Techniques for Neuromotor Assessment in Rehabilitative Applications: A Systematic Review." *Sensors* 21 (21): 7014. https://doi.org/10.3390/s21217014.

Brand, Yonatan E., Dafna Schwartz, Eran Gazit, Aron S. Buchman, Ran Gilad-Bachrach, and Jeffrey M. Hausdorff. 2022. "Gait Detection from a Wrist-Worn Sensor Using Machine Learning Methods: A Daily Living Study in Older Adults and People with Parkinson's Disease." *Sensors* 22 (18): 7094. https://doi.org/10.3390/s22187094.

Callejas-Cuervo, Mauro, Aura Ximena González-Cely, and Teodiano Bastos-Filho. 2020. "Control Systems and Electronic Instrumentation Applied to Autonomy in Wheelchair Mobility: The State of the Art." *Sensors* 20 (21): 6326. https://doi.org/10.3390/s20216326.

Campagnini, Silvia, Chiara Arienti, Michele Patrini, Piergiuseppe Liuzzi, Andrea Mannini, and Maria Chiara Carrozza. 2022. "Machine Learning Methods for Functional Recovery Prediction and Prognosis in Post-Stroke Rehabilitation: A Systematic Review." *Journal of NeuroEngineering and Rehabilitation* 19 (1): 54. https://doi.org/10.1186/s12984-022-01032-4.

Chatterjee, Soumya, Kaniska Samanta, Niladri Ray Choudhury, and Rohit Bose. 2019. "Detection of Myopathy and ALS Electromyograms Employing Modified Window Stockwell Transform." *IEEE Sensors Letters* 3 (7): 1–4. https://doi.org/10.1109/LSENS.2019.2921072.

Chen, Chengjun, Kai Huang, Dongnian Li, Yong Pan, Zhengxu Zhao, and Jun Hong. 2021. "Assembly Torque Data Regression Using SEMG and Inertial Signals." *Journal of Manufacturing Systems* 60 (July): 1–10. https://doi.org/10.1016/j.jmsy.2021.04.011.

Chen, Jian-Wen, Chun-Ju Wu, Yi-Tseng Lin, Yu-Cheng Kuo, and Chung-Hsien Kuo. 2020. "Mechatronic Implementation and Trajectory Tracking Validation of a BCI-Based Human-Wheelchair Interface." In *2020 8th IEEE RAS/EMBS International Conference for Biomedical Robotics and Biomechatronics (BioRob)*, 304–309. IEEE. https://doi.org/10.1109/BioRob49111.2020.9224373.

Chen, Wen, Shih-Kang Chen, Yi-Hung Liu, Yu-Jen Chen, and Chin-Sheng Chen. 2022. "An Electric Wheelchair Manipulating System Using SSVEP-Based BCI System." *Biosensors* 12 (10): 772. https://doi.org/10.3390/bios12100772.

Chen, Xiaogang, Bing Zhao, Yijun Wang, and Xiaorong Gao. 2019. "Combination of High-Frequency SSVEP-Based BCI and Computer Vision for Controlling a Robotic Arm." *Journal of Neural Engineering* 16 (2): 026012. https://doi.org/10.1088/1741-2552/aaf594.

Chen, Xiaoshi, Li Gong, Lirong Zheng, and Zhuo Zou. 2020. "Soft Exoskeleton Glove for Hand Assistance Based on Human-Machine Interaction and Machine Learning." In *2020 IEEE International Conference on Human-Machine Systems (ICHMS)*, 1–6. IEEE. https://doi.org/10.1109/ICHMS49158.2020.9209381.

Chen, Yan, Song Yu, Ke Ma, Shuangyuan Huang, Guofeng Li, Siqi Cai, and Longhan Xie. 2019. "A Continuous Estimation Model of Upper Limb Joint Angles by Using Surface Electromyography and Deep Learning Method." *IEEE Access* 7: 174940–174950. https://doi.org/10.1109/ACCESS.2019.2956951.

Chen, Yuyang, Chenyun Dai, and Wei Chen. 2020. "Cross-Comparison of EMG-to-Force Methods for Multi-DoF Finger Force Prediction Using One-DoF Training." *IEEE Access* 8: 13958–13968. https://doi.org/10.1109/ACCESS.2020.2966007.

Choi, Hongyoon, Seunggyun Ha, Hyejin Kang, Hyekyoung Lee, and Dong Soo Lee. 2019. "Deep Learning Only by Normal Brain PET Identify Unheralded Brain Anomalies." *EBioMedicine* 43 (May): 447–453. https://doi.org/10.1016/j.ebiom.2019.04.022.

Christodoulou, Evangelia, Jie Ma, Gary S. Collins, Ewout W. Steyerberg, Jan Y. Verbakel, and Ben van Calster. 2019. "A Systematic Review Shows No Performance Benefit of Machine Learning Over Logistic Regression for Clinical Prediction Models." *Journal of Clinical Epidemiology* 110 (June): 12–22. https://doi.org/10.1016/j.jclinepi.2019.02.004.

Ertel, Wolfgang. 2017. *Introduction to Artificial Intelligence*. Cham: Springer International Publishing. https://doi.org/10.1007/978-3-319-58487-4.

Fahrmeir, Ludwig, Thomas Kneib, Stefan Lang, and Brian D. Marx. 2021. *Regression*. Berlin, Heidelberg: Springer Berlin Heidelberg. https://doi.org/10.1007/978-3-662-63882-8.

Fang, Chaoming, Bowei He, Yixuan Wang, Jin Cao, and Shuo Gao. 2020. "EMG-Centered Multisensory Based Technologies for Pattern Recognition in Rehabilitation: State of the Art and Challenges." *Biosensors* 10 (8): 85. https://doi.org/10.3390/bios10080085.

Fernandes, Felipe, Ingridy Barbalho, Daniele Barros, Ricardo Valentim, César Teixeira, Jorge Henriques, Paulo Gil, and Mário Dourado Júnior. 2021. "Biomedical Signals and Machine Learning in Amyotrophic Lateral Sclerosis: A Systematic Review." *BioMedical Engineering OnLine* 20 (1): 61. https://doi.org/10.1186/s12938-021-00896-2.

Fitter, Naomi T., Rebecca Funke, Jose Carlos Pulido, Maja J. Mataric, and Beth A. Smith. 2020. "Toward Predicting Infant Developmental Outcomes from Day-Long Inertial Motion Recordings." *IEEE Transactions on Neural Systems and Rehabilitation Engineering* 28 (10): 2305–2314. https://doi.org/10.1109/TNSRE.2020.3016916.

Gao, Shuo, Yixuan Wang, Chaoming Fang, and Lijun Xu. 2020. "A Smart Terrain Identification Technique Based on Electromyography, Ground Reaction Force, and Machine Learning for Lower Limb Rehabilitation." *Applied Sciences* 10 (8): 2638. https://doi.org/10.3390/app10082638.

Gautam, Arvind, Madhuri Panwar, Dwaipayan Biswas, and Amit Acharyya. 2020. "MyoNet: A Transfer-Learning-Based LRCN for Lower Limb Movement Recognition and Knee Joint Angle Prediction for Remote Monitoring of Rehabilitation Progress from SEMG." *IEEE Journal of Translational Engineering in Health and Medicine* 8: 1–10. https://doi.org/10.1109/JTEHM.2020.2972523.

Giarmatzis, Georgios, Evangelia I. Zacharaki, and Konstantinos Moustakas. 2020. "Real-Time Prediction of Joint Forces by Motion Capture and Machine Learning." *Sensors* 20 (23): 6933. https://doi.org/10.3390/s20236933.

Gilja, Vikash, Chethan Pandarinath, Christine H. Blabe, Paul Nuyujukian, John D. Simeral, Anish A. Sarma, Brittany L. Sorice, et al. 2015. "Clinical Translation of a High-Performance Neural Prosthesis." *Nature Medicine* 21 (10): 1142–1145. https://doi.org/10.1038/nm.3953.

Guerrero-Mendez, Cristian David, Cristian Felipe Blanco-Diaz, and Andres Felipe Ruiz-Olaya. 2021a. "Identification of Motor Imagery Tasks Using Power-Based Connectivity Descriptors from EEG Signals." In *2021 XXIII Symposium on Image, Signal Processing and Artificial Vision (STSIVA)*, 1–6. IEEE. https://doi.org/10.1109/STSIVA53688.2021.9591997.

Guerrero-Mendez, Cristian David, Cristian Felipe Blanco-Diaz, and Andres Felipe Ruiz-Olaya. 2021b. "How Do Factors of Comfort, Concentration, and Eye Fatigue Affect the Performance of a BCI System Based on SSVEP?" In *2021 IEEE 2nd International Congress of Biomedical Engineering and Bioengineering (CI-IB&BI)*, 1–4. IEEE. https://doi.org/10.1109/CI-IBBI54220.2021.9626107.

Guerrero-Mendez, Cristian David, Moreno Brayan, Ramirez-Ruiz Valery, Duarte-Gonzales Mario, Ruiz-Olaya Andres Felipe, and Jaramillo-Isaza Sebastian. 2021. "Comparison of the Muscular Electrical Activity and Hip–Knee Joint Amplitude during Bent-Knee Sit-up Movement and Abdominal Exercises Using a Five-Minute Shaper Device: A Case Study on an Unconditioned Subject." *Journal of Physical Education and Sport* 21 (6).

Guerrero-Méndez, Cristian David, Brayan Sneider Moreno-Arévalo, Valery Ramírez-Ruiz, Mario Enrique Duarte-González, Andrés Felipe Ruiz-Olaya, and Sebastián Jaramillo-Isaza. 2021. "Análisis Cinemático de Movimientos Realizados En Dispositivos de Acondicionamiento Físico Tipo Five Minutes Shaper." *Revista Ontare* 9 (October). https://doi.org/10.21158/23823399.v9.n0.2021.3027.

Guerrero-Mendez, Cristian D., and Andres F. Ruiz-Olaya. 2022. "Coherence-Based Connectivity Analysis of EEG and EMG Signals during Reach-to-Grasp Movement Involving Two Weights." *Brain-Computer Interfaces* 9 (3): 140–154. https://doi.org/10.1080/2326263X.2022.2029308.

Hamidah, A., T. Adiono, I. Syafalni, Herianto, M. Andriana, M. Kurnia, S. Ratunanda, and Vitriana. 2019. "Review on Machine Learning Applications in Assisted Treadmill for Stroke Rehabilitation." In *2019 International Symposium on Electronics and Smart Devices (ISESD)*, 1–5. IEEE. https://doi.org/10.1109/ISESD.2019.8909416.

Hashmi, Mohammad Farukh, Jagdish D. Kene, Deepali M. Kotambkar, Praveen Matte, and Avinash G. Keskar. 2022. “An Efficient P300 Detection Algorithm Based on Kernel Principal Component Analysis-Support Vector Machine.” *Computers & Electrical Engineering* 97 (January): 107608. https://doi.org/10.1016/j.compeleceng.2021.107608.

He, Yongtian, Trieu Phat Luu, Kevin Nathan, Sho Nakagome, and Jose L. Contreras-Vidal. 2018. “A Mobile Brain-Body Imaging Dataset Recorded during Treadmill Walking with a Brain-Computer Interface.” *Scientific Data* 5 (1): 180074. https://doi.org/10.1038/sdata.2018.74.

Herbert, Cornelia, and Michael Munz. 2020. “Measuring Gait-Event-Related Brain Potentials (GERPs) during Instructed and Spontaneous Treadmill Walking: Technical Solutions and Automated Classification through Artificial Neural Networks.” *Applied Sciences* 10 (16): 5405. https://doi.org/10.3390/app10165405.

Hooda, Neha, Ratan Das, and Neelesh Kumar. 2020. “Fusion of EEG and EMG Signals for Classification of Unilateral Foot Movements.” *Biomedical Signal Processing and Control* 60 (July): 101990. https://doi.org/10.1016/j.bspc.2020.101990.

Hu, Yu, Yongkang Wong, Wentao Wei, Yu Du, Mohan Kankanhalli, and Weidong Geng. 2018. “A Novel Attention-Based Hybrid CNN-RNN Architecture for SEMG-Based Gesture Recognition.” *PLoS ONE* 13 (10): e0206049. https://doi.org/10.1371/journal.pone.0206049.

Hua, Shaoyang, Congqing Wang, and Xuewei Wu. 2022. “A Novel SEMG-Based Force Estimation Method Using Deep-Learning Algorithm.” *Complex & Intelligent Systems* 8 (3): 1949–1961. https://doi.org/10.1007/s40747-021-00338-5.

Hwang, Yi-Ting, Wei-An Lu, and Bor-Shing Lin. 2022. “Use of Functional Data to Model the Trajectory of an Inertial Measurement Unit and Classify Levels of Motor Impairment for Stroke Patients.” *IEEE Transactions on Neural Systems and Rehabilitation Engineering* 30: 925–935. https://doi.org/10.1109/TNSRE.2022.3162416.

Imamura, Keiko, Yuichiro Yada, Yuishin Izumi, Mitsuya Morita, Akihiro Kawata, Takayo Arisato, Ayako Nagahashi, et al. 2021. “Prediction Model of Amyotrophic Lateral Sclerosis by Deep Learning with Patient Induced Pluripotent Stem Cells.” *Annals of Neurology* 89 (6): 1226–1233. https://doi.org/10.1002/ana.26047.

Irshad, Muhammad Tausif, Muhammad Adeel Nisar, Philip Gouverneur, Marion Rapp, and Marcin Grzegorzek. 2020. “AI Approaches Towards Prechtl’s Assessment of General Movements: A Systematic Literature Review.” *Sensors* 20 (18): 5321. https://doi.org/10.3390/s20185321.

Ishii, Chiharu, Shunsuke Murooka, and Minato Tajima. 2016. “Navigation of an Electric Wheelchair Using Electromyograms, Electrooculograms, and Electroencephalograms.” *International Journal of Mechanical Engineering and Robotics Research* 7 (2): 143–149. https://doi.org/10.18178/ijmerr.7.2.143-149.

Jang, Sang Jin, Yu Jin Yang, Seokyun Ryun, June Sic Kim, Chun Kee Chung, and Jaeseung Jeong. 2022. “Decoding Trajectories of Imagined Hand Movement Using Electrocorticograms for Brain–Machine Interface.” *Journal of Neural Engineering* 19 (5): 056011. https://doi.org/10.1088/1741-2552/ac8b37.

Jiang, Shuo, Peiqi Kang, Xinyu Song, Benny Lo, and Peter Shull. 2022. “Emerging Wearable Interfaces and Algorithms for Hand Gesture Recognition: A Survey.” *IEEE Reviews in Biomedical Engineering* 15: 85–102. https://doi.org/10.1109/RBME.2021.3078190.

Juan, Javier V., Luis de la Ossa, Eduardo Iáñez, Mario Ortiz, Laura Ferrero, and José M. Azorín. 2022. “Decoding Lower-Limbs Kinematics from EEG Signals While Walking with an Exoskeleton.” In *Artificial Intelligence in Neuroscience: Affective Analysis and Health Applications*, 615–624. https://doi.org/10.1007/978-3-031-06242-1_61.

Kandel, Eric R., James H. Schwartz, Thomas M. Jessell, Steven Siegelbaum, A. James Hudspeth, Sarah Mack and others. 2000. *Principles of Neural Science*. Vol. 4. New York: McGraw-Hill.

Khan, Rayyan Azam, Noman Naseer, Nauman Khalid Qureshi, Farzan Majeed Noori, Hammad Nazeer, and Muhammad Umer Khan. 2018. "FNIRS-Based Neurorobotic Interface for Gait Rehabilitation." *Journal of NeuroEngineering and Rehabilitation* 15 (1): 7. https://doi.org/10.1186/s12984-018-0346-2.

Kong, Wanzeng, Shijie Guo, Yanfang Long, Yong Peng, Hong Zeng, Xinyu Zhang, and Jianhai Zhang. 2018. "Weighted Extreme Learning Machine for P300 Detection with Application to Brain Computer Interface." *Journal of Ambient Intelligence and Humanized Computing* (May). https://doi.org/10.1007/s12652-018-0840-1.

Korik, Attila, Ronen Sosnik, Nazmul Siddique, and Damien Coyle. 2018. "Decoding Imagined 3D Hand Movement Trajectories from EEG: Evidence to Support the Use of Mu, Beta, and Low Gamma Oscillations." *Frontiers in Neuroscience* 12, March. https://doi.org/10.3389/fnins.2018.00130.

Krizhevsky, Alex, Ilya Sutskever, and Geoffrey E. Hinton. 2017. "ImageNet Classification with Deep Convolutional Neural Networks." *Communications of the ACM* 60 (6): 84–90. https://doi.org/10.1145/3065386.

Kumarasinghe, Kaushalya, Nikola Kasabov, and Denise Taylor. 2021. "Brain-Inspired Spiking Neural Networks for Decoding and Understanding Muscle Activity and Kinematics from Electroencephalography Signals during Hand Movements." *Scientific Reports* 11 (1): 2486. https://doi.org/10.1038/s41598-021-81805-4.

Kundu, Sourav, and Samit Ari. 2020. "P300 Based Character Recognition Using Convolutional Neural Network and Support Vector Machine." *Biomedical Signal Processing and Control* 55 (January): 101645. https://doi.org/10.1016/j.bspc.2019.101645.

Lee, Hyeon Kyu, and Young-Seok Choi. 2018. "A Convolution Neural Networks Scheme for Classification of Motor Imagery EEG Based on Wavelet Time-Frequecy Image." In *2018 International Conference on Information Networking (ICOIN)*, 906–909. IEEE. https://doi.org/10.1109/ICOIN.2018.8343254.

Lee, Min-Ho, O-Yeon Kwon, Yong-Jeong Kim, Hong-Kyung Kim, Young-Eun Lee, John Williamson, Siamac Fazli, and Seong-Whan Lee. 2019. "EEG Dataset and OpenBMI Toolbox for Three BCI Paradigms: An Investigation into BCI Illiteracy." *GigaScience* 8 (5). https://doi.org/10.1093/gigascience/giz002.

Lee, Seulah, Minchang Sung, and Youngjin Choi. 2020. "Wearable Fabric Sensor for Controlling Myoelectric Hand Prosthesis via Classification of Foot Postures." *Smart Materials and Structures* 29 (3): 035004. https://doi.org/10.1088/1361-665X/ab6690.

Li, Xin, Jinkang Liu, Yijing Huang, Donghao Wang, and Yang Miao. 2022. "Human Motion Pattern Recognition and Feature Extraction: An Approach Using Multi-Information Fusion." *Micromachines* 13 (8): 1205. https://doi.org/10.3390/mi13081205.

Liu, Haoyan, Atiyehsadat Panahi, David Andrews, and Alexander Nelson. 2022. "An FPGA-Based Upper-Limb Rehabilitation Device for Gesture Recognition and Motion Evaluation Using Multi-Task Recurrent Neural Networks." *IEEE Sensors Journal* 22 (4): 3605–3615. https://doi.org/10.1109/JSEN.2022.3141659.

Lu, Lin, Jiayao Zhang, Yi Xie, Fei Gao, Song Xu, Xinghuo Wu, and Zhewei Ye. 2020. "Wearable Health Devices in Health Care: Narrative Systematic Review." *JMIR MHealth and UHealth* 8 (11): e18907. https://doi.org/10.2196/18907.

Lu, Yanzheng, Hong Wang, Bin Zhou, Chunfeng Wei, and Shiqiang Xu. 2022. "Continuous and Simultaneous Estimation of Lower Limb Multi-Joint Angles from SEMG Signals Based on Stacked Convolutional and LSTM Models." *Expert Systems with Applications* 203 (October): 117340. https://doi.org/10.1016/j.eswa.2022.117340.

Luu, Trieu Phat, David Eguren, Manuel Cestari, and Jose L. Contreras-Vidal. 2019. "EEG-Based Neural Decoding of Gait in Developing Children." In *2019 IEEE International Conference on Systems, Man and Cybernetics (SMC)*, 3608–3612. IEEE. https://doi.org/10.1109/SMC.2019.8914380.

Maitin, Ana M., Juan Pablo Romero Muñoz, and Álvaro José García-Tejedor. 2022. "Survey of Machine Learning Techniques in the Analysis of EEG Signals for Parkinson's Disease: A Systematic Review." *Applied Sciences* 12 (14): 6967. https://doi.org/10.3390/app12146967.

Meattini, Roberto, Alessandra Bernardini, Gianluca Palli, and Claudio Melchiorri. 2022. "SEMG-Based Minimally Supervised Regression Using Soft-DTW Neural Networks for Robot Hand Grasping Control." *IEEE Robotics and Automation Letters* 7 (4): 10144–10151. https://doi.org/10.1109/LRA.2022.3193247.

Mercado, Luis, Lucero Alvarado, Griselda Quiroz-Compean, Rebeca Romo-Vazquez, Hugo Vélez-Pérez, M.A. Platas-Garza, Andrés A. González-Garrido, et al. 2021. "Decoding the Torque of Lower Limb Joints from EEG Recordings of Pre-Gait Movements Using a Machine Learning Scheme." *Neurocomputing* 446 (July): 118–129. https://doi.org/10.1016/j.neucom.2021.03.038.

Montolío, Alberto, Alejandro Martín-Gallego, José Cegoñino, Elvira Orduna, Elisa Vilades, Elena Garcia-Martin, and Amaya Pérez del Palomar. 2021. "Machine Learning in Diagnosis and Disability Prediction of Multiple Sclerosis Using Optical Coherence Tomography." *Computers in Biology and Medicine* 133 (June): 104416. https://doi.org/10.1016/j.compbiomed.2021.104416.

Morbidoni, Christian, Alessandro Cucchiarelli, Sandro Fioretti, and Francesco di Nardo. 2019. "A Deep Learning Approach to EMG-Based Classification of Gait Phases during Level Ground Walking." *Electronics* 8 (8): 894. https://doi.org/10.3390/electronics8080894.

Mulfari, Davide, Donatella la Placa, Chiara Rovito, Antonio Celesti, and Massimo Villari. 2022. "Deep Learning Applications in Telerehabilitation Speech Therapy Scenarios." *Computers in Biology and Medicine* 148 (September): 105864. https://doi.org/10.1016/j.compbiomed.2022.105864.

Myszczynska, Monika A., Poojitha N. Ojamies, Alix M.B. Lacoste, Daniel Neil, Amir Saffari, Richard Mead, Guillaume M. Hautbergue, Joanna D. Holbrook, and Laura Ferraiuolo. 2020. "Applications of Machine Learning to Diagnosis and Treatment of Neurodegenerative Diseases." *Nature Reviews Neurology* 16 (8): 440–456. https://doi.org/10.1038/s41582-020-0377-8.

Nakagome, Sho, Trieu Phat Luu, Yongtian He, Akshay Sujatha Ravindran, and Jose L. Contreras-Vidal. 2020. "An Empirical Comparison of Neural Networks and Machine Learning Algorithms for EEG Gait Decoding." *Scientific Reports* 10 (1): 4372. https://doi.org/10.1038/s41598-020-60932-4.

National Institute of Biomedical Imaging and Bioengineering (NIBIB). 2013. "Rehabilitation Engineering". Available online: https://www.nibib.nih.gov/sites/default/files/Rehabilitation%20Engineering%20Fact%20Sheet_0.pdf (accessed on 15 September 2022).

Nizamis, Kostas, Alkinoos Athanasiou, Sofia Almpani, Christos Dimitrousis, and Alexander Astaras. 2021. "Converging Robotic Technologies in Targeted Neural Rehabilitation: A Review of Emerging Solutions and Challenges." *Sensors* 21 (6): 2084. https://doi.org/10.3390/s21062084.

Nusinovici, Simon, Yih Chung Tham, Marco Yu Chak Yan, Daniel Shu Wei Ting, Jialiang Li, Charumathi Sabanayagam, Tien Yin Wong, and Ching-Yu Cheng. 2020. "Logistic Regression Was as Good as Machine Learning for Predicting Major Chronic Diseases." *Journal of Clinical Epidemiology* 122 (June): 56–69. https://doi.org/10.1016/j.jclinepi.2020.03.002.

Ommeren, A.L. van, B. Sawaryn, G.B. Prange-Lasonder, J.H. Buurke, J.S. Rietman, and P.H. Veltink. 2019. "Detection of the Intention to Grasp During Reaching in Stroke Using Inertial Sensing." *IEEE Transactions on Neural Systems and Rehabilitation Engineering* 27 (10): 2128–2134. https://doi.org/10.1109/TNSRE.2019.2939202.

Padfield, Natasha, Jaime Zabalza, Huimin Zhao, Valentin Masero, and Jinchang Ren. 2019. "EEG-Based Brain-Computer Interfaces Using Motor-Imagery: Techniques and Challenges." *Sensors* 19 (6): 1423. https://doi.org/10.3390/s19061423.

Pancotti, Corrado, Giovanni Birolo, Cesare Rollo, Tiziana Sanavia, Barbara di Camillo, Umberto Manera, Adriano Chiò, and Piero Fariselli. 2022. "Deep Learning Methods to Predict Amyotrophic Lateral Sclerosis Disease Progression." *Scientific Reports* 12 (1): 13738. https://doi.org/10.1038/s41598-022-17805-9.

Pei, Dingyi, Parthan Olikkal, Tülay Adali, and Ramana Vinjamuri. 2022. "Reconstructing Synergy-Based Hand Grasp Kinematics from Electroencephalographic Signals." *Sensors* 22 (14): 5349. https://doi.org/10.3390/s22145349.

Pfurtscheller, G., and F.H. Lopes da Silva. 1999. "Event-Related EEG/MEG Synchronization and Desynchronization: Basic Principles." *Clinical Neurophysiology* 110 (11): 1842–1857. https://doi.org/10.1016/S1388-2457(99)00141-8.

Pfurtscheller, Gert, and Christa Neuper. 2003. "Movement and ERD/ERS." In *The Bereitschaftspotential*, 191–206. Boston, MA: Springer US. https://doi.org/10.1007/978-1-4615-0189-3_12.

Picton, Terence W. 1992. "The P300 Wave of the Human Event-Related Potential." *Journal of Clinical Neurophysiology* 9 (4): 456–479. https://doi.org/10.1097/00004691-199210000-00002.

Robinson, Neethu, Ravikiran Mane, Tushar Chouhan, and Cuntai Guan. 2021. "Emerging Trends in BCI-Robotics for Motor Control and Rehabilitation." *Current Opinion in Biomedical Engineering* 20 (December): 100354. https://doi.org/10.1016/j.cobme.2021.100354.

Rodríguez-Ugarte, Marisol, Eduardo Iáñez, Mario Ortíz, and Jose M. Azorín. 2017. "Personalized Offline and Pseudo-Online BCI Models to Detect Pedaling Intent." *Frontiers in Neuroinformatics* 11 (July). https://doi.org/10.3389/fninf.2017.00045.

Romero-Laiseca, Maria Alejandra, Denis Delisle-Rodriguez, Vivianne Cardoso, Dharmendra Gurve, Flavia Loterio, Jorge Henrique Posses Nascimento, Sridhar Krishnan, Anselmo Frizera-Neto, and Teodiano Bastos-Filho. 2020. "A Low-Cost Lower-Limb Brain-Machine Interface Triggered by Pedaling Motor Imagery for Post-Stroke Patients Rehabilitation." *IEEE Transactions on Neural Systems and Rehabilitation Engineering* 28 (4): 988–996. https://doi.org/10.1109/TNSRE.2020.2974056.

Romijnders, Robbin, Elke Warmerdam, Clint Hansen, Gerhard Schmidt, and Walter Maetzler. 2022. "A Deep Learning Approach for Gait Event Detection from a Single Shank-Worn IMU: Validation in Healthy and Neurological Cohorts." *Sensors* 22 (10): 3859. https://doi.org/10.3390/s22103859.

Russell, Stuart J., and Peter Norvig. 2003. *Artificial Intelligence: A Modern Approach*. 2nd ed. Upper Saddle River, New Jersey: Prentice Hall.

Saha, Olimpiya, and Prithviraj Dasgupta. 2018. "A Comprehensive Survey of Recent Trends in Cloud Robotics Architectures and Applications." *Robotics* 7 (3): 47. https://doi.org/10.3390/robotics7030047.

Schalk, Gerwin, and Eric C. Leuthardt. 2011. "Brain-Computer Interfaces Using Electrocorticographic Signals." *IEEE Reviews in Biomedical Engineering* 4: 140–154. https://doi.org/10.1109/RBME.2011.2172408.

Sivaranjini, S., and C.M. Sujatha. 2020. "Deep Learning Based Diagnosis of Parkinson's Disease Using Convolutional Neural Network." *Multimedia Tools and Applications* 79 (21–22): 15467–15479. https://doi.org/10.1007/s11042-019-7469-8.

Sosnik, Ronen, and Li Zheng. 2021. "Reconstruction of Hand, Elbow and Shoulder Actual and Imagined Trajectories in 3D Space Using EEG Current Source Dipoles." *Journal of Neural Engineering* 18 (5): 056011. https://doi.org/10.1088/1741-2552/abf0d7.

Sui, Xiuwu, Kaixin Wan, and Yang Zhang. 2019. "Pattern Recognition of SEMG Based on Wavelet Packet Transform and Improved SVM." *Optik* 176 (January): 228–235. https://doi.org/10.1016/j.ijleo.2018.09.040.

Tanna, S. Rashmin, and Chandulal H. Vithalani. 2022. "Classification of Lower Limb Rehabilitation Exercises with Multiple and Individual Inertial Measurement Units." *Indonesian Journal of Electrical Engineering and Computer Science* 28 (2): 840. https://doi.org/10.11591/ijeecs.v28.i2.pp840-849.

Too, Jingwei, A.R. Abdullah, Norhashimah Mohd Saad, N. Mohd Ali, and H. Musa. 2018. "A Detail Study of Wavelet Families for EMG Pattern Recognition." *International Journal of Electrical and Computer Engineering (IJECE)* 8 (6): 4221. https://doi.org/10.11591/ijece.v8i6.pp4221-4229.

Too, Jingwei, Abdul Abdullah, Norhashimah Mohd Saad, and Weihown Tee. 2019. "EMG Feature Selection and Classification Using a Pbest-Guide Binary Particle Swarm Optimization." *Computation* 7 (1): 12. https://doi.org/10.3390/computation7010012.

Tortora, Stefano, Luca Tonin, Carmelo Chisari, Silvestro Micera, Emanuele Menegatti, and Fiorenzo Artoni. 2020. "Hybrid Human-Machine Interface for Gait Decoding Through Bayesian Fusion of EEG and EMG Classifiers." *Frontiers in Neurorobotics* 14 (November). https://doi.org/10.3389/fnbot.2020.582728.

Usakli, A.B., S. Gurkan, F. Aloise, G. Vecchiato, and F. Babiloni. 2010. "On the Use of Electrooculogram for Efficient Human Computer Interfaces." *Computational Intelligence and Neuroscience* 2010: 1–5. https://doi.org/10.1155/2010/135629.

Wang, Tingting, Shengzhi Du, and Enzeng Dong. 2021. "A Novel Method to Reduce the Motor Imagery BCI Illiteracy." *Medical & Biological Engineering & Computing* 59 (11–12): 2205–2217. https://doi.org/10.1007/s11517-021-02449-0.

Williams, Heather, Ahmed W. Shehata, Michael Dawson, Erik Scheme, Jacqueline Hebert, and Patrick Pilarski. 2022. "Recurrent Convolutional Neural Networks as an Approach to Position-Aware Myoelectric Prosthesis Control." *IEEE Transactions on Biomedical Engineering* 69 (7): 2243–2255. https://doi.org/10.1109/TBME.2022.3140269.

World Health Organization (WHO). 2011. "World Report on Disability." Gevene.

World Health Organization (WHO). 2013. "Guidelines on Health-Related Rehabilitation (Rehabilitation Guidelines)."

Xiong, Dezhen, Daohui Zhang, Xingang Zhao, and Yiwen Zhao. 2021. "Deep Learning for EMG-Based Human-Machine Interaction: A Review." *IEEE/CAA Journal of Automatica Sinica* 8 (3): 512–533. https://doi.org/10.1109/JAS.2021.1003865.

Xu, Yue, Qingcong Wu, Bai Chen, and Xi Chen. 2022. "SSVEP-Based Active Control of an Upper Limb Exoskeleton Using a Low-Cost Brain–Computer Interface." *Industrial Robot: The International Journal of Robotics Research and Application* 49 (1): 150–159. https://doi.org/10.1108/IR-03-2021-0062.

Yang, Geng, Jia Deng, Gaoyang Pang, Hao Zhang, Jiayi Li, Bin Deng, Zhibo Pang, et al. 2018. "An IoT-Enabled Stroke Rehabilitation System Based on Smart Wearable Armband and Machine Learning." *IEEE Journal of Translational Engineering in Health and Medicine* 6: 1–10. https://doi.org/10.1109/JTEHM.2018.2822681.

Yang, Nachuan, Juncheng Li, Pengpeng Xu, Ziniu Zeng, Siqi Cai, and Longhan Xie. 2022. "Design of Elbow Rehabilitation Exoskeleton Robot with SEMG-Based Torque Estimation Control Strategy." In *2022 6th International Conference on Robotics and Automation Sciences (ICRAS)*, 105–113. IEEE. https://doi.org/10.1109/ICRAS55217.2022.9842264.

Yeom, Hong Gi, June Sic Kim, and Chun Kee Chung. 2013. "Estimation of the Velocity and Trajectory of Three-Dimensional Reaching Movements from Non-Invasive Magnetoencephalography Signals." *Journal of Neural Engineering* 10 (2): 026006. https://doi.org/10.1088/1741-2560/10/2/026006.

Yu, Kun-Hsing, Andrew L. Beam, and Isaac S. Kohane. 2018. "Artificial Intelligence in Healthcare." *Nature Biomedical Engineering* 2 (10): 719–731. https://doi.org/10.1038/s41551-018-0305-z.

Yu, Yang, Chen Chen, Xinjun Sheng, and Xiangyang Zhu. 2020. "Multi-DoF Continuous Estimation for Wrist Torques Using Stacked Autoencoder." *Biomedical Signal Processing and Control* 57 (March): 101733. https://doi.org/10.1016/j.bspc.2019.101733.

Yuk, Do-Gyeong, and Jung Woo Sohn. 2022. "User Independent Hand Motion Recognition for Robot Arm Manipulation." *Journal of Mechanical Science and Technology* 36 (6): 2739–2747. https://doi.org/10.1007/s12206-022-0507-x.

Zandonà, Alessandro, Rosario Vasta, Adriano Chiò, and Barbara di Camillo. 2019. "A Dynamic Bayesian Network Model for the Simulation of Amyotrophic Lateral Sclerosis Progression." *BMC Bioinformatics* 20 (S4): 118. https://doi.org/10.1186/s12859-019-2692-x.

Zhang, Jing. 2017. "Multivariate Analysis and Machine Learning in Cerebral Palsy Research." *Frontiers in Neurology* 8 (December). https://doi.org/10.3389/fneur.2017.00715.

Zhang, Rui, Fali Li, Tao Zhang, Dezhong Yao, and Peng Xu. 2020. "Subject Inefficiency Phenomenon of Motor Imagery Brain-Computer Interface: Influence Factors and Potential Solutions." *Brain Science Advances* 6 (3): 224–241. https://doi.org/10.26599/BSA.2020.9050021.

Zhao, Aite, Lin Qi, Junyu Dong, and Hui Yu. 2018. "Dual Channel LSTM Based Multi-Feature Extraction in Gait for Diagnosis of Neurodegenerative Diseases." *Knowledge-Based Systems* 145 (April): 91–97. https://doi.org/10.1016/j.knosys.2018.01.004.

Zhu, Yuanlu, Ying Li, Jinling Lu, and Pengcheng Li. 2021. "EEGNet with Ensemble Learning to Improve the Cross-Session Classification of SSVEP Based BCI from Ear-EEG." *IEEE Access* 9: 15295–15303. https://doi.org/10.1109/ACCESS.2021.3052656.

11 Emerging Computational Methods Applied to BCI Systems for Restoring Motor Functions

Andrés Felipe Ruiz-Olaya,†, Javier M. Antelis**, Alexander Cerquera***, and Sebastián Jaramillo-Isaza**

*Antonio Nariño University, Faculty of Mechanical, Electronic and Biomedical Engineering, Bogotá, Colombia; **Tecnologico de Monterrey, Escuela de Ingeniería y Ciencias, Monterrey, Mexico; ***Department of Engineering, Neuro Wave Systems, Beachwood, OH, USA

†Corresponding Author: andresru@uan.edu.co

ABBREVIATIONS

AI	Artificial intelligence
ANN	Artificial neural network
BCI	Brain–computer interface
CAR	Common average reference
CCA	Canonical correlation analysis
CMRR	Common mode rejection ratio
CNN	Convolutional neural network
CNS	Central nervous system
CSP	Common spatial pattern
DSF	Dynamic spatial filter
DL	Deep learning
EcoG	Electrocorticogram
EEG	Electroencephalography
EMG	Electromyography
ERD	Event-related desynchronization
ERP	Event-related potential
ErrP	Error-related potential
ERS	Event-related synchronization
FBCSSP	Filter bank common spatio-spectral patterns
FES	Functional electrical stimulation

DOI: 10.1201/9781032699882-11

FIR	Finite impulse response
fNIRS	Functional near-infrared spectroscopy
GMM	Gaussian mixture model
hBCI	Hybrid brain–computer interface
ICA	Independent component analysis
LDA	Linear discriminant analysis
LSTM	Long short-term memory
MI	Motor imagery
ML	Machine learning
NIRS	Near-infrared spectroscopy
NP	Neuroprostheses
PCA	Principal component analysis
RDA	Regularized discriminant analysis
RNN	Recurrent neural network
SBCSP	Sub-band common spatial pattern
SCP	Slow cortical potential
SMR	Sensorimotor rhythm
SNR	Signal-to-noise ratio
SSVEP	Steady-state visually evoked potentials
SVM	Support vector machine

11.1 INTRODUCTION

The electroencephalogram (EEG) is the measurement of the electrical activity at cortical brain regions, originated by flowing currents through the layer of pyramidal neurons in the cerebral cortex (Tong and Thankor, 2009). The magnitude of these currents is very small, but the sum of the simultaneous activity of many neurons generates an electric field that can be measured on the scalp surface. EEG signals reflect mental tasks (Padfield et al., 2019), which can be classified into six main bands according to the frequency content, as seen in Figure 11.1, which are: delta (0.5–4Hz), theta (4–8Hz), alpha (8–13Hz), beta (14–30Hz), and gamma (>30Hz) (Tong and Thankor, 2009). Mu (μ) rhythms consist of EEG activity with a falling alpha frequency band, acquired over the sensorimotor cortex. The increase and decrease in power are specific to the frequency band, and it has been reported that the different frequency bands are related to different neurobiological mechanisms (Neuper and Pfurtscheller, 2001).

During the last few years, great attention has been given to brain–computer interfaces (BCIs) because these systems could be used for restoring control and communication functions in people with disabilities. An open problem in implementing a BCI interface lies in identifying the user's intention, which can be performed by recording EEG activity to control a machine without using the neuromuscular pathway (McFarland and Wolpaw, 2011). BCI systems use signal processing techniques to classify "patterns" in EEG signals, which are modulated by the user when performing a mental task or in response to a specific event (Abiri et al., 2019). EEG signal acquisition could be performed by placing small metal discs denominated "electrodes", usually made of stainless steel, gold, tin, or silver covered with a silver chloride coating. These electrodes on the surface of the skull provide a non-invasive way to quantify brain function and regional brain activity. Electrodes are located according to anatomical references for their distribution and location, as defined by the international 10–20 standard (Tong and Thankor, 2009).

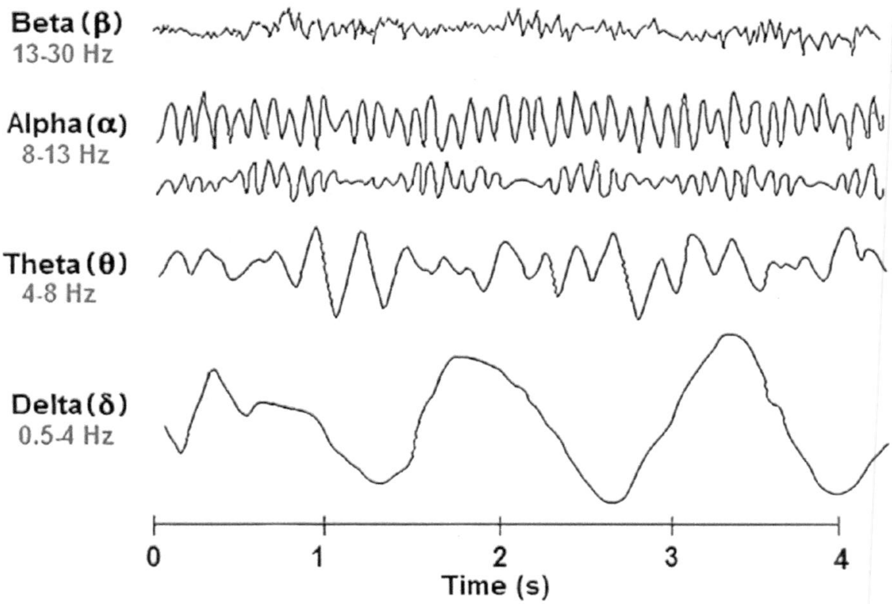

FIGURE 11.1 Representation of the main bands of EEG according to the frequency content.

An interface BCI can record and measure brain activity, process it, and identify commands that are delivered to external devices or applications to carry out a user's desired action. EEG-based BCIs provide the brain with alternate output channels to peripheral nerves and muscles based on the user's EEG signals. BCIs could replace, restore, or improve the human central nervous system (CNS) output, enhancing its interactions with the external or internal environment (Wolpaw, 2013).

The interaction between a person and a BCI can be implemented through mental tasks performed by the user (such as motor imagination, mathematical calculations, etc.) and through selective attention tasks (for example using evoked potentials, event-related potentials (ERP), etc.), the latter through the presentation of external stimuli (Abiri et al., 2019). A widely used interaction mechanism corresponds to motor imagination, which consists of imagining the "visualization" or execution of some movement, for example of the lower or upper limb, without actually executing it. It has been shown that motor imagination can modify neural activities in motor-sensory areas of the cerebral cortex in a similar way to executing a real movement, which is known as synchronization- or desynchronization-related (ERS/ERD) events, mainly reflected in the power of the EEG signal at different time points, represented in different frequency bands. Another widely used BCI user–system interaction mechanism corresponds to steady-state visual evoked potentials (SSVEP), which generate natural responses at the brain level (specifically in the occipital area of visual processing) to visual stimuli presented repetitively at different frequencies.

Thus, BCIs are an emerging technology that could facilitate the recovery of affected functions by serving as training tools to induce brain plasticity and compensating lost motor functions. BCIs have effectively been used for rehabilitation (Brambilla et al., 2021) and for controlling electric wheelchairs (Chen et al., 2022), exoskeletons (Juan et al., 2022), and arm robots (Chen et al., 2019).

EEG signal processing techniques are important for BCI systems because they provide methods to identify or classify cognitive tasks from the brain electrical activity recorded at the skull. During the last few years, multiple computational and EEG signal processing methods have been reported focused on increasing the effectiveness of recognizing mental states in BCI interfaces. Widely used computational methods applied for EEG signal processing include independent component analysis (ICA), principal component analysis (PCA), common spatial patterns (CSPs), and canonical correlation analysis (CCA), among others (Padfield et al., 2019; Aggarwal and Chugh, 2022). Furthermore, different temporal, spectral, and spatial filtering methods has been explored, aimed to choose the most discriminating features from EEG data for motor intention decoding (Blanco-Diaz et al., 2022). Feature extraction allows for data characterization through representations in the temporal, frequency, and time-frequency domains; techniques widely used include power spectral density, coherence, phase coupling (phase lock value), and complexity measures, among others (Aggarwal and Chugh, 2022).

Identification of a movement or its intention requires methods that interpret data features and translate them into outputs within a classification or regression problem. Widely used methods are artificial neural networks (ANNs), support vector machines (SVMs), regularized discriminant analysis (RDA), filter bank common spatio-spectral patterns (FBCSSPs), sub-band common spatial patterns (SBCSPs), and clustering algorithms, among others (Padfield et al., 2019). In addition, with the fast advances in artificial intelligence (AI), which include machine learning (ML) and deep learning (DL) techniques, there are potential novel applications in EEG-based BCI systems for restoring human motor functions.

This chapter focuses on reviewing the background, applications, and reported effectiveness of novel and emerging computational methods applied to BCI systems to restore motor functions, in which two approaches will be further explored:

- Deep-learning-based methods
- Fusion of multimodal information

Traditionally, the use of artificial neural networks (ANNs) requires selecting specific weights according to performance criteria, which is a drawback for implementation in EEG-BCI. Recently, deep learning has successfully been used in multiple areas (such as computer vision), providing high performance. Deep learning methods, including deep neural networks, have also been applied for decoding a subject's intention in BCI systems.

Thus, in recent years, with the advent of DL algorithms including transfer learning, ensemble learning, reinforcement learning, multitask learning, recurrent neural networks (RNNs), convolutional neural networks (CNNs), and transformers (Krizhevsky et al., 2017; Kundu and Ari, 2020), an increased performance has been obtained when applied to BCI applications. Algorithms such as EEGNet, Deep-ConvNet, and Shallow-ConvNet have been proposed in BCI applications (Fujiwara and Ushiba, 2022). Mean accuracy at the group level of 96.36% for motor imagery (MI) classification has been reported, quantifying differences in left and right hemispheric EEG with the implementation of a dual CNN (Lun et al., 2022).

Secondly, decoding user intention from multimodal information sources, such as electromyography (EMG) and functional near-infrared spectroscopy (fNIRS), has improved BCI systems' performance (Liu et al., 2021). These advanced hybrid brain–computer interfaces (hBCIs) require novel information fusion methods from two or more sources and must be developed and validated so that they allow the user to conduct a more accurate classification/translation. Recent studies have concluded that coherence between EEG and EMG does not only have an efferent origin (neuronal activity that would go from the brain or spinal cord to the periphery) but also an afferent origin, in such a way that it would also depend on the information sent back from the periphery to the brain (Fauvet et al., 2021). This fact suggests the importance of providing sensory feedback in BCI systems, which has important implication for restoring motor functions. Additionally, several authors have implemented BCI systems combining different paradigms using EEG, including motor imagery and steady-state visually evoked potential, among others.

11.2 EEG-BASED BCI FOR REHABILITATION

The implementation of an EEG-based BCI requires of three modules: an EEG signal acquisition module, a signal processing module (pre-processing, feature extraction, and classification/translation), and an application module. Figure 11.2 shows the components of an EEG-based BCI and their interactions.

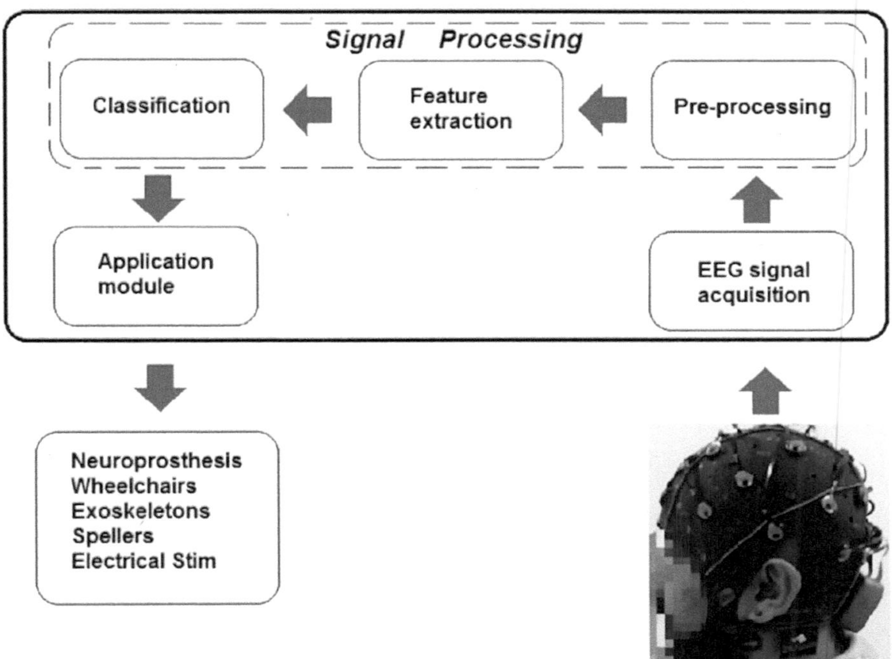

FIGURE 11.2 Diagram of an EEG-based BCI system using computational methods.

Interaction with a BCI system, as shown in Figure 11.2, could include two steps: 1) a training step focused on calibrating the system and 2) an online operating stage focused on recognizing EEG signal patterns and translating them into commands to control an external system. Taking into account that EEG signals are user-sensitive, most of the implemented BCIs have been calibrated specifically for each person.

11.2.1 Acquisition of EEG Signals for BCI

The EEG signal acquisition module aims to detect brain or neuronal activity. In the literature, it has been reported that BCI systems can record electrophysiological signals using invasive techniques such as electrocorticogram (EcoG) and using non-invasive techniques, including scalp electroencephalogram (EEG) and near-infrared spectroscopy (NIRS). EcoG provides a good signal quality, but it is a high-risk method for the user. Taking into account the spatial resolution parameter, EEG and NIRS have a spatial resolution of centimeters, while EcoG has a spatial resolution of millimeters. On the other hand, EEG and EcoG have a high temporal resolution while NIRS has moderate resolution in time.

Before being detected by the EEG electrodes, the currents from the brain cortical regions have gone through the meninges, skull, and scalp. Therefore, their amplitude is considerably attenuated, characterized by very low signal-to-noise ratios (SNR). Accordingly, EEG signal acquisition systems must have a very high common-mode rejection ratio (CMRR > 90dB) to attenuate noise sources. Furthermore, as the recorded signals are in the order of ±100μV, acquired EEG values must be amplified before the analogue-to-digital conversion. Figure 11.3 describes the locations of EEG electrodes according to the 10–20 International System.

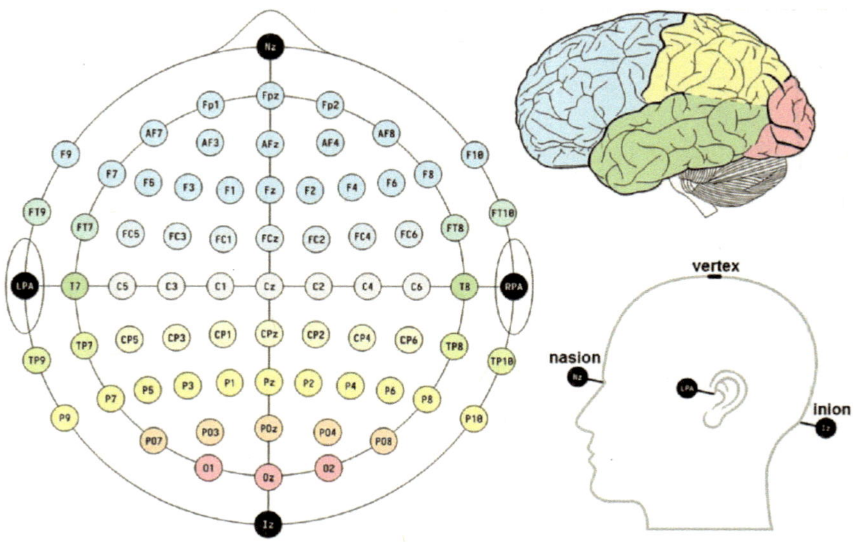

FIGURE 11.3 Acquisition of EEG signals according to the 10–20 International System of electrode placement.

11.2.2 Paradigms for Restoring Motor Functions

Several brain potentials can be used to implement EEG-based BCI systems, including steady-state visual evoked potential, event-related potential, cerebral oscillatory activity, and slow cortical potential, among others (Abiri et al., 2019). Herein, a description of neurophysiological signals most widely used in the implementation of BCI systems for restoring motor functions is provided:

- Steady-state visually evoked potentials (SSVEP): These are potentials that are neural responses elicited by visual stimulation at different frequencies. A brain electrical activity arises at the same (or harmonic) frequency of the visual stimulus. These potentials can be measured on the EEG after a sensory visual stimulation. Figure 11.4 presents a diagram of a SSVEP-based BCI.
- Event-related potentials (ERPs): These are potentials that are generated in response to a stimulus. These potentials can be measured on the EEG before, during, and after a psychological, motor, or sensory event. The most widely used ERP in BCI applications is P300, which consists of a positive deflection in the EEG signal that appears 300 ms after stimulation (visual, auditory, somatosensory) of a rare event. Error-related potentials (ErrPs) are variations of the well-known ERPs, described as neurophysiological signals associated with error processing (Aggarwal and Chugh, 2022). An

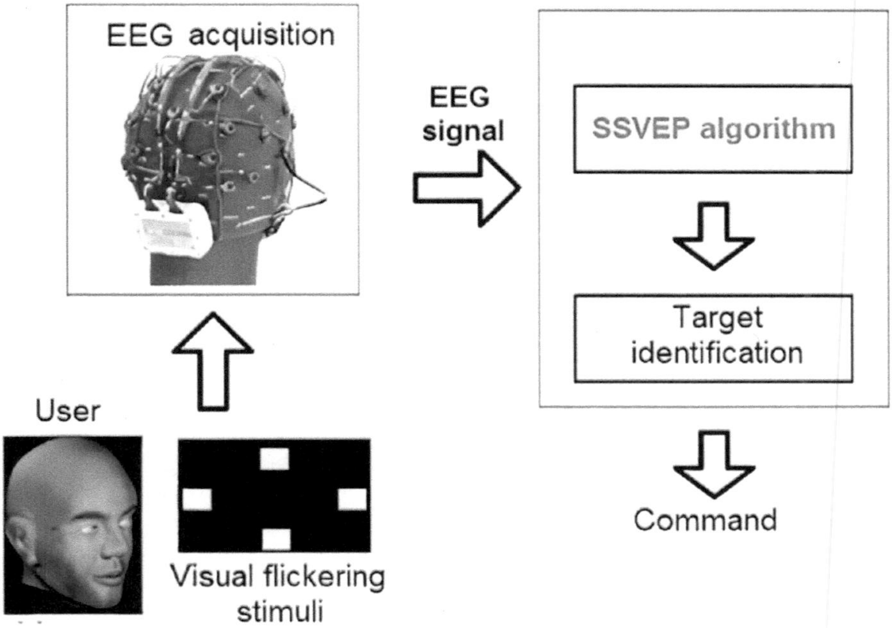

FIGURE 11.4 Block diagram of a SSVEP-based BCI for identification of a user's commands.

ErrP is triggered when wrong actions are perceived between the patient's target and the BCI output. Physiologically, frontal and central brain regions evoke ERP responses with greater amplitude.

- Sensorimotor rhythm (SMR): These are cerebral oscillatory activity that appear in the different frequency bands (μ, β) associated with real and imagined movement. To control a BCI interface using SMR, the user must concentrate on imagining a specific movement. This yields a desynchronization in the specific bands representing the imagined movement, which is interpreted by the computer interface executing a predefined action. Figure 11.5 shows the development of a BCI system that uses brain oscillatory activity through motor imagery (MI) as input. MI is defined as the mental task of representing a corporal motion without executing it.
- Slow cortical potentials (SCPs): These are low-frequency potentials that the user can learn to control through biofeedback. With training, the user can modulate positive or negative changes in the signal, which allows the control of devices that allow the user to communicate with the environment.

Table 11.1 presents some reported works of BCI systems for restoring motor function, according to used computational methods and taking into account the used paradigms.

11.2.3 Application Module: Case Studies

The use of computational methods based on artificial intelligence have been reported in BCI systems to restore lost motor functions. These applications include motor neuroprostheses, virtual reality systems, robotic arms, prostheses, and exoskeletons, among others.

TABLE 11.1
EEG-Based BCI for Restoring Motor Function by Paradigm and Used Methods

Reference	Methods	Paradigm	Application
Benzy et al., 2020	Phase locking value (PLV)	MI	Control of motorized arm support
Kwak et al., 2017	Convolutional neural network (CNN)	SSVEP	Exoskeleton control
Okahara et al., 2017	LDA	P300	Spinocerebellar ataxia
Ang and Guan, 2017	FBCSP	MI	Stroke rehabilitation
Delijorge et al., 2020	Regularized LDA	P300	Robotic hand orthosis
Chen et al., 2019	CCA	SSVEP	Robotic arm
Savic et al., 2021		SCP	Assistive active glove
Lopes-Dias et al., 2019		ErrP	Robot control

11.2.3.1 Controlling Motor Neuroprostheses

Neuroprostheses (NP) are systems that permit the electrical stimulation of nerves, aimed to furnish sensory input to the nervous system (sensory NPs), or to innervate the muscle fiber (motor NPs), (Prochazka, 2018). Functional electrical stimulation (FES) is focused on using timed and synchronized electrical stimulations to artificially elicit a functional motor response, for example to compensate for drop-foot during the swing phase of the gait. Figure 11.5 shows a diagram of a BCI-controlled motor neuroprosthesis using motor imagery.

BCI systems allow synchronizing cortical commands and movements generated by FES, providing a mechanism to induce neuroplasticity. In the literature, it has been reported how neural mechanisms underlying the use of a BCI-triggered FES could enhance neuromotor rehabilitation processes (Milosevic et al., 2020). In addition, to command a BCI-controlled motor neuroprosthesis, active participation by the user is required. Thus, the integration of neural afferents with cognitive, attentional, volitional, and motivational components has been reported to enhance plasticity processes at the synaptic level.

11.2.3.2 Controlling Virtual Reality Systems

Virtual reality systems enable the use of an immersive environment for restoring motor functions, which enhances intervention therapies of disabled subjects when controlling a BCI interface (Kong et al., 2015). However, various problems arise in a clinical scenario when applying the new technology for motor rehabilitation,

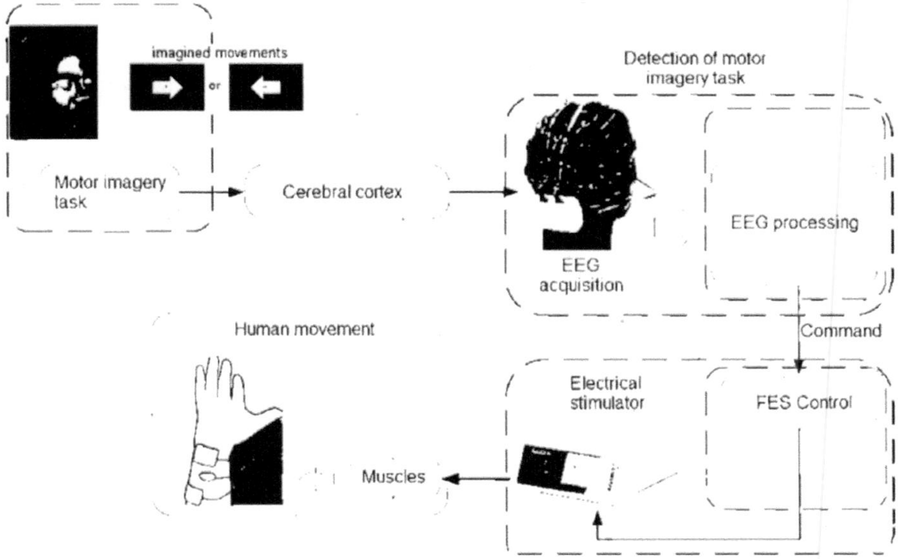

FIGURE 11.5 Block diagram of a BCI-controlled motor neuroprosthesis using a motor imagery task.

including real-time implementation, intra- and inter-subject variability, and user engagement (Wen et al., 2020).

11.2.3.3 Controlling Robotic Arms, Orthoses, and Prostheses

The precise manipulation of robotic prosthesis and exoskeletons using a BCI involves addressing different issues focused on decoding dynamic, continuous, and real-time control commands from the patient's electrical brain signals (Vilela and Hochberg, 2020; Ruiz-Olaya et al., 2019).

The integration of BCI and robotic systems for motor rehabilitation and assistance relies on the identification of a user's intention to execute a motor task using electrical brain activity in such a way that the robotic device provides assistive forces during therapy sessions (Baniqued et al., 2021; Robinson et al., 2021).

11.3 PIPELINES FOR EEG SIGNAL PROCESSING

The EEG signal processing module of a BCI includes multiple stages such as pre-processing, feature extraction, and classification/translation, as seen in Figure 11.2.

Pre-processing aims at conditioning acquired EEG data by using artifact detection and applying spectral and spatial filtering, among other techniques (Padfield et al., 2019). The feature extraction stage provides task-specific features of the EEG signal in both the spectral domain and the spatial domain. EEG signal techniques, including wavelet transform, spectral power, autoregressive models, and common spatial patterns (CSPs), have been reported in the literature to obtain descriptors from EEG data. The CSP algorithm is a high-performance technique for MI task decoding in BCI, considering its high identification rate and low computational cost (Aggarwal and Chugh, 2022).

The main techniques used in the analysis of EEG signals and the emerging methods that are currently being used to improve performance are described herein.

11.3.1 Artifact Detection, Rejection, and Correction

In BCI implementation, artifact detection, rejection, and correction in EEG signals plays a fundamental step to reach a good performance. Electrodes used in EEG recording do not discriminate the electrical signals they receive; therefore, one of the biggest challenges when processing EEG signals is artifact recognition and elimination. As seen in Figure 11.6, an acquired EEG signal could be represented as a sum of electrical brain activity (EEG) and biological artifacts (i.e., electrical muscle activity and electrical activity from eye movement, among others).

Pre-processing includes removing artifacts from EEG signals. Widely used methods include principal component analysis (PCA), independent component analysis (ICA), regression, filters, EEG signal decomposition, and wavelets, among others. According to Figure 11.6, acquired EEG signal $x(n)$ results of the sum of the brain activity $s(n)$ and the artifacts $a(n)$. Considering the assumption that neural

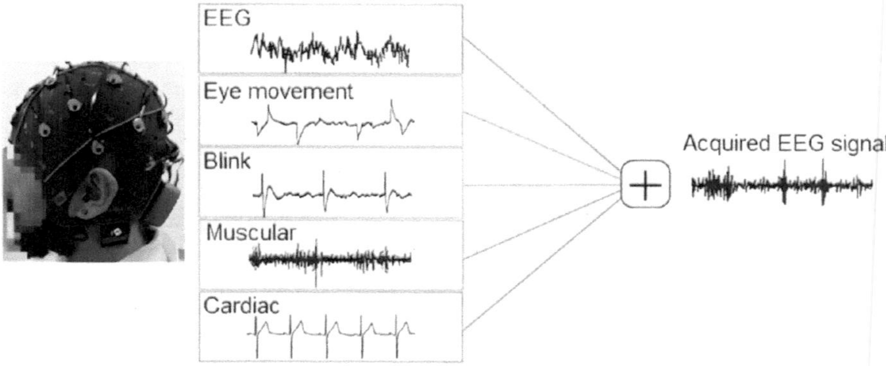

FIGURE 11.6 Representation of the acquired EEG signal as a sum of electrical brain activity (EEG) and biological artifacts.

activity and non-brain sources are linearly combined, these can be modeled in the equation:

$$x(s) = A \cdot s(n) + a(n) \tag{1}$$

where: $x(n) = \left[x_1(n), x_2(n), x_3(n), \ldots, x_p(n)\right]^T$ is the recorded p-channel EEG data at the n-th sample and T represents the transpose operation; $s(n) = \left[s_1(n), s_2(n), s_3(n), \ldots, s_q(n)\right]^T$ is the unknown source data, where each row represent brain activity or non-brain source; A represents a p × q unknown mixing matrix; and $a(n) = \left[a_1(n), a_2(n), a_3(n), \ldots, a_p(n)\right]^T$ is the is the p additive zero-mean noise data. Most of the implemented artifact rejection methods focus on obtaining the demixing matrix, W, to estimate sources from observed EEG data:

$$\hat{s}(n) = W \cdot x(n) \tag{2}$$

According to Minguillon et al. (2017), new applications of ambulatory BCI applications using low-cost wearable EEG headsets to restore motor functions at home (unrestricted experimental condition) include multiple kinds of artifacts. Current methods of artifact identification and rejection in EEG signals have to be improved to be implemented under unrestricted conditions.

Recently, emerging computational methods has been reported for artifact detection, rejection and/or correction, taking into account that traditional methods to artifact detection require a specialized person to manually explore and identify artifacts in segments. The work in Saba-Sadiya et al. (2021) proposes a method based on representation learning for implementing artifact detection and correction in EEG signals. The pipeline uses a deep learning network. The work in Mathe et al. (2021) describes a hybrid meta-heuristic-based deep learning method for the removal of artifacts from EEG. The model uses one-dimensional convolution neural networks that permit rejecting artifacts from EEG data.

11.3.2 Spectral and Spatial Filtering

Spatial filtering is implemented in EEG processing to discriminate important spatial information in the EEG data by weighting the contributions from multiple EEG electrodes. Thus, spatial filters permit the use of signals from various EEG electrodes to enhance the EEG information. Optimizing spatial filters have become an important step in BCI classification that could be implemented with artifact detection, rejection, and correction in EEG signals. There is a set of spatial filtering techniques applied for EEG pre-processing in BCI systems. Common average referencing (CAR) and Laplacian spatial filtering are techniques to average values of a set of electrodes that are subtracted from the EEG channel of interest, which have been implemented to remove the common-mode signals (i.e., those that appear simultaneously, such as power line noise). Furthermore, spatial filtering can be implemented using data-driven and unsupervised techniques that include principal component analysis (PCA) and independent component analysis (ICA).

The most used method to obtain spatial filters for MI tasks is CSP. This method calculates spatial filters for maximizing the variance of EEG signals from one class while the variance from the other class is minimized (Mishuhina and Jiang, 2021). Although CSP provides excellent performance, it does have some drawbacks, which include overfitting and sensitivity to artifacts. In order to increase the performance of CSP, multiple variants of this technique have been reported. The common spatio-spectral patterns (CSSP) technique uses CSP combined with a finite impulse response (FIR) filter. Sub-band CSP and filter bank CSP (FBCSP) decompose the EEG signal into a set of sub-bands (Blanco-Diaz and Ruiz-Olaya, 2020).

Furthermore, CCA allows implementing spatial filters to improve the functionality of EEG-based BCIs. CCA is based on finding linear combinations of two vectors of random variables, which have a maximum correlation with each other, when there are correlations among the variables (Mishuhina and Jiang, 2021). Principle component analysis (PCA) is used to decompose an EEG signal into several components. The effect of variants for spectral and temporal parameters have been reported for decoding hand motor imagery mental tasks using CSP-based methods (Blanco-Diaz et al., 2022).

The work reported in (Banville et al., 2022) describes dynamic spatial filtering (DSF), a technique that enhances the robustness against EEG signal contamination in prediction tasks. The authors report that the method obtains a similar performance to baseline methods if no noise is added, outperforming baselines methods (over 29.4%) if there is significant channel corruption.

11.3.3 Epoching and Feature Extraction

Electroencephalogram (EEG) signals are non-stationary, indicating that statistical characteristics of the features used in an EEG-based BCI to decode mental tasks could be continuously changing. Therefore, considering that the EEG signal is non-stationary, conventional or linear methods may not be suitable for obtaining features.

EEG epoching is a technique based on extracting specific time-windows, named "epochs", from the ongoing recorded EEG signal. Epochs are time-locked according to a specific event or stimulus, e.g., a visual stimulus. The length of actual epochs should be chosen very carefully and is strongly related to the aims of each study.

Feature extraction focuses on selecting discriminative data for subsequent classification or detection methods. Despite the availability of several metrics in which EEG signals can be represented, the most widely used features correspond to frequency band power features and time point features. In fact, band spectral features are the gold standard to identify mental task of MI for BCI. For example, a spectral analysis of EEG using fast Fourier transform (FFT) can be performed using Equation 3:

$$X(k) = \sum_{n=1}^{N} x(n) \exp\left(-j\frac{2\pi}{N}\right)^{nk}, \quad k = 0,\ldots,N-1 \tag{3}$$

where $X(k)$ represents the discrete Fourier coefficients, N is the length of the transform, and $x(n)$ corresponds to an EEG signal of one channel in time.

In the scientific literature, multiple features for design of EEG-based BCIs have been reported, including amplitude of EEG signals, power spectral density, and time-frequency features from wavelets, among others.

Additionally, a feature selection procedure could be implemented focused on selecting a subset of extracted features from EEG, considering that those features might contain redundant information. Furthermore, selecting a smaller number of features provide a faster parameter optimization by the classifier.

11.3.4 Classification, Regression, and Clustering

Machine learning methods can be divided into supervised learning and unsupervised learning. The classification/translation component, as seen in Figure 11.2, aims to interpret or classify the features provided by the feature extraction step in a command. According to ML, in supervised learning, the data is frequently divided into two subsets: the training and testing sets. Instead, unsupervised learning includes multiple algorithms focused on handling unlabeled data (i.e. data without prior knowledge about its class). Clustering relates to several algorithms for unsupervised learning, aimed at identifying groups of observations in a dataset that are similar to one another according to some kind of metric. Some reported clustering algorithms for BCI are k-means and the Gaussian mixture model (GMM) (Padfield et al., 2019; Kulkarni et al., 2022).

In the area of brain–computer interfaces to restore motor functions, the most used techniques for classification are linear discriminant analysis (LDA), support vector machines (SVMs), and artificial neural networks (ANNs).

11.3.4.1 Linear Discriminant Analysis

This is a statistical technique that allows the user to classify "elements" into a set of groups that are mutually exclusive (classes) based on measurable characteristics in each of these objects. When implementing linear discriminant analysis, the challenge is selecting the function or rule that best separates the classes. When the number of classes is two, the separation is a line. If the number of classes is three, the discriminant function is a plane, and for more than three dimensions, the separation is performed by a hyper-plane.

11.3.4.2 Support Vector Machines

Given a group of separable samples, support vector machines (SVMs) identify a plane or hyper-plane that separates the groups. Taking into account that it could be many planes that permit separability between groups, the SVM determines the plane that provides the optimal separation, i.e., the plane that permits the maximum distance between the most distant samples of each group.

11.3.4.3 Artificial Neural Networks

Artificial neural networks (ANNs) simulate the properties found in natural brain neurons to solve problems, with the aim to obtain the generality and robustness provided by a biological neural network (Aggarwal and Chugh, 2022). Unlike traditional system modeling methods, where it is necessary to formulate or define mathematical equations to generate a set of instructions, neural networks are trained by applying input characteristics with known outputs.

Neural networks have been relevant as a computational method for classification of EEG signals. Currently, multiple variants of ANNs allow an adequate classification of EEG signals to recognize patterns related to the user's intention for motor rehabilitation. The main advantage of neural networks compared to other classifiers such as LDA is that the ANNs do not require the user to know the probability model of the process, as the ANN can fit the data without any specification of the process that generates the data. However, ANNs have the disadvantage of requiring large computing resources, which does not make them appropriate when such resources are limited.

11.4 TRENDS IN EEG SIGNAL PROCESSING FOR BCI

The emerging development of artificial intelligence (AI) technology and other computational methods has allowed the use MI techniques, deep learning (DL), and data fusion methods to face problems in classifying EEG-based BCI.

11.4.1 Deep Learning and Clustering Methods

A few years ago, with the fast evolution of deep learning, outstanding outcomes of using convolution neural networks (CNN) for EEG-based BCI were reported. CNN and CNN-based algorithms, including EEGNet and CNN-stacked autoencoders (CNN-SAE), showed adequate performance for motor imagery decoding tasks (Wang et al., 2018; Zhu et al., 2022). Other algorithms reported focused on Long short-term memory (LSTM)-based models for feature extraction of EEG for motor imagery (Wang et al., 2018). A major drawback of deep learning supervised models is that they require high volumes of EEG data during the training step.

On the other hand, to implement the classification of unlabeled EEG data in BCI applications, algorithms using clustering have been reported (Kulkarni et al., 2022).

Clustering for BCI applications focuses on separating EEG samples into a reduced set in such a way that EEG samples belong to the same groups. Several methods have been reported for EEG source decomposition, which permits grouping the EEG data (Frolov et al., 2020).

Table 11.2 presents recent deep learning methods implemented for EEG-based BCI systems.

11.4.2 Fusion of Multimodal Brain Signals

In the literature, hybrid or multimodal BCI (hBCI) systems have been implemented to include multiple biosignals, paradigms, and/or multisensory stimuli. Considering the difficulties in identifying user intent using EEG, it has been proposed to complement the information of EEG to decode the intention of movement by recording and processing information from other sources of information, for instance electromyography (EMG), which is related to neural activity to execute a motor task (López-Larraz et al., 2018; Balasubramanian et al., 2018). Several techniques have been

TABLE 11.2
Deep Learning Methods Implemented for EEG-Based BCI Systems

Reference	Dataset	Deep Learning Method	Paradigm	Performance
Luo and Chao, 2018	BCI Competition IV 2a and 2b	Deep RNN, sliding window cropping strategy (SWCS)	MI	Error rate: Dataset 2a: 26.44 ± 4.38, Dataset 2b:17.25 ± 3.84
Uyulan, 2021	BCI Competition IV Dataset A	LSTM, CNN	MI	Accuracy: 95.62%
Zhu et al., 2021		CNN–EEGNet	SSVEP	81.74%
Kumar et al., 2019	BCI Competition IV Dataset I and GigaDB dataset	Long short-term memory (LSTM) network	MI	Error rate: BCI Competition IV Dataset I: 3.09%, GigaDB: 2.07%
Kundu and Ari, 2020	BCI Competition II Dataset IIb and BCI Competition III Dataset II	Multiscale CNN and ensemble of SVMs	P300	Accuracy: 96%, Correctly recognized characters: 31
Li et al., 2020	Owner	Convolutional neural network	P300	Average accuracy: 97%
Podmore et al., 2019		Deep convolutional neural networks (DCNN)	SSVEP	Accuracy: 86%
Li, Xiang, and Kesavadas, 2020		Convolutional correlation analysis (Conv-CA)	SSVEP	ITR: 226.19 bits/min

Recurrent neural network (RNN), support vector machine (SVM)

reported for the analysis of EEG and EMG signals. The processing of EMG signals has been performed mainly using the time domain, identifying onsets, extracting onsets features, and calculating envelopes, while frequency analysis focused mainly on analyzing muscle fatigue (Asghar et al., 2022). However, the analysis and mechanism for the combined use or "fusion" of multimodal information EEG–EMG continues in research.

Multimodal BCI could be implemented by recording brain activity from other sources different to EEG, such as fNIRS, to increase quality of the signals. An fNIRS-based BCI can be used for recording the hemodynamic signals from target brain regions, which allows localizing and classifying a specific brain activity. Therefore, the simultaneous use of EEG and NIRS permits to implement a multimodal hybrid BCI, which have been proven to improve the performance of a BCI system compared to the use of an independent modality (i.e., EEG or NIRS) (Ruhunage et al., 2019; Zhu et al., 2017). An open source dataset for a hybrid EEG–NIRS fusion BCI system, implemented using a linear discriminant analysis classifier for the data classifications, has been reported in Liu et al. (2021). Emerging methods, such as deep learning classification, can significantly improve performance of BCI systems (Chiarelli et al., 2018).

In addition, various authors have reported the implementation of hybrid BCIs that use multiple paradigms simultaneously, for example, MI and P300 jointly (Pfurtscheller et al., 2010). Those systems improve classification accuracy better than using a single-modality method (Zuo et al., 2020). Table 11.3 shows some reported works that use the fusion of multimodal signals to implement EEG-based BCI systems.

TABLE 11.3
Fusion of Multimodal Signals Implemented for EEG-Based BCI Systems

Reference	Multimodal Signals	Application	ML Method
Ruhunage et al., 2019	EEG, EMG	Transhumeral prosthesis	Neural network
Guerrero-Mendez and Ruiz-Olaya, 2022	EEG–EMG	Reach-to-grasp movement	Coherence
Hooda et al., 2020	EEG, EMG	Foot movements	MAV, ZC, WL, and SSC for EMG. Power change of ERD/ERS for EEG. SVM for classification.
Zhu et al., 2017	EEG, fNIRS	Left-right hand grasping	Wavelet, slope information, SVM, LDA
Chiarelli et al., 2018	EEG, fNIRS	Left and right hand MI	DNN
Zuo et al., 2020	EEG: P300 and MI	Writing imagery	PLV, SFBCSP, BLDA
Luo et al., 2022	EEG: SSVEP and MI	MI: grasping movement SSVEP: four stimuli	TSCNN

Mean absolute value (MAV), zero crossing (ZC), waveform length (WL), slope sign change (SSC), sparse filter band common spatial pattern (SFBCSP), phase locking value (PLV), Bayesian linear discriminant analysis (BLDA), two-stream convolutional neural network (TSCNN)

11.5 FUTURE PROSPECTS AND LIMITATIONS

Considering that brain networks work at multiple spatial and temporal scales, connectivity analysis can provide new approaches for implementation of BCI systems for the restoration of lost motor functions (Gonzalez-Astudillo et al., 2021). Frequently used brain connectivity measures are bivariate, representing interactions between two brain regions or signals. Some computational methods to obtain connectivity include coherence, transfer entropy, complexity measures, Granger causality, and mutual information, among others (Bastos and Schoffelen, 2016).

The use of personalized methods adapted to the patient needs could provide a solution to the situations arising during interaction with a BCI application, including requirements of a user's learning with the interface, specific response to stimuli, and usability, using machine learning (ML) methods (Zhang et al., 2020). However, some techniques, like supervised deep learning models, need a huge amount of labeled data during the training step. Furthermore, deep learning models are sensitive to the quality of the training data to obtain discriminatory outcomes.

Finally, most of the reported computational methods in the scientific literature rely on linear methods, under the supposition of stationarity when using short-time segments (Samek et al., 2012). Linear methods of EEG signal analysis extract a limited amount of information from brain activity. EEG signals show nonlinear dynamics and chaotic behavior (Tong and Thankor, 2009; Maksimenko, 2018). Therefore, additional features obtained by methods from nonlinear dynamics have provided discriminative information to identify user's intent. The literature has reported BCI applications based on nonlinear dynamic features, such as mutual information, entropy, and complexity measures, including Shannon entropy, Lempel–Ziv complexity, Lyapunov exponent, and Kolmogorov entropy (Hosni et al., 2022; Wang et al., 2022; Tortora et al., 2019).

11.6 CONCLUSIONS

An alternative for restoring lost motor functions relies on using a BCI system. The effectiveness of an EEG-based BCI is based on several aspects that include: 1) producing stable and repeatable patterns in EEG signal according to specific mental tasks; 2) enhancing the signal quality of the recorded EEG; and 3) using decoding methods to translate EEG patterns into control commands. The main drawbacks of using EEG-based BCIs relate to the low SNR of EEG signals, contamination by internal and external artifacts, non-stationarity, and intra and inter-subject variability. Therefore, the performance and classification accuracy of an EEG-based BCI to restore motor functions depends on the implementation of adequate computational methods in the pipelines for EEG signal processing (i.e., pre-processing, feature extraction, and classification/translation). The most used machine learning algorithms for decoding user intention are LDA and SVM classifiers. However, state-of-the-art EEG decoding methods for BCI are benchmarked on EEG datasets acquired under controlled conditions. These models could have a low performance in real-world contexts, including applications for restoring motor function and rehabilitation at home.

Furthermore, considering that brain signals are high-dimensional, noisy, and non-stationary, emerging ML techniques could increase the performance of BCI systems aimed to restore motor function, including deep learning algorithms and the fusion of multimodal signals. Among reported EEG-based BCI applications, DL has been used to extract EEG features and has been combined with the traditional ML technology to perform a classification or regression task.

On the other hand, using multimodal signals, such as the P300 and SCPs, would offer a superior performance in specific applications where the user must select multiple options and where algorithms should recognize a command.

11.7 ACKNOWLEDGMENT

Authors thank the Universidad Antonio Nariño (Colombia) for funding under the project number 2021020 "Model based on multimodal EEG-EMG information to improve motion intention decoding for the control of a BCI system".

REFERENCES

Abiri, R., S. Borhani, E. Sellers, Y. Jiang, and X. Zhao. 2019. A Comprehensive Review of EEG-Based Brain–Computer Interface Paradigms. *J Neural Eng.* 16:011001.

Aggarwal, S., and N. Chugh. 2022. Review of Machine Learning Techniques for EEG Based Brain Computer Interface. *Arch Comput Methods Eng.* 29(5):3001–3020.

Ang, K.K., and C. Guan. 2017. EEG-Based Strategies to Detect Motor Imagery for Control and Rehabilitation. *IEEE Trans Neural Syst Rehabil Eng.* 25(4):392–401.

Asghar, A., S. Jawaid Khan, F. Azim, C.S. Shakeel, A. Hussain, and I.K. Niazi. 2022. Review on Electromyography Based Intention for Upper Limb Control Using Pattern Recognition for Human-Machine Interaction. *Proc Inst Mech Eng H.* 236(5):628–645.

Balasubramanian, S., E. Garcia-Cossio, N. Birbaumer, E. Burdet, and A. Ramos-Murguialday. 2018. Is EMG a Viable Alternative to BCI for Detecting Movement Intention in Severe Stroke? *IEEE Trans Biomed Eng.* 65(12):2790–2797.

Baniqued, P.D.E., E.C. Stanyer, M. Awais, A. Alazmani, A.E. Jackson, and M.A. Mon-Williams. 2021. Brain–Computer Interface Robotics for Hand Rehabilitation after Stroke: A Systematic Review. *J Neuro Eng Rehabil.* 18:15.

Banville, H., S. Wood, C. Aimone, D.A. Engemann, and A. Gramfort. 2022. Robust Learning from Corrupted EEG with Dynamic Spatial Filtering. *NeuroImage* 251:118994.

Bastos, A.M., and J.M. Schoffelen. 2016. A Tutorial Review of Functional Connectivity Analysis Methods and Their Interpretational Pitfalls. *Front Syst Neurosci.* 9:175, eCollection 2015.

Benzy, V.K., A.P. Vinod, R. Subasree, S. Alladi, and K. Raghavendra. 2020. Motor Imagery Hand Movement Direction Decoding Using Brain Computer Interface to Aid Stroke Recovery and Rehabilitation. *IEEE Trans Neural Syst Rehabil Eng.* 28(12):3051–3062.

Blanco-Diaz, C.F., J.M. Antelis, and A.F. Ruiz-Olaya. 2022. Comparative Analysis of Spectral and Temporal Combinations in CSP-Based Methods for Decoding Hand Motor Imagery Tasks. *J Neurosci Methods.* 371(April):109495.

Blanco-Diaz, C.F., and A.F. Ruiz-Olaya. 2020. A Novel Method Based on Regularized Logistic Regression and CCA for P300 Detection Using a Reduced Number of EEG Trials. *IEEE Lat Am Trans.* 18(12):2147–2154.

Brambilla, C., I. Pirovano, R.M. Mira, G. Rizzo, A. Scano, and A. Mastropietro. 2021. Combined Use of EMG and EEG Techniques for Neuromotor Assessment in Rehabilitative Applications: A Systematic Review. *Sensors.* 21(21):7014.

Chen, Wen, Shih-Kang Chen, Yi-Hung Liu, Yu-Jen Chen, and Chin-Sheng Chen. 2022. An Electric Wheelchair Manipulating System Using SSVEP-Based BCI System. *Biosensors.* 12(10):772.

Chen, Xiaogang, B. Zhao, Y. Wang, and X. Gao. 2019. Combination of High-Frequency SSVEP-Based BCI and Computer Vision for Controlling a Robotic Arm. *J Neural Eng.* 16(2):026012.

Chiarelli, A.M., et al. 2018. Deep Learning for Hybrid EEG-fNIRS Brain-Computer Interface: Application to Motor Imagery Classification. *J Neural Eng.* 15(3):036028.

Delijorge, J., O. Mendoza-Montoya, J.L. Gordillo, R. Caraza, H.R. Martinez, and J.M. Antelis. 2020. Evaluation of a P300-Based Brain-Machine Interface for a Robotic Hand-Orthosis Control. *Front Neurosci.* 14:589659.

Fauvet, M., D. Gasq, A. Chalard, J. Tisseyre, and D. Amarantini. 2021. Temporal Dynamics of Corticomuscular Coherence Reflects Alteration of the Central Mechanisms of Neural Motor Control in Post-Stroke Patients. *Front Hum Neurosci.* 15:682080.

Frolov, A., et al. 2020. Using Multiple Decomposition Methods and Cluster Analysis to Find and Categorize Typical Patterns of EEG Activity in Motor Imagery Brain–Computer Interface Experiments. *Front Robot AI, Sec Biomed Robot.* 7.

Fujiwara, Y., and J. Ushiba. 2022. Deep Residual Convolutional Neural Networks for Brain–Computer Interface to Visualize Neural Processing of Hand Movements in the Human Brain. *Front Comput Neurosci.* 16:882290.

Gonzalez-Astudillo, J., T. Cattai, G. Bassignana, M.C. Corsi, and F. Fallani. 2021. Network-Based Brain–Computer Interfaces: Principles and Applications. *J Neural Eng.* 18(1).

Guerrero-Mendez, C.D., and A.F. Ruiz-Olaya. 2022. Coherence-Based Connectivity Analysis of EEG and EMG Signals During Reach-to-Grasp Movement Involving Two Weights. *Brain Comp Int.* 9(3):140–154.

Hooda, N., R. Das, and N. Kumar 2020. Fusion of EEG and EMG Signals for Classification of Unilateral Foot Movements. *Biomed Signal Process Control.* 60:101990.

Hosni, S.M.I., S.B. Borgheai, J. McLinden, S. Zhu, X. Huang, S. Ostadabbas, and Y. Shahriari. 2022. A Graph-Based Nonlinear Dynamic Characterization of Motor Imagery Toward an Enhanced Hybrid BCI. *Neuroinformatics.* 20(4):1169–1189.

Juan, J.V., L. Ossa, E. Iáñez, M. Ortiz, L. Ferrero, and J.M. Azorín. 2022. Decoding Lower-Limbs Kinematics from EEG Signals While Walking with an Exoskeleton. *Lect Notes Comput Sci.* 13258:615–624.

Kong, L., Z. Xue, L. Chen, F. He, H. Qi, B. Wan, et al. 2015. Research Progress of Brain-Computer Interface Technology Based on Virtual Reality Environment. *J Electron Meas Instrum.* 29:317–327.

Krizhevsky, A., I. Sutskever, and G.E. Hinton. 2017. ImageNet Classification with Deep Convolutional Neural Networks. *Commun ACM.* 60(6):84–90.

Kulkarni, V., Y. Joshi, and R. Manthalkar. 2022. A Clustering Approach for Sensory-Motor Cortex Signal Classification Using Electroencephalogram Signal for Brain-Computer Interface. *Lect Notes Electr Eng.* 911:277–291.

Kumar, S., A. Sharma, and T. Tsunoda. 2019. Brain Wave Classification Using Long Short-Term Memory Network Based OPTICAL Predictor. *Sci Rep.* 9(1):1–13.

Kundu, S., and S. Ari. 2020. P300 Based Character Recognition Using Convolutional Neural Network and Support Vector Machine. *Biomed Signal Process Control.* 55(January):101645.

Kwak, N.S., K.R. Müller, and S.W. Lee. 2017. A Convolutional Neural Network for Steady State Visual Evoked Potential Classification Under Ambulatory Environment. *PLoS ONE* 12(2):e0172578

Li, F., X. Li, F. Wang, D. Zhang, Y. Xia, and F. He. 2020. A Novel P300 Classification Algorithm Based on a Principal Component Analysis Convolutional Neural Network. *Appl Sci.* 10(4):1546.

Li, Y., J. Xiang, and T. Kesavadas. 2020. Convolutional Correlation Analysis for Enhancing the Performance of SSVEP-Based Brain-Computer Interface. *IEEE Trans Neural Syst Rehabil Eng.* 28(12):2681–2690.

Liu, Z., J. Shore, M. Wang, F. Yuan, A. Buss, and X. Zhao. 2021. A Systematic Review on Hybrid EEG/fNIRS in Brain-Computer Interface. *Biomed Signal Process Control.* 68:102595.

Lopes-Dias, C., A.I. Sburlea, and G.R. Müller-Putz. 2019. Online Asynchronous Decoding of Error-Related Potentials During the Continuous Control of a Robot. *Sci Rep.* 9:Article 17596.

López-Larraz, E., N. Birbaumer, and A. Ramos-Murguialday. 2018. A Hybrid EEG-EMG BMI Improves the Detection of Movement Intention in Cortical Stroke Patients with Complete Hand Paralysis. In *Annual International Conference of the IEEE Engineering in Medicine and Biology Society*, Honolulu, HI, USA, 2018, pp. 2000–2003.

Lun, X., J. Liu, Y. Zhang, Z. Hao, and Y. Hou. 2022. Motor Imagery Signals Classification Method via the Difference of EEG Signals Between Left and Right Hemispheric Electrodes. *Front Neurosci.* 16:Article 865594.

Luo, T.J., and F. Chao. 2018. Exploring Spatial-Frequency-Sequential Relationships for Motor Imagery Classification with Recurrent Neural Network. *BMC Bioinform.* 19(1):1–18.

Luo, W., W. Yin, Q. Liu, and Y. Qu. 2022. A Hybrid Brain-Computer Interface Using Motor Imagery and SSVEP Based on Convolutional Neural Network. *arXiv 2212.05289.*

Maksimenko, V.A. 2018. Nonlinear Analysis of Brain Activity, Associated with Motor Action and Motor Imaginary in Untrained Subjects. *Nonlinear Dyn.* 91:2803–2817.

Mathe, M., M. Padmaja, and B.T. Krishna. 2021. Intelligent Approach for Artifacts Removal from EEG Signal Using Heuristic-Based Convolutional Neural Network. *Biomed Signal Process Control.* 70(102935).

McFarland, D.J., and J.R. Wolpaw. 2011. Brain-Computer Interfaces for Communication and Control. *Commun ACM.* 54(5):60–66.

Milosevic, M., C. Marquez-Chin, K. Masani, M. Hirata, T. Nomura, M.R. Popovic, and K. Nakazawa. 2020. Why Brain-Controlled Neuroprosthetics Matter: Mechanisms Underlying Electrical Stimulation of Muscles and Nerves in Rehabilitation. *Biomed Eng Online.* 19(1):81.

Minguillon, J., M.A. Lopez-Gordo, and F. Paleo. 2017. Trends in EEG-BCI for Daily-Life: Requirements for Artifacts Removal. *Biomed Signal Process Control.* 31:407–418.

Mishuhina, V., and X. Jiang. 2021. Complex Common Spatial Patterns on Time-Frequency Decomposed EEG for Brain-Computer Interface. *Pattern Recognit.* 115:107918.

Neuper, C., and G. Pfurtscheller. 2001. Event-Related Dynamics of Cortical Rhythms: Frequency-Specific Features and Functional Correlates. *Int JPsychophysiol.* 43(1):41–58.

Okahara, Y., K. Takano, T. Komori, M. Nagao, Y. Iwadate, and K. Kansaku. 2017. Operation of a P300-Based Brain-Computer Interface by Patients with Spinocerebellar Ataxia. *Clin Neurophysiol Pract.* 2:147–153.

Padfield, N., J. Zabalza, H. Zhao, V. Masero, and J. Ren. 2019. EEG-Based Brain-Computer Interfaces Using Motor-Imagery: Techniques and Challenges. *Sensors.* 19(6):1423.

Pfurtscheller, G., et al. 2010. The Hybrid BCI. *Front Neurosci.* 4:42.

Podmore, J.J., T.P. Breckon, N.K. Aznan, and J.D. Connolly. 2019. On the Relative Contribution of Deep Convolutional Neural Networks for SSVEP-Based Bio-Signal Decoding in BCI Speller Applications. *IEEE Trans Neural Syst Rehabil Eng.* 27(4):611–618.

Prochazka, A. 2018. Motor Neuroprostheses. *Compr Physiol.* 9(1):127–148.

Robinson, N., R. Mane, T. Chouhan, and C. Guan. 2021. Emerging Trends in BCI-Robotics for Motor Control and Rehabilitation. *Curr Opin Biomed Eng.* 20(December):100354.

Ruhunage, I., et al. 2019. Hybrid EEG-EMG Signals Based Approach for Control of Hand Motions of a Transhumeral Prosthesis. *IEEE 1st Global Conference on Life Sciences and Technologies Osaka*, Japan, 12–14 March 2019:50–53.

Ruiz-Olaya, A.F., A. Lopez-Delis, and A.F. Da Rocha. 2019. Upper and Lower Extremity Exoskeletons. In *The Book Handbook of Biomechatronics*, Elsevier, pp. 283–317.

Saba-Sadiya, S., E. Chantland, T. Alhanai, T. Liu, and M.M. Ghassemi. 2021. Unsupervised EEG Artifact Detection and Correction. *Front Digit Health.* 2:608920.

Samek, W., K.R. Muller, M. Kawanabe, and C. Vidaurre. 2012. Brain-Computer Interfacing in Discriminative and Stationary Subspaces. *Annu Int Conf IEEE Eng Med Biol Soc.* 2012:2873–2876.

Savić, A.M., S. Aliakbaryhosseinabadi, J.U. Blicher, D. Farina, N. Mrachacz-Kersting, and S. Došen. 2021. Online Control of an Assistive Active Glove by Slow Cortical Signals in Patients with Amyotrophic Lateral Sclerosis. *J Neural Eng.* 18(4).

Tong, S., and N.V. Thankor. 2009. Quantitative EEG Analysis Methods and Clinical Applications. *Artech House.* Boston MA.USA.

Tortora, S., G. Beraldo, L. Tonin, and E. Menegatti. 2019. Entropy-based Motion Intention Identification for Brain-Computer Interface. In *IEEE International Conference on Systems, Man, and Cybernetics,* Bari, Italy October 2019.

Uyulan, C. 2021. Development of LSTM&CNN Based Hybrid Deep Learning Model to Classify Motor Imagery Tasks. *Commun Math Biol Neurosci.* 2021:4.

Vilela, M., and L.R. Hochberg. 2020. Applications of Brain-Computer Interfaces to the Control of Robotic and Prosthetic Arms. *Handb Clin Neurol.* 168:87–99.

Wang, J., L. Bi, and W. Fei. 2022. Using Non-linear Dynamics of EEG Signals to Classify Primary Hand Movement Intent Under Opposite Hand Movement. *Front Neurorobot.* 16:845127.

Wang, P., A. Jiang, X. Liu, J. Shang, and L. Zhang. 2018. LSTM-based EEG Classification in Motor Imagery Tasks. *IEEE Trans Neural Syst Rehabil Eng.* 26(11):2086–2095.

Wen, D., Y. Fan, S.H. Hsu, J. Xu, Y. Zhou, J. Tao, X. Lan, and F. Li. 2020. Combining Brain-Computer Interface and Virtual Reality for Rehabilitation in Neurological Diseases: A Narrative Review. *Ann Phys Rehabil Med.* 64(1):101404.

Wolpaw, J.R. 2013. Chapter 6 – Brain–Computer Interfaces. *Handbook Clin Neurol* 110:67–74.

Zhang, R., F. Li, T. Zhang, D. Yao, and P. Xu. 2020. Subject Inefficiency Phenomenon of Motor Imagery Brain-Computer Interface: Influence Factors and Potential Solutions. *Brain Sci Adv.* 6(3):224–241.

Zhu, G., et al. 2017. A Simplified Hybrid EEG-fNIRS Brain-Computer Interface for Motor Task Classification. *International IEEE/EMBS Conference on Neural Engineering, NER,* Shanghai, China, May 2017.

Zhu, H., D. Forenzo, and B. He. 2022. On the Deep Learning Models for EEG-Based Brain-Computer Interface Using Motor Imagery. *IEEE Trans Neural Syst Rehabil Eng.* 30:2283–2291.

Zhu, Y., Y. Li, J. Lu, and P. Li. 2021. EEGNet With Ensemble Learning to Improve the Cross-Session Classification of SSVEP Based BCI from Ear-EEG. *IEEE Access.* 9:15295–15303.

Zuo, C., et al. 2020. Novel Hybrid Brain–Computer Interface System Based on Motor Imagery and P300. *Cogn Neurodyn.* 14(2):253–265.

12 Enhancing Telerehabilitation Using Wearable Sensors and AI-Based Machine Learning Methods

Sebastián Jaramillo-Isaza[*,†],
Alberto López Delis[**], *Edith Pulido Herrera*[***],
and *Andrés Felipe Ruiz-Olaya*[*]

*Antonio Nariño University, Faculty of Mechanical, Electronic and Biomedical Engineering, Bogotá, Colombia; **Centro de Biofìsica Médica, Universidad de Oriente, Santiago de Cuba, Cuba; ***Escuela Militar de Cadetes General "José María Córdova", Engineering and Simulation Research Group (GINSI), Bogotá, Colombia
†Corresponding Author: sebastian.jaramilloi@outlook.com

ABBREVIATIONS

3D-CNN	3D Convolution Neural Network
ADLs	Activities of daily living
AFE	Analog Front-End
AI	Artificial intelligence
ANN	Artificial neural network
ASR	Automatic Speech Recognition
asynch-TR	Asynchronous Telerehabilitation
BIA	Bioelectrical Impedance Analyzer
BLE	Bluetooth Low-Energy
CNNs	Convolutional Neural Networks
COCO	Common Objects in Context
CV	Computer Vision
DL	Deep learning
DTs	Decision Trees
ECG	Electrocardiogram ECG
EEG	Electroencephalography
eHealth	Electronic Health
EMG	Electromyography
EOG	Electrooculography

DOI: 10.1201/9781032699882-12

FNNs	Feedforward Neural Networks
GCG	Gyrocardiography
HAR	Human Activity Recognition
IC	Integrated Circuit
ICT	Information and Communications Technology
IMU	Inertial Measurement Units
IoMT	Internet of Medical Things
IoT	Internet of Things
IPG	Impedance Photoplethysmography
k-NN	k-Nearest Neighbors
LNA	Low-Noise Amplifier
mHealth	Mobile Health
ML	Machine Learning
MLP	Multilayer Perceptron
NIH	National Institutes of Health
NM	Nearest Mean
NNs	Neural Networks
PD	Parkinson's Disease
PGA	Programmable Gain Amplifier
PPG	Photoplethysmography
PSD	Power Spectral Density
PT	Physical Therapy
R-CNN	Region-based Convolutional Neural Networks
RFs	Random Forests
SCG	Seismocardiography
SOM	Self-Organizing Map
SVMs	Support Vector Machines
synch-TR	Synchronous Telerehabilitation
TR	Telerehabilitation
WHO	World Health Organization

12.1 INTRODUCTION

Telerehabilitation (TR) focuses on providing rehabilitation services through information and communications technology (ICT), which includes processes and services for diagnostics, follow-up, training, intervention, orientation, advisement, and telemonitoring, among others (Fiani et al., 2020; Shem et al., 2022). In addition, TR has been developed for allowing users to continue with patient healthcare processes from home, look for their wellness, and reduce patient hospitalization times and costs to healthcare providers and healthcare systems (Peretti et al., 2017).

Telerehabilitation is a field that has contributed to the solution to longstanding limitations on therapy services faced by people with limited mobility or difficulties accessing healthcare facilities. Furthermore, it is a facilitator to remove geographical and time barriers. Recently, telerehabilitation was intensely used in the response to the COVID pandemic, showing important benefits related to widely used face-to-face rehabilitation services and reducing in-person contact between patient and clinician (Michell et al., 2022; Vieira et al., 2022).

With increasing age, people are more prone to bodily dysfunction and are victims of chronic diseases; this further increases the need for medical assistance with quality services. The services offered by telerehabilitation have a high quality standard and facilitate access to rehabilitation services, especially for the geriatric population, eliminating the access barrier that mobility limitations represent for this age group (Anton et al., 2018). As reported by the World Health Organization, the population that will cross the age of 60 will be approximately 1.2 billion by 2025 and will continue to rise to 2 billion by 2050.

The great challenge ahead for remote rehabilitation platforms is the heterogeneity of rehabilitation techniques, the specificities of the physiological-metabolic-biomechanical processes involved in each of them, the heterogeneity of the measurement systems that can be used, the procedural analysis, and decision making. This means that the design and development of platforms that integrate specific solutions for each of these techniques require a disruptive vision that encompasses different design approaches, techniques, and methodologies.

Some of the emerging technologies that enable the use of telerehabilitation are those based on images and video, those based on wearable sensors, and those based on virtual technologies. In addition, AI-based methods have been used in a complementary way, so that these technologies motivate greater motor development and retention of skills already learned. Thus, machine learning (ML) and deep learning (DL) methods for telerehabilitation applications have been reported (Hospodarskyy & Tsvyakh, 2020; Mulfari et al., 2022; Abbas et al., 2021). Figure 12.1 shows an example of emerging technologies and AI-based methods that enable the use for telerehabilitation.

Wearable sensors are devices that are integrated into accessories, clothes, or directly with the body for monitoring health and/or providing clinically important data for care (Cheng et al., 2021). Those devices record biomedical signals including electrocardiogram, electromyogram, photoplethysmogram, glucose levels, cardiac frequency, respiratory frequency, electroencephalogram, electrodermal activity, skin temperature, and accelerometry, among others. The use of the signals from wearable sensors and machine learning methods could improve telerehabilitation services for

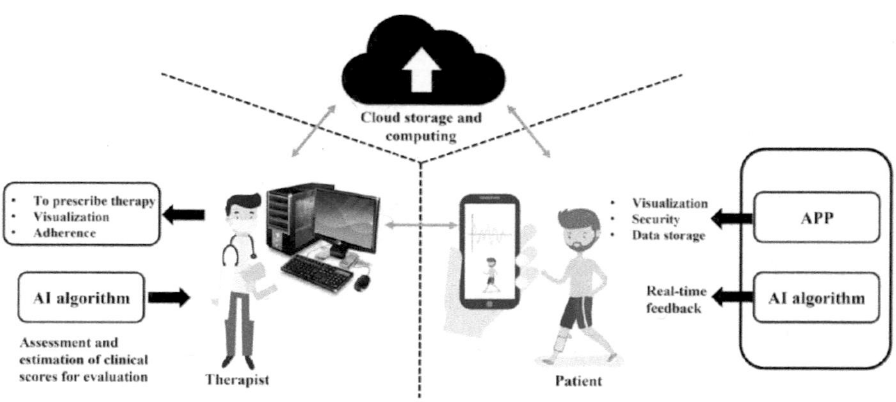

FIGURE 12.1 Example of emerging technologies and AI-based methods that enable the use for telerehabilitation.

diseases including stroke, diabetes, hypertension, heart failure, musculoskeletal disorders, etc., providing processed information about adherence to therapy, assessment of function, and evolution of therapy (Boukhennoufa et al., 2022; Adans-Dester et al., 2020).

Considering that acquired data from wearable sensors could be highly noisy due to several artifacts, such as internal and external factors, their raw recorded signals must be processed using methods ranging from traditional to algorithms based on artificial intelligence and machine learning. Artifacts include motion, power lines, electromagnetic interferences, and physical conditions, among others. Signal processing includes filtering, transformation, normalization, decomposition, feature extraction and selection, machine learning-based techniques, and deep learning-based algorithms. Feature extraction methods using data from wearable devices are sensitive to signal quality, which has been addressed using multiple signal processing computational methods (Vijayan et al., 2021). An analysis of potential applications of AI-based machine learning methods for diagnosis, clinical evaluation, personalized care, treatment responsiveness, telemonitoring, and adherence evaluation will be presented, analyzing case studies in telerehabilitation.

12.2 FUNDAMENTALS OF TELEREHABILITATION

The World Health Organization (WHO) defines rehabilitation as "a set of interventions designed to optimize functioning and reduce disability in individuals with health conditions in interaction with their environment" (WHO, 2013). It is estimated that between 76% and 85% of people with disabilities in developing countries have not accessed diagnostic, treatment, or follow-up programs (WHO, 2013). Traditional rehabilitation processes currently are increasing public health costs due to increased demand. Rehabilitation can be a time-consuming process, requiring that it be carried out after an initial phase of intervention (Calvaresi et al., 2017). Thus, telerehabilitation has become a complementary tool to traditional processes of rehabilitation. Furthermore, to provide personalized therapy and improve outcomes of the therapeutic process, telerehabilitation should not be based uniquely on a remote observational analysis of the patient. The TR should also opportunely provide a response to factors that include the physical (e.g., rigidity, spasticity, fatigue, pain), psychological, and cognitive (e.g., engagement, cognitive affectation) factors. In that context, telerehabilitation using AI-based methods has become a potential solution.

12.2.1 Barriers, Challenges, and Facilitators

Currently, accessibility to professionals in the area of physical rehabilitation is not easy for people who are in places far from health centers that provide the service. There are still access barriers to services such as healthcare, for which the populations furthest away from the country present the greatest problems, as the quality of the service and inaccessibility are precarious conditions (WHO, 2017).

People residing in rural areas encounter additional barriers in their therapy process, reflected in the displacement of their meetings with specialists, for example.

This can affect the performance of a user in the physiotherapeutic procedure and therefore inhibit adequate rehabilitation (Nuara et al., 2022). Many patients not only do not attend the meeting but also do not comply with the home plan for fear of doing it wrong or doing inappropriate exercises for their condition; this is an important factor that can influence the outcome of the rehabilitation.

One of the potential benefits of telerehabilitation is an increase in therapeutic adherence, taking into account that it allows monitoring of the therapy carried out by the patient (Gaboury et al., 2021). In addition, there is a decrease in economic cost that encourages this type of patient to comply with their rehabilitation, given that public transport in a developing country represents a physical access barrier for a person with motor disorders.

Telerehabilitation can become a profitable alternative in terms of the provision of physiotherapy services at a distance because of the difficulties that a patient may have in accessing or approaching a health center (Seron et al., 2021). Based on this, concerns have arisen that put on the table the efficiency of telerehabilitation over face-to-face physical therapy, where a variety of results have been found that make telerehabilitation a more effective modality than face-to-face therapy.

TR has been widely used for motor and neurological rehabilitation of patients affected by accidents, diseases, lifestyle, or environmental health problems (Dierick et al., 2021; Vellata et al., 2021). In addition, a wide variety of healthcare professionals ranging from doctors and physical therapists to speech-language therapists also give the TR (Shem et al., 2022).

12.2.2 Synchronous and Asynchronous Telerehabilitation

TR could be implemented to be delivered using several synchronous/interactive and asynchronous/non-interactive interventions (Vieira et al., 2022). In synchronous telerehabilitation (synch-TR), both the user and the health professional interactively communicate through a technological system in real time (i.e., teleconsultation). Asynchronous telerehabilitation (asynch-TR) allows the user to interact remotely, recording relevant data/signals about the intervention processes, which is carried out without a real-time interaction. ICTs that support the use of synch-TR include videocalls, audio calls, and real-time "smartphone" applications, among others. ICTs that support the use of asynch-TR include web-based platforms for "storing and forwarding" patient data examination, motion capture in situ using markerless tools, non-real-time "smartphone" applications, and so on.

Telemonitoring is the relationship between health personnel and a user where biomedical information is collected and transmitted through a technological infrastructure so that health personnel carry out their analysis. Telemonitoring could be used for telerehabilitation programs, allowing remote monitoring of the rehabilitation intervention, and could include cardiovascular parameters (electrocardiogram [ECG], blood pressure, oxygen saturation), respiratory parameters, kinematics information, and kinetics information, among others. The Internet of Medical Things (IoMT) incorporates wireless sensors into biomedical equipment combined with the internet. The advantage of the IoMT is that there is a possibility to carry out daily tasks while the patient is under continuous health monitoring or in rehabilitation processes. In addition, through IoMT, some problems with the portability of usual medical monitoring devices are solved since ultra-low-power and fast communication sensor devices are presented (Vishnu et al., 2020).

12.2.3 On the Use of AI-Based Methods for Telerehabilitation

Artificial intelligence (AI) is a research field that permits the machine simulation of human intelligence and behaviors ranging from learning to problem solving (Ertel, 2017; Dzobo et al., 2020). Machine learning (ML) is an area of artificial intelligence that, among all AI-based techniques, allows computers to gather data autonomously and learn from the experience of the issues or situations they have faced (Kolanovic & Krishnamachari, 2017). Figure 12.2 shows differences between AI-based methods for telerehabilitation.

ML algorithms employ statistics to detect patterns in data that range in size from small to enormous. ML was created on the principle that computers can utilize data to demonstrate organization without knowing a priori what the structure is like. The concept of data encompasses a wide range of elements, including words, numbers, photos, clicks, and many more. As a result, a machine learning algorithm can use anything stored digitally for optimizing a parameter based on previously stored data, which permits ML algorithms to "learn" from available data and provide models. Those models could be used to identify the underlying structure (through unsupervised learning) or to predict output variables data (i.e., to categorize data or predict outcomes). ML-based methods have been used for classification, regression, clustering, and reinforcement learning applications. Most commonly supervised learning for telerehabilitation includes k-nearest neighbors (k-NN), support vector machines

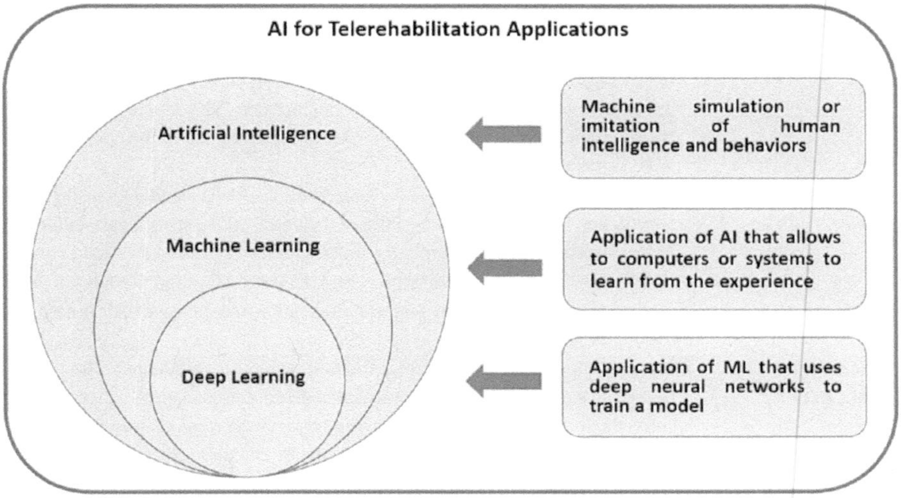

FIGURE 12.2 Differences between AI-based methods for telerehabilitation.

(SVMs), decision trees (DTs), random forests (RFs), and multiple variants of neural networks (NNs) such as feedforward neural networks (FNNs) and multilayer perceptron (MLP). Unsupervised learning permits the identification of patterns in datasets, such as k-means, nearest mean (NM), and self-organizing map (SOM).

ML algorithms have been used in combination with wearable human activity recognition (HAR) systems for telerehabilitation systems. Most HAR systems use inertial measurement units (IMU). On the other hand, deep learning (DL) algorithms are commonly used to learn and make decisions based on a large dataset, without being explicitly programmed to perform the task. Table 12.1 shows an overview of the use of ML and DL in telerehabilitation.

TABLE 12.1
Overview of Some ML and DL Applications in Telerehabilitation

ML Applications	
Wei et al., 2019	Implemented an ML-based virtual physical therapy (PT) focused on treatment of Parkinson's disease (PD). The proposed algorithm includes hidden Markov models to detect repetitions from Kinect data and an SVM classifier to identify correctly and incorrectly performed movements, previously classified by the therapist.
Nasrabadi et al., 2022	Reported a ML-based algorithm for HAR that includes NM, k-NN, MLP, and SVM. Features were in the time domain (average, skewness, and kurtosis), frequency domain (power spectral density—PSD and entropy), and time-frequency domain (wavelet coefficients).
Khanghah et al., 2023	Proposed a 3D convolution neural network (3D-CNN) aimed at classifying physical therapy videos, providing information to the patients on the correct execution of the prescribed exercise to enhance the rehabilitation process.
DL Applications	
Rosique et al., 2021	Present a telerehabilitation system called ExerCam, which uses an augmented reality mirror application to create gamified exergames for the remote rehabilitation of patients with mobility impairments. This system uses convolutional neural networks (CNNs) to estimate the 2D human pose from RGB camera images.
Mulfari et al., 2022	Proposed the use of automatic speech recognition (ASR) technology using DL approaches. The application consists of the creation of a speech dataset for Italian speakers with dysarthria, the training of a convolutional neural network (CNN) for isolated word recognition, and the potential of mobile speech therapy apps to help patients practice articulation and improve their speech therapy progress.
Ramírez-Sanz et al., 2023	Presented a low-cost home telerehabilitation system for individuals with Parkinson's disease. To assist therapists in determining whether patients are correctly conducting their exercises, the system makes use of deep neural networks and big data technologies. The major articulations of a human body were identified using models that were trained using common objects in context (COCO) and region-based convolutional neural networks (R-CNN).

DL and ML are often used interchangeably, but they have some differences (see Figure 12.2). Both are subfields of artificial intelligence, and DL comprises neural networks that use multiple layers in the network. Wearable technologies, the Internet of Things (IoT), video-based sensors, and other sources of information can be utilized by AI-based algorithms to develop data-driven decision-making methods that can enhance treatment outcomes for patients undergoing telerehabilitation.

12.3 WEARABLES AND SENSOR-BASED TECHNOLOGY

In the past, health assessments were typically conducted in clinical settings like hospitals and doctor's offices. However, recent advancements in health monitoring and assistance technologies have led to a revolution in health services. Electronic devices have allowed users to improve their quality of life in multiple activities of daily life (Mukhopadhyay et al., 2022). As wearable and sensor-based technology continues to advance and become more accessible, devices are capable of much more than just tracking activity levels. In fact, the data produced by sensors can provide valuable insights into a person's well-being and offer novel applications in telerehabilitation that can greatly benefit healthcare services.

12.3.1 Biomedical Signals for Telerehabilitation

The rapid development of telerehabilitation technologies is increasingly focused on the integration of a greater number of devices for the measurement of biopotential signals. Wearable sensors provide physiological measurements of signals such as electrocardiography (ECG), impedance photoplethysmography (IPG), photoplethysmography (PPG), seismocardiography (SCG), electrooculography (EOG), electromyography (EMG), and electroencephalography (EEG) (Seshadri et al., 2019; Palumbo et al., 2020; Qureshi & Krishnan, 2018; Castaneda et al., 2018). Figure 12.3 illustrates different biomedical signal forms from various parts of the body. The monitoring of electrophysiological events in sport, clinical, and telerehabilitation contexts has been made possible by integrated circuit (IC) technologies and portable devices.

Wearable sensors offer diverse applications for diagnostics and monitoring, as demonstrated by preceding research (Postolache et al., 2016; Palumbo et al., 2009). These applications include detecting movement disorders, assisting with rehabilitation and fall prevention through home-based motion sensing, evaluating athletes' performance and physical condition, correcting postural control for better stability, monitoring physical activity during rehabilitation, assessing the effectiveness of interventions, and tracking physical activity after surgery, among others.

Biomedical wearable devices involve a three-step process that includes (i) acquiring and preprocessing data, (ii) transmitting it, and (iii) analyzing and classifying the acquired data. The information recorded by biomedical wearable sensors could be used for continuous monitoring of the patient's health, improve diagnosis, and evaluate therapeutic processes. Through the use of these wearable devices, healthcare professionals can access real-time data to monitor the patient's rehabilitation process. Zhao et al. (2020) developed a wearable monitoring system that integrates ECG/EMG sensors for upper limb rehabilitation. By tracking hand movements and changes in

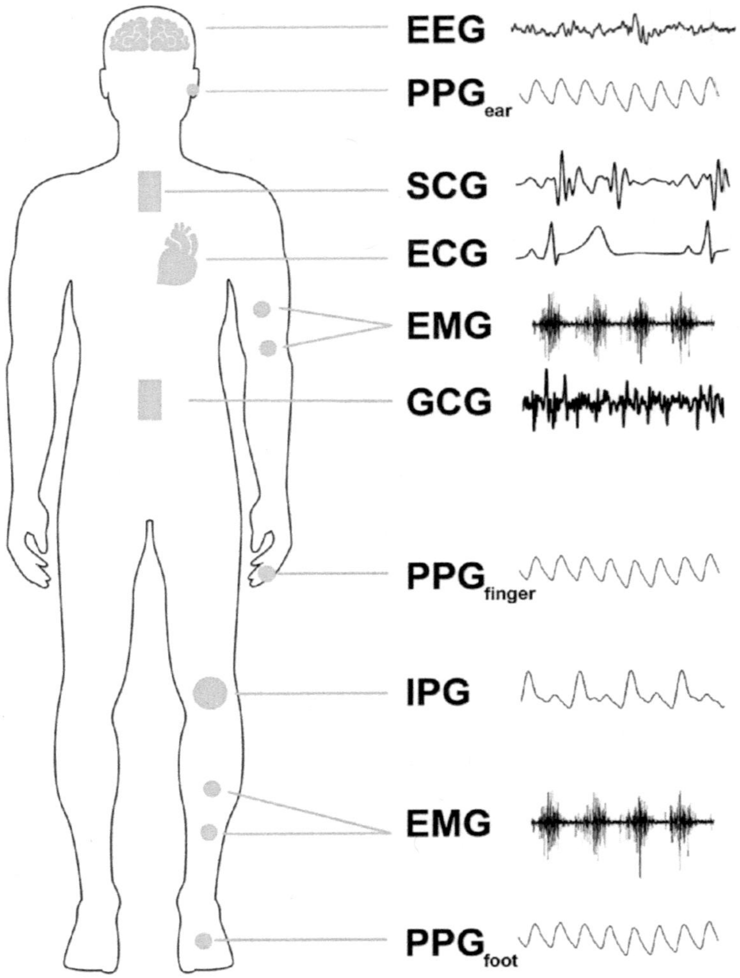

FIGURE 12.3 Scheme of some biological signals: electrocardiography (ECG), impedance photoplethysmography (IPG), photoplethysmography (PPG), gyrocardiography (GCG), seismocardiography (SCG), electromyography (EMG), and electroencephalography (EEG)

physiological state during robotic glove-assisted training, the device helps the subject with rehabilitation. A portable system with eight acquisition channels, a potent microcontroller unit, and Bluetooth 3.0 data transmission was suggested by Liu et al. (2019) for real-time signal measurement. This method assists doctors and scientists in gathering physiological signals for study. A wearable data acquisition system for multiple signals was suggested by Kast et al. (2017). The system also includes a synchronization module to reliably synchronize all acquired signals. These proposed devices have the potential to enhance the monitoring and rehabilitation of physiological signals. The proposed system can record up to 64 bipolar channels in real time. Tran and Cha (2021) designed, fabricated and verified an ultra-low power four-channel neural recording analog front-end (AFE) IC comprised of a low-noise amplifier (LNA), a programmable gain amplifier (PGA), and buffers. Sarker et al. (2017) designed and implemented a wearable biosignal acquisition system to record ECG and EMG signals using eight channels with a 24-bit resolution per channel at a sampling frequency of 500 Hz. Mazzetta et al. (2018) proposed a wearable sEMG device for monitoring muscle activity in real time from the detection of muscle activation potentials, which could provide the biomedical information of patients when performing activities of daily life (ADLs). The study achieved a specificity and sensitivity of over 87% and 82%, respectively, in recognizing the exact activity timing. The system integrates an AFE, a sensor for electrodermal activity, inertial measurement units (IMU), and a Bluetooth low-energy (BLE) element for real-time monitoring. Kim et al. (2016) presented a novel system architecture based on a multimodal analog front-end for low power consumption. The design integrates three sensors for biopotentials, PPG, and a bioelectrical impedance analyzer (BIA). Li and Sun (2017) proposed a small, wearable, wireless non-contact device for continuous biomedical signal monitoring, including ECG, EMG, and EEG. The device features an ultra-high input impedance AFE, allowing non-skin contact detection. Senapati et al. (2017) designed a wearable sensor for monitoring ECG, EMG, EEG, and EOG signals to allow disease diagnosis and management.

Numerous commercial products for collecting and processing health data have been developed in the area of wearable portable sensors, allowing for the early detection of pathological symptoms and ongoing disease tracking. In wireless, portable, and lab configurations, Biometrics Ltd. (2022) offers a variety of signal acquisition devices that gather data from different sensors. Shimmer offers customized ECG and EMG signal sensors for monitoring various factors (Individual Sensors, 2022). For EEG, ECG, and EMG records, BioSemi Instrumentation provides the ActiveTwo biopotential measurement system, with graphical programming available in LabVIEW (Biosemi Products, 2022). Delsys offers mobile systems, EMG sensors, and software for device integration to provide comprehensive wireless EMG-based solutions for tracking human activity in contexts such as sports, study, clinical, and educational situations (Delsys, 2022).

12.3.2 Internet of Medical Things (IoMT)

Smart healthcare aims to utilize technology for disease prevention, diagnosis, and treatment. One such technology is the Internet of Things (IoT), which interconnects various monitoring devices over a network with a decision support system, leading to more accurate disease diagnosis. The Internet of Medical Things (IoMT) is a type of IoT aimed at connecting medical devices and systems with others over a network and exchanging data to healthcare IT systems (Noor & Tantawy, 2019; Wang et al., 2020). Some IoMT applications are: telemonitoring for tracking patients with chronic or long-term conditions, monitoring medication orders, locating patients admitted to hospitals, and providing telerehabilitation services that use wearable m-health devices to send information to caregivers. Figure 12.4 presents a schematic

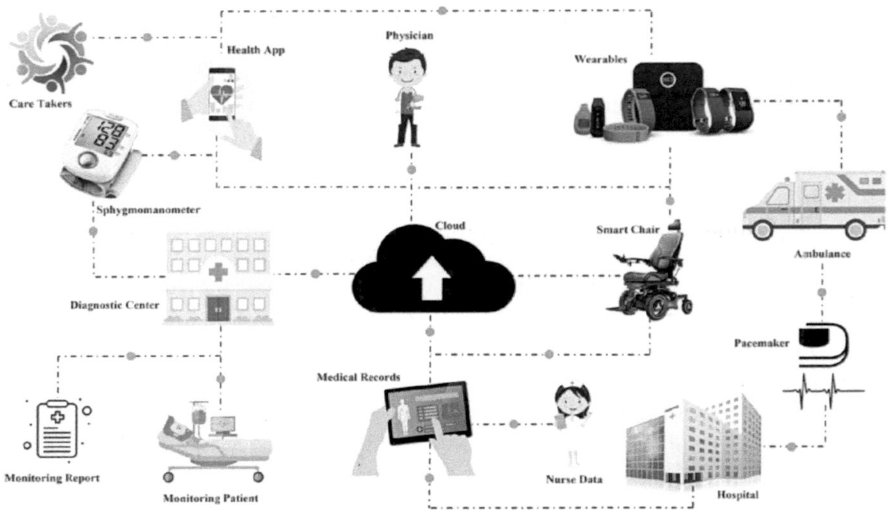

FIGURE 12.4 Structure of the Internet of Medical Things (IoMT).

representation of the structure of IoMT. By leveraging these technologies, healthcare providers can access and monitor real-time health data and deliver personalized care to patients.

The monitoring of the heart is considered a crucial area of focus for IoMT devices, as vital signs can reveal hidden illnesses such as arrhythmia. Various studies have presented the development of real-time signal monitoring through vital signal sensing with internet connectivity. For instance, Malasinghe et al. (2019) and Szydlo and Konieczny (2015) presented android-based remote monitoring systems that use pulsometer and pedometer sensors, respectively. Ramesh et al. (2012) developed a wireless corporal sensor and ECG monitoring system for heart patients, while Tan et al. (2017) presented a multi-parameter monitoring system with a defibrillator device. Additionally, Otoom et al. (2015) created a platform-dependent heart rate detection system based on a plug-and-play Pulse Sensor Amped.

IoMT devices have numerous applications in monitoring brain and neurological signals associated with conditions such as epilepsy, Alzheimer's, dementia, stroke, and Parkinson's. These systems represent a significant advancement in patient behavior monitoring (Adams et al., 2017). For instance, in (Abramiuc et al., 2015), a camera-based system using the HC-V720 high-definition camera is developed to monitor neurodegenerative diseases by capturing the patient's movement. In (Sarma et al., 2016), a stress level monitoring system that uses blood pressure information is reported. Devices used for the telemonitoring of brain and neurological diseases include those based on textile autonomic nervous systems (Kozlovszky et al., 2014), a t-shirt with embedded sensors (Casacci et al., 2015), and a wireless sensor tag-based wristwatch (Karakostas et al., 2015).

The IoMT facilitates real-time monitoring of patients' glucose levels through mobile or web applications utilizing smart and low-power devices. Ali et al. (2011) proposed a Bluetooth-based glucose monitoring system that connects the sensor node to a smartphone via Bluetooth. In a study by Lucisano et al. (2016), a long-term monitoring system with an implanted sensor was designed for diabetic patients, with glucose level updates sent to a remote server every 2 minutes. Menon et al. (2013) explained a near-infrared-based non-invasive glucose monitoring system that measures the variations in received signal intensity from the NIR sensor.

The use of ingestible sensors in IoT is an innovative solution to monitor the digestive system in a non-invasive manner. Capsule endoscopy is one application where the sensors can provide images of the interior of the human body, as described by Yuce and Dissanayake (2013). Ingestible sensors can also measure the formation of gases during the digestion process, as demonstrated by Yu et al. (2012). Such capabilities enable a better understanding of the digestive system and may lead to improvements in diagnosis and treatment of digestive disorders.

IoMT applications for fall detection in elderly patients use a variety of sensors, including gyroscopes, accelerometers, vibration sensors, and single- or multi-channel cameras, to form a data acquisition system. These sensors are connected to a smart platform and network, enabling signals to be sent to a central server and an alarm system to be established to alert clinicians or home nurses to a patient's fall. Yu et al. (2012) used a local processing device with an accelerometer to monitor patients' movements in their homes, while Pinheiro et al. (2013) developed wheelchair-based monitoring systems to track patients' physical condition and movement. In addition to monitoring tasks, several systems have an extra sensor node set up for fall detection, with accelerometers, breathing rate sensors (Sannino et al., 2015), and wireless wearable motes (Paoli et al., 2012) among the commonly used sensors.

12.3.3 Applications of AI-Based Methods Using Wearable Sensors

The characteristics of wearable sensors used in telerehabilitation studies are categorized according to the main purpose: activity recognition, movement classification, and clinical assessment emulation (Boukhnnoufa et al., 2022). Activity recognition systems recognize specific movements of rehabilitation patients for record and monitoring purposes, with a focus on activities of daily living (ADLs), including standing, sitting, lying down, standing up, and sitting down (Meng et al., 2021). Movement classification systems that quantify limb use to classify tasks have been also reported by Meng et al. (2021). Clinical assessment emulation systems focus on quantifying the quality in the execution of the prescribed exercises using post-stroke assessment scoring systems (Adans-Dester et al., 2020). Support Vector Machines (SVMs) were the most commonly used classifier, primarily for activity recognition purposes but also in regression problems for medical assessments where users are given a clinical score (Park et al., 2020; Khera & Kumar, 2020; Bobin et al., 2018; Capela et al., 2015; Wang & Oates, 2015). Decision Trees (DTs) were also widely implemented (O'Brien et al., 2017; Chen et al., 2021). Artificial Neural Networks (ANNs), including multilayer perceptron (MLP) and Convolutional Neural Network (CNN) architecture, were common choices for post-stroke rehabilitation assessment (Bisio et al.,

2019; Butt et al., 2019; Boukhennoufa et al., 2021; Kaku et al., 2020). k-Nearest Neighbor (kNN) was also used in several studies (Balestra et al., 2021; Meng et al., 2021; Tran et al., 2018) due to its suitability for real-time applications and lack of underlying assumptions about the dataset distribution.

12.3.4 Future Prospects and Limitations

Wearable sensors are small devices integrated into accessories or clothing or directly attached to the human body to monitor health and provide clinically important data for care. These sensors have a variety of diagnostic and monitoring applications. For example, Postolache et al. (2016) and Palumbo et al. (2009) used movement detection sensors in home-care studies to evaluate patient performance in rehabilitation, physical therapies (such as postural stability control), and post-surgery monitoring. Wearable sensors can record a range of biomedical signals, including electrocardiogram, electromyogram, photoplethysmogram, glucose levels, cardiac frequency, respiratory frequency, electroencephalogram, electrodermal activity, skin temperature, and accelerometry. By using artificial intelligence methods to analyze the data collected from wearable sensors, telerehabilitation services could be improved. This technology could provide assessments and estimations of clinical scores, evaluate the progress of therapy, and predict the long-term dynamics of patient recovery.

In the future, wearable sensors will facilitate physiological data acquisition in home settings, including preventive health programs and rehabilitation protocols. The next steps involve developing small and affordable devices that can be used on a large population and in communities. With the advantages of new IoT-based technology, home rehabilitation and telerehabilitation can be enhanced remarkably by including machine learning and deep learning studies to assess and treat rehabilitation exercises. Additionally, investigating multisensory fusion and human–computer interaction applications is suggested. New trends based on the automation of rehabilitation strategies and plans could be further investigated, which could enable the sharing and optimization of similar applications for patients worldwide (Boukhennoufa et al., 2022; Palumbo et al., 2021; Razfar et al., 2021).

Several studies have demonstrated that effective health monitoring systems can be designed with only a few sensors, making them user-friendly by incorporating visual cues such as avatars and positive feedback. Such systems can monitor changes in health and alert users to potential threats. By clouding data, the system can analyze medication usage and recovery rates. To this end, there is a growing trend in using deep learning algorithms, which require less signal processing expertise and provide better accuracy than conventional machine learning algorithms. Specifically, 1D time series deep learning algorithms have emerged as a popular option due to their speed and improved performance (Boukhennoufa et al., 2022; Palumbo et al., 2021; Razfar et al., 2021).

12.4 VIDEO-BASED TECHNOLOGY

Emerging technologies, such as low-cost markerless motion capture systems, medical applications using mobile phones, and gaming technologies (including video game consoles, Wii, Xbox, virtual reality, and Kinect), are revolutionizing the recording of biomedical information and enabling remote rehabilitation processes. Through the use of artificial intelligence algorithms, this information can be analyzed and processed, facilitating the deployment of telerehabilitation health services both in clinical environments and patients' homes. In the following sections, we will provide an in-depth overview of each of these technologies and their roles in advancing telerehabilitation.

12.4.1 Markerless Motion Capture and m-Health for Telerehabilitation

Motion capture and analysis systems are extensively employed in clinical and physical rehabilitation settings to study two- and three-dimensional movements. These tools aid in determining the underlying reasons for changes in movement patterns, which helps prevent, identify, monitor, and rehabilitate different musculoskeletal conditions, disabilities, and injuries. (Hill et al., 2022; Wade et al., 2022).

Today, three-dimensional motion capture using multiple camera systems alongside optical marker-based tracking is the most accurate method to compute kinematic data due to their high "resolution." However, traditional marker-based approaches have significant environmental constraints (Nakano et al., 2020). Therefore, optical markerless tracking has appeared as a new option that could be more suitable for specific applications and conditions, for example, in situ data acquisition. A brief comparison between both systems is shown in Figure 12.5.

Markerless motion capture systems have emerged as a result of advancements in computer vision and machine learning, leading to a growing interest in computer analysis of human actions and behavior. When compared to marker-based methods, markerless motion capture enables movement analysis with a lower requirement for data gathering and processing time (Wade et al., 2022).

Many applications have been made using markerless technology for pose estimation and detection. Those applications span from body, hand, and food tracking to face recognition (see Figure 12.6) for sports, fitness, rehabilitation, cinema, and 3D animation purposes (Knippenberg et al., 2017; Pueo & Jimenez-Olmedo, 2017; Armstrong et al., 2022; Needham et al., 2022; Wade et al., 2022). Many software alternatives exist in the market for markerless applications. These software programs include payment and free-access options, including OpenPose, MediaPipe, AlphaPose, Sonar, and Freemocap.

The term "mobile health" (mHealth) has been defined by The World Health Organization (WHO) as the "use of mobile and wireless technologies to support the achievement of health objectives" (Rehman, 2017; WHO, 2018). Likewise, the National Institutes of Health (NIH) defines m-health as "the use of mobile and wireless devices (cell phones, tablets, etc.) to improve health outcomes, health care services, and health research" (Ruotsalainen & Blobel, 2022; NIH - Department of Health and Human Services, 2018). This term generally refers to the collection, transmission, storage, and interaction with healthcare providers of health-related data through the use of mobile devices, cellphone applications, and web-based platforms.

The use of information and communication technology in a safe and economical manner for health and health-related purposes is known as electronic health (eHealth). It involves the application of wireless mobile technologies for public health.

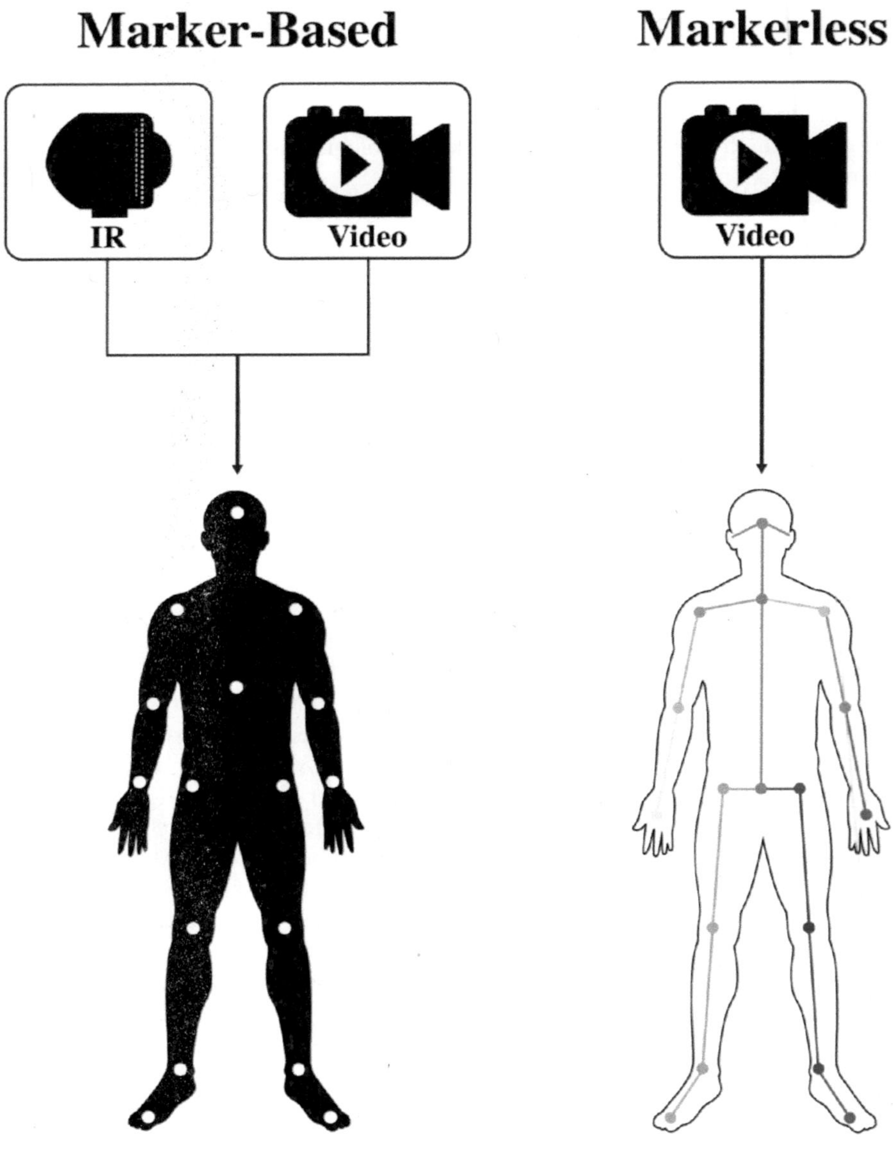

FIGURE 12.5 Configuration of the camera setup for marker-based and markerless technologies.

The goal of combining markerless motion capture tools with mobile technology services for telerehabilitation (TR) is to offer a service that is both affordable and accessible for a large number of people, as well as to make it easier for experts, healthcare professionals, and patients to coordinate and securely transmit knowledge. Figure 12.7 shows a representation of a TR system architecture including motion capture tools and mobile technology.

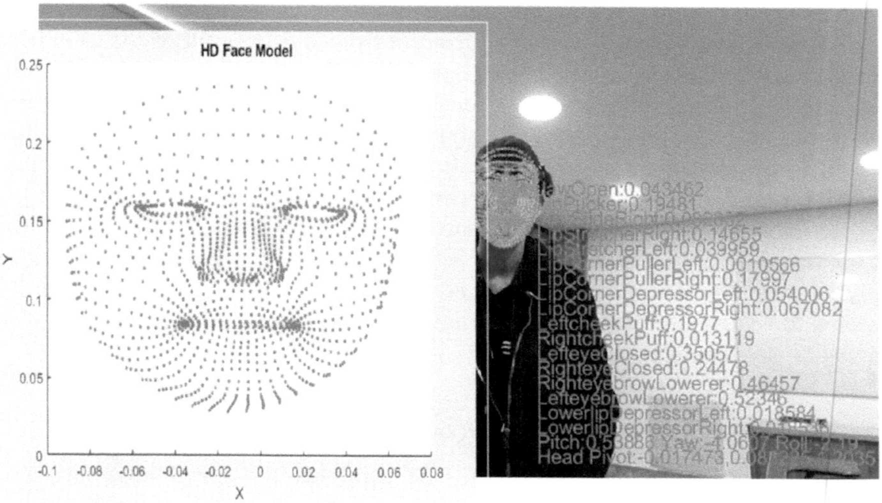

FIGURE 12.6 Example of face tracking using a Kinect device (Plazas-Molano et al., 2020).

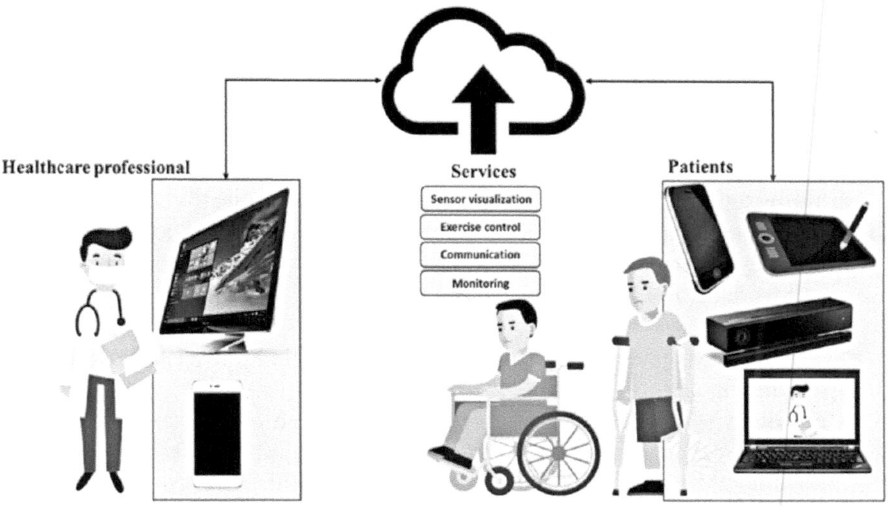

FIGURE 12.7 Representation of a telerehabilitation system architecture.

Markerless motion capture and m-health technologies leverage telecommunication tools to provide assistive services and care for individuals who require acute or subacute care, as well as long-term follow-up during and after rehabilitation. In addition to supporting patients with disabilities, these tools also empower individuals without disabilities to proactively manage their healthcare using low-cost and readily available technology, which ultimately helps to reduce healthcare costs.

Costs of healthcare have increased recently all over the world. Global government expenditure on healthcare has been further restricted as a result of the COVID-19 pandemic and the ensuing economic recession, aggravating the problem (Fiani et al., 2020). However, if illnesses were identified, evaluated, and dealt with at an early stage through a focus on prevention and health promotion, many healthcare costs could be avoided. This renewed interest in self-care could help reduce healthcare costs by promoting early disease detection and treatment.

Recently, digital health programs are emerging as a solution to reduce healthcare cost. Those programs encourage people to use computers and mobile devices to access health information and services. As a consequence, and aiming to increase access to healthcare services, various mobile-based programs and innovative technologies have been developed.

12.4.2 Computer Game-Based Therapy

"Serious games" is an umbrella term for any game-based tool with a "serious" purpose. These games are aimed toward problem solving rather than entertainment or fun (Smith, 2012; Caserman et al., 2020). Using controlled and corrective feedback, the main goal is teaching, learning, communicating, or providing an opportunity to practice or refine a new skill with the enjoyable aspects of video games. For instance, in therapy practice, serious games could assist patients by improving adherence and effectiveness of existing therapy methods, as well as dealing with limitations affecting the achievement of activities of daily living (ADLs).

According to (Caserman et al., 2020), the quality criteria for effective and attractive serious games should be based on the following concepts:

- Top-notch serious games should keep the defining objective in mind and employ techniques suited for the target audience and application area.
- For players (patients), caregivers, and therapists to evaluate their progress and work toward the primary goal, serious games should offer appropriate feedback.
- The efficacy of serious games should be proven through scientific studies or winning game awards.
- Fun and enjoyment are essential components of high-quality serious games, as are player engagement and flow maintenance (ability vs. skills).
- It is important to balance the serious and the playful elements.
- To be more engaging, serious games must be able to integrate the characterizing goal into the gameplay.
- The interface and nature of the technology must be appropriate for the game's target audience and objective.

Computer game-based rehabilitation emerged in the late 1990s when researchers recognized the benefits of using this technology in various controlled conditions (Kato, 2010). In the last decade, several studies have demonstrated the advantages and effectiveness of using challenging games through video consoles and virtual reality in rehabilitation (Lohse et al., 2013; Taylor & Griffin, 2015; Seo et al., 2016;

Cano-Mañas et al., 2020; Gandhi et al., 2021). Therefore, computer game-based therapy has become a component of many rehabilitation programs.

The exponential development of gaming technologies (e.g., video game consoles such as PlayStation, Wii, Xbox, Virtual Reality [VR], or motion sensors, Kinect) is allowing researchers, therapies, engineers, and some companies in the field of technology design for rehabilitation to engage in the exploration of a variety of new agreeable, commercially available, and highly motivating challenging games that can be used by younger populations and older adults as well. Figure 12.8 presents some of the gaming technologies commercially available.

Tools based on computer games are frequently utilized for rehabilitation and motor/cognitive skill training. However, their success is founded on neuroplasticity, driven by focused, intense, and motivated practice. Therefore, there is a need for efficient rehabilitation protocols using this simple tool to increase patient compliance and unlock the potential of neuroplasticity, which will ultimately result in an enhanced quality of life (Gandhi et al., 2020; Gandhi et al., 2021). As mentioned earlier, efficient and appealing serious game requirements can help achieve this.

Computer game-based technologies can be adapted for patient-specific needs. They can also collect some parameters associated with therapy, helping the specialist objectively assess the patient's progress. Recent experimental evidence suggests that computer game-based technologies hold tremendous promise in the neurological rehabilitation of patients experiencing movement and balance disorders. This is due to their ability to induce neuroplasticity and promote recovery.

Most clinical hypotheses and findings indicate that integrating specialized computer games with physical therapy exercises can be an effective approach to generating patient interest, increasing motivation, and promoting the proper execution of movements during training. Furthermore, this approach can help maintain a positive emotional state during rehabilitation.

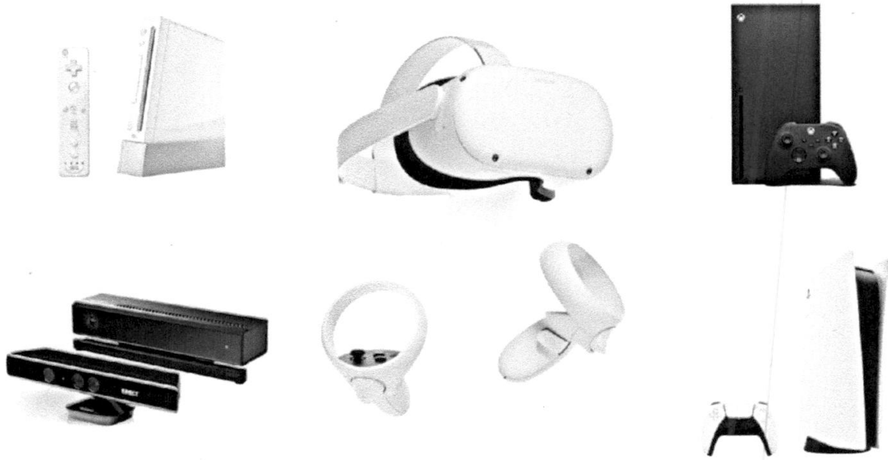

FIGURE 12.8 Different gaming technologies used in computed game-based therapy.

12.4.3 Applications of AI-Based Methods Using Video-Based Technology

Video footage is widely utilized in various disciplines, including the development and validation of medical equipment, rehabilitation, and biomechanics. This technology is often employed for tasks such as monitoring, analysis, assessment, and workflow management. However, processing and analyzing video-based technology data requires a large workforce to evaluate different parameters. While reducing the effort for video analysis, artificial intelligence (AI)-based techniques improve the accuracy of tasks like detection and classification. As a result, video-based technology has increasingly incorporated AI-based techniques. AI possesses different subfields with diverse characteristics and applications. Figure 12.9 shows some of the most popular and commonly used AI subfields.

Precisely, AI-based resources can be integrated into clinical, sports, and rehabilitation biomechanics to help avoid errors in data analysis due to failed marker positions or data missing due to occlusion and lighting, or to obtain new information (patrons, optimal and critical values, alternatives for data visualization) from motion data.

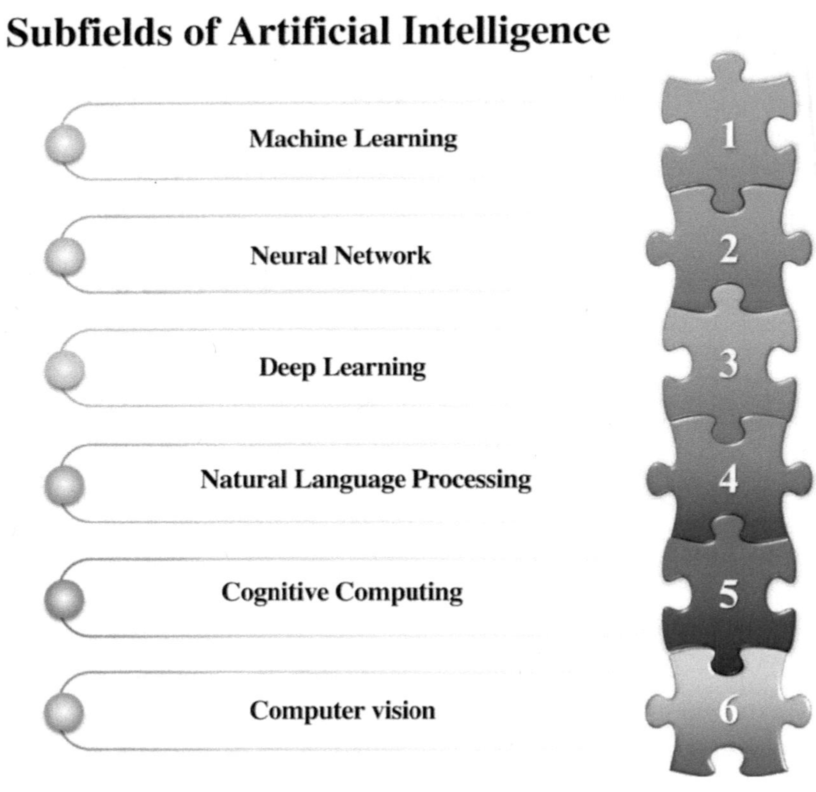

FIGURE 12.9 Some of the most popular artificial intelligence subfields.

The concept of data encompasses a wide range of elements, including words, numbers, photos, clicks, and many more. As a result, a machine learning algorithm can use anything stored digitally.

- As digital data, videos can be processed using ML algorithms by treating each video as a collection of images. There are numerous applications of ML for video that are currently under development. These include cognitive systems that use object identification, video segmentation, assistive robots, and self-driving cars.
- Metadata recognition, which involves identifying content compliance and recognizing video metadata.
- Intelligent surveillance, which includes automatic alarming and monitoring of patients.

ML techniques can be applied to video-based applications to detect, classify, and track people, animals, and robotics, as well as multiple objects. These applications can be used for various purposes, including security, entertainment, and object recognition.

Artificial neural networks (ANNs) are another AI tool used in biomechanics and rehabilitation that gain knowledge by processing various training examples obtained from motion (kinematics) data. This data is mainly obtained from video-based technologies such as MoCap systems and some wearables. For example, ANNs have been used to estimate humans' limbs angle amplitudes during the execution of different tasks, along with gait characterization and the estimation of ground reaction forces (Komaris et al., 2019; Stetter et al., 2019; Mundt et al., 2020; Blanco-Díaz et al., 2021).

Video-based AI is connected to computer vision (CV), a required field that uses artificial intelligence to describe an image or video's visual components. The notion of CV in artificial intelligence enables the computer to automatically identify, examine, and interpret visual information from real-world images. Additionally, it lays the groundwork for cutting-edge technological applications like face recognition and self-driving cars.

The following broad steps can describe traditional computer vision algorithms for video-based AI:

- To obtain either a dense or sparse set of interest points to extract the local high-dimensional visual attributes that describe a specific area of the video.
- To compile the retrieved characteristics into a description at the fixed-size video level.
- To conduct a final prediction or train a classifier, such as a support vector machine (SVM) or random forest (RF), on a collection of visual words.

When the amount of data is significantly large, another AI method, denominated deep learning (DL), is used. By processing and analyzing the input data using a variety of techniques until the computer finds the single desired output, DL employs neural networks with numerous layers to find patterns in datasets. Most DL applications aim to produce predictive analysis that can be used to improve performance or predict some response of the analyzed system. In recent years, DL approaches have been integrated into video-based technologies for applications in biomechanics, rehabilitation, clinical assessments, and sports (Kidziński et al., 2020; Zhang et al., 2021; Bicer et al., 2022).

By using AI-based methods on video-based technologies, the following benefits can be obtained:

- The reliability will be more remarkable since the human components can be entirely or partially removed from data processing.
- Time will be reduced. By utilizing ML techniques, researchers and users can process large amounts of data in a shorter amount of time, while also reducing the likelihood of errors.
- More information can be obtained. For example, video-based technologies can extract patron recognition and other features directly.

12.4.4 Future Prospects and Limitations

The delivery of healthcare services and the creation of universal public health coverage depend increasingly on digital technologies. Digital health, particularly mobile health, has demonstrated its ability to enhance the accessibility of health information, services, and skills and improve the quality and scope of care. It has also been shown to encourage healthy behavior changes that delay the onset of acute and chronic diseases.

Mobile wireless technologies are particularly pertinent owing to their ease of use, extensive coverage, and widespread acceptance. In addition, disruptive technologies (wearables, motion capture using markerless methods, computer game-based technologies) have become more and more common due to their relatively low-cost and flexible use in health applications. These technologies can revolutionize how populations interact with national health services.

Implementing m-health services in telerehabilitation programs has been widely investigated in many countries and under different patients' conditions (Baldazzi et al., 2020; Pastora-Bernal et al., 2021; Lin et al., 2022). However, many countries, most in the low- and middle-income categories, may still need to overcome technological, political, social, religious, and economic challenges before its implementation.

The WHO advocates for the development of mobile health programs that are based on scientifically verified knowledge, as many m-health tools or apps are currently lacking in this area. This lack of scientific evidence may put the health of the users at risk. WHO non-profit enterprises provide economic and, in some cases, technological resources to the countries to impulse research programs in health tech.

Several factors take time to assess, scale up, and integrate m-health services and new technologies into public health programs. Most of these factors include:

- The capacity to use digital health methods and solutions to deal with the wide range of patient populations and the numerous pilot initiatives that lack a scale-up strategy.

- A lack of interaction with current national eHealth plans, health information systems, and connectivity between specific apps.
- A lack of normative guidance due to a lack of standards and methods for comparing and evaluating rapidly growing digital health systems' functionality, scalability, and relative worth.
- The absence of a multisectoral strategy within the government and among donor organizations, particularly concerning the use of ICTs by ministries of health and churches, and suggested guidelines for interactions with mobile network providers and the business sector.

The standard MoCap systems, including cameras and markers, are the gold standard in motion capture. Despite this, many researchers, hospitals, and universities around the world have yet to be able to afford these systems. Therefore, there is a particular interest in developing new motion capture technology alternatives that are accessible, simple to use, and accurate enough to measure motor performance in human movement sciences and rehabilitation engineering (Nakano et al., 2020).

Compared to marker-based methods, markerless motion capture has the advantage of requiring fewer technological resources and having shorter data collection and processing times for movement analysis. However, advanced computational methods and complex information processing technology are essential to creating a reliable algorithm that can identify human positions or skeletons from video-based technology. Users of these markerless systems must be aware of their promise and limitations, as this technology is already beginning to be used for sporting, rehabilitation, and entertainment applications. The use of WiFi antennae for body tracking, segmentation, and key-point body recognition is a recent development in markerless technologies and posture estimation (Geng et al., 2022). This might significantly advance motion capture technology.

Computer-based solutions have the potential to improve rehabilitation protocols by enhancing standardization, increasing activity intensity and frequency, providing services tailored to demographic diversity, and enabling creative treatment delivery. Computer-based therapy has frequently been applied via commercial gaming consoles like the Sony PlayStation, Nintendo Wii, Microsoft Kinect, and virtual reality. Those consoles require video games specific for therapy, known as serious games. However, one of the most common challenges for using computer game-based in rehabilitation is the difficulty of engaging young and older adults in repetitive, tedious therapy. Therefore, there is a particular need for innovative approaches and tools to motivate these populations and improve adherence to the rehabilitation processes. Commercial video games that can be utilized in treatment are one suggested option. However, more research is needed to gather sufficient data to support their efficacy. The analysis of the feedback and opinions from both the participants and therapists will provide valuable insights into the perceived health benefits of exercise, potential challenges related to technology and activity, the motivational value of computer games, individual and environmental factors that may affect exercise, and recommendations for enhancing rehabilitation programs.

Apart from adherence, computer game-based treatment presents others challenges that must be considered in future research programs. These challenges include:

- Developing computer skills in therapists and patients (mainly in the elderly population).
- Providing support infrastructure in patients' homes, especially in eHealth applications.
- Financial of the initial investment for consoles.
- Integration of user feedback in the design of serious games.
- Quantification of wellness data.

AI-based video analytics solutions support us in our daily tasks. This technology has applicability across many industries, especially with the recent rise in application sophistication. As an example, the biomedical field is currently focusing on video analytics solutions to identify when a patient requires examination and alert healthcare workers. Additionally, efforts are being made to reduce wait times and provide direct access to emergency services, allocate hospital beds efficiently, track patient and visitor flow, and integrate eHealth apps to improve clinical and hospital services.

The main challenges of video-based AI applications in the biomedical field include the following:

- Reducing computational cost.
- Speeding up real-time video analytics.
- Considering spatiotemporal context across frames for accurate video recognition tasks.
- Building extensive and deeper knowledge of AI techniques to appropriately construct applications and reveal the desired benefits in patients and health systems.
- Creating new international standards and regulations.
- Developing patient- and clinician-oriented applications.
- Providing understandable data analysis for both medical specialists and patients.
- Ensuring the amount of data available for new robust AI-based computer approaches.

12.5 CONCLUSIONS

The emerging research on wearable sensing technologies, video-based sensors, and AI methods allows us to overcome some of the limitations of telerehabilitation, such as enhancing adherence, improving usability, and providing customized care. It is important to note that telerehabilitation, when combined with emerging technologies and AI-based methods, is not meant to replace traditional rehabilitation but to complement it. Telerehabilitation offers several benefits, such as promoting the continuity of therapies for patients with motor limitations, enhancing therapeutic adherence, and providing patient-centered intervention.

To provide personalized therapy and improve therapeutic outcomes, TR must address physical factors such as rigidity, spasticity, and pain, as well as psychological and cognitive factors such as engagement and cognitive affectation. In this context, telerehabilitation using AI-based methods has the potential to offer a solution. For instance, TR systems that provide real-time biofeedback to patients about the quality of their personalized therapy routines and exercises could significantly impact rehabilitation outcomes.

Moreover, combining technologies such as serious videogames and virtual reality can enhance TR outcomes by recreating realistic environments where patients can perform their therapy while wearable, video-based, and other sensors record the quality of their movements or exercises. Data analysis and AI-based methods can then provide an assessment, estimation of clinical scores, and evaluation of the progress of therapy, enabling a prediction of the effectiveness of patient recovery.

In conclusion, telerehabilitation using emerging technologies and AI-based methods has enormous potential for improving the quality of patient care, enhancing therapeutic outcomes, and providing patient-centered intervention.

12.6 ACKNOWLEDGMENT

The authors thank the Universidad Antonio Nariño (Colombia) for funding, under the "Support for the Assessment and Telerehabilitation of People with Motor Functional Diversity Using an E-Health Platform" project number 2019213.

REFERENCES

Abbas, M., Somme, D., & Le Bouquin Jeannès, R. (2021). D-SORM: A digital solution for remote monitoring based on the attitude of wearable devices. *Computer Methods and Programs in Biomedicine*, 208. https://doi.org/10.1016/j.cmpb.2021.106247

Abramiuc, B., Zinger, S., de With, P. H. N., de Vries-Farrouh, N., van Gilst, M. M., Bloem, B., & Overeem, S. (2015). Home video monitoring system for neurodegenerative diseases based on commercial HD cameras. *IEEE 5th International Conference on Consumer Electronics-Berlin (ICCE-Berlin)* (pp. 489–492). IEEE Xplore. https://doi.org/10.1109/ICCE-Berlin.2015.7391318

Adams, Z. W., McClure, E. A., Gray, K. M., Danielson, C. K., Treiber, F. A., & Ruggiero, K. J. (2017). Mobile devices for the remote acquisition of physiological and behavioral biomarkers in psychiatric clinical research. *Journal of Psychiatric Research*, 85, 1–14. https://doi.org/10.1016/j.jpsychires.2016.10.019

Adans-Dester, C., Hankov, N., O'Brien, A., Vergara-Diaz, G., Black-Schaffer, R., Zafonte, R., Dy, J., Lee, S. I., & Bonato, P. (2020). Enabling precision rehabilitation interventions using wearable sensors and machine learning to track motor recovery. *NPJ Digital Medicine*, 3(1), 121. https://doi.org/10.1038/s41746-020-00328-w

Ali, M., Albasha, L., & Al-Nashash, H. (2011). A Bluetooth low energy implantable glucose monitoring system. In *2011 8th European Radar Conference* (pp. 377–380). IEEE Xplore. Available online: https://ieeexplore.ieee.org/document/6101073

Anton, D., Berges, I., Bermúdez, J., Goñi, A., & Illarramendi, A. (2018). A telerehabilitation system for the selection, Evaluation and remote management of therapies. *Sensors*, 18, 1459. https://doi.org/10.3390/s18051459

Armstrong, K., Wen, Y., Zhang, L., Ye, X., Lee, P., & Armstrong, K. (2022). Novel clinical applications of marker-less motion capture as a low-cost human motion analysis method in the detection and treatment of knee osteoarthritis. *Journal of Arthritis*, *11*(1). https://doi.org/10.4172/2167-7921.2022.11.053

Baldazzi, G., Masciavè, G. K., Gusai, E., Spanu, S., Sulas, E., Raffo, L., & Pani, D. (2020). A plantar pressure biofeedback M-health system for stroke patients. *IEEE International Symposium on Medical Measurements and Applications (MeMeA)* (pp. 1–5). IEEE Xplore. https://doi.org/10.1109/MeMeA49120.2020.9137172.

Balestra, N., Sharma, G., Riek, L. M., & Busza, A. (2021). Automatic identification of upper extremity rehabilitation exercise type and dose using body-worn sensors and machine learning: A pilot study. *Digital Biomarkers*, 5(2), 158–166. https://doi.org/10.1159/000516619

Bicer, M., Phillips, A. T. M., Melis, A., McGregor, A. H., & Modenese, L. (2022). Generative deep learning applied to biomechanics: A new augmentation technique for motion capture datasets. *Journal of Biomechanics*, 144, 111301. https://doi.org/10.1016/j.jbiomech.2022.111301

Biometrics Ltd. Available online: www.biometricsltd.com/index.htm (accessed on 24 August 2022).

BioSemi Products. Available online: www.biosemi.com/products.htm (accessed on 05 December 2022).

Bisio, I., Garibotto, C., Lavagetto, F., & Sciarrone, A. (2019). When eHealth meets IoT: A smart wireless system for post-stroke home rehabilitation. *IEEE Wireless Communications*, 26(6), 24–29. IEEE Xplore. https://doi.org/10.1109/MWC.001.1900125

Blanco-Diaz, C. F., Guerrero-Méndez, C. D., Duarte-González, M. E., & Jaramillo-Isaza, S. (2021). Estimation of limbs angles amplitudes during the use of the five-minute shaper device using artificial neural networks. In: Figueroa-García, J. C., Díaz-Gutierrez, Y., Gaona-García, E. E., & Orjuela-Cañón, A. D. (eds) *Applied Computer Sciences in Engineering. WEA 2021. Communications in Computer and Information Science*, vol. 1431. Springer, Cham. https://doi.org/10.1007/978-3-030-86702-7_19

Bobin, M., Amroun, H., Boukalle, M., Anastassova, M., & Ammi, M. (2018). Smart cup to monitor stroke patients activities during everyday life. In *2018 IEEE International Conference on Internet of Things (iThings) and IEEE Green Computing and Communications (GreenCom) and IEEE Cyber, Physical and Social Computing (CPSCom) and IEEE Smart Data (SmartData)* (pp. 189–195). IEEE Xplore. https://doi-org/10.1109/Cybermatics_2018.2018.00062

Boukhennoufa, I., Zhai, X., McDonald-Maier, K. D., Utti, V., & Jackson, J. (2021). Improving the activity recognition using GMAF and transfer learning in post-stroke rehabilitation assessment. In *2021 IEEE 19th World Symposium on Applied Machine Intelligence and Informatics (SAMI)* (pp. 000391–000398). IEEE Xplore. https://doi.org/10.1109/SAMI50585.2021.9378670

Boukhennoufa, I., Zhai, X., Utti, V., Jackson, J., & McDonald-Maier, K. D. (2022). Wearable sensors and machine learning in post-stroke rehabilitation assessment: A systematic review. *Biomedical Signal Processing and Control*, 71, Part B. https://doi.org/10.1016/j.bspc.2021.103197

Butt, A. H., Zambrana, C., Idelsohn-Zielonka, S., Claramunt-Molet, M., Ugartemendia-Etxarri, A., Rovini, E., & Cavallo, F. (2019). Assessment of purposeful movements for post-stroke patients in activites of daily living with wearable sensor device. In *2019 IEEE Conference on Computational Intelligence in Bioinformatics and Computational Biology (CIBCB)* (pp. 1–8). IEEE Xplore. https://doi.org/10.1109/CIBCB.2019.8791470

Calvaresi, D., Schumacher, M., Marinoni, M., Hilfiker, R., Dragoni, A. F., & Buttazzo, G. (2017). Agent-based systems for telerehabilitation: Strengths, limitations and future challenges. *X Workshop on Agents Applied in Health Care*. https://doi.org/10.1007/978-3-319-70887-4_1

Cano-Mañas, M. J., Colldo-Vázquez, S., Rodríguez Hernández, J., Muñoz Villena, A. J., & Cano-De-La-Cuerda, R. (2020). Effects of video-game based therapy on balance, postural control, functionality, and quality of life of patients with subacute stroke: A randomized controlled trial. *Journal of Healthcare Engineering*, 2020. https://doi.org/10.1155/2020/5480315

Capela, N. A., Lemaire, E. D., & Baddour, N. (2015). Feature selection for wearable smartphone-based human activity recognition with able bodied, elderly, and stroke patients. *PLoS ONE*, 10(4), e0124414. https://doi.org/10.1371/journal.pone.0124414

Casacci, P., Pistoia, M., Leone, A., Caroppo, A., & Siciliano, P. (2015). Alzheimer patient's home rehabilitation through ICT advanced technologies: The ALTRUISM project. In *Ambient Assisted Living: Italian Forum 2014* (pp. 377–385). Springer International Publishing. https://doi.org/10.1007/978-3-319-18374-9_35

Caserman, P., Hoffmann, K., Müller, P., Schaub, M., Straßburg, K., Wiemeyer, J., Bruder, R., & Göbel, S. (2020). Quality criteria for serious games: Serious part, game part, and balance. *JMIR Serious Games*, 8(3), 1–14. https://doi.org/10.2196/19037

Castaneda, D., Esparza, A., Ghamari, M., Soltanpur, C., & Nazeran, H. (2018). A review on wearable photoplethysmography sensors and their potential future applications in health care. *International Journal of Biosensors & Bioelectronics*, 4(4), 195–202. https://doi.org/10.15406/ijbsbe.2018.04.00125

Chen, P. W., Baune, N. A., Zwir, I., Wang, J., Swamidass, V., & Wong, A. W. (2021). Measuring activities of daily living in stroke patients with motion machine learning algorithms: A pilot study. *International Journal of Environmental Research and Public Health*, 18(4), 1634. https://doi.org/10.3390/ijerph18041634

Cheng, S., Gu, Z., Zhou, L., Hao, M., An, H., Song, K., Wu, X., Zhang, K., Zhao, Z., Dong, Y., & Wen, Y. (2021). Recent progress in intelligent wearable sensors for health monitoring and wound healing based on biofluids. *Frontiers in Bioengineering and Biotechnology*, 9(November), 1–21. https://doi.org/10.3389/fbioe.2021.765987

Delsys. Available online: https://delsys.com/ (accessed on 3 November 2022).

Dierick, F., Pierre, A., Profeta, L., Telliez, F., & Buisseret, F. (2021). Perceived usefulness of telerehabilitation of musculoskeletal disorders: A belgium–france pilot study during the second wave of Covid-19 pandemic. *Healthcare (Switzerland)*, 9(11), 1–12. https://doi.org/10.3390/healthcare9111605

Dzobo, K., Adotey, S., Thomford, N. E., & Dzobo, W. (2020). Integrating artificial and human intelligence: A partnership for responsible innovation in biomedical engineering and medicine. *OMICS A Journal of Integrative Biology*, *24*(5), 247–263. https://doi.org/10.1089/omi.2019.0038

Ertel, W. (2017). Introduction to artificial intelligence. In *Smart Systems for Industrial Applications*. Springer International Publishing. https://doi.org/10.1007/978-3-319-58487-4

Fiani, B., Siddiqi, I., Lee, S. C., & Dhillon, L. (2020). Telerehabilitation: Development, application, and need for increased usage in the COVID-19 era for patients with spinal pathology. *Cureus*, 12(9). https://doi.org/10.7759/cureus.10563

Gaboury, I., Tousignant, M., Corriveau, H., Menear, M., Le Dorze, G., Rochefort, C., Vachon, B., Rochette, A., Gosselin, S., Michaud, F., Bollen, J., & Dean, S. (2021). Effects of telerehabilitation on patient adherence to a rehabilitation plan: Protocol for a mixed methods trial. *JMIR Research Protocols*, 10(10), e32134. https://doi.org/10.2196/32134

Gandhi, D. B. C., Pandian, J. D., Szturm, T., Kanitkar, A., Kate, M. P., & Bhanot, K. (2021). A computer-game-based rehabilitation platform for individuals with fine and gross motor upper extremity deficits post-stroke (CARE fOR U)—Protocol for a randomized controlled trial. *European Stroke Journal*, 6(3), 291–301. https://doi.org/10.1177/2396987321994293

Gandhi, D. B. C., Sterba, A., Khatter, H., & Pandian, J. D. (2020). Mirror therapy in stroke rehabilitation: Current perspectives. *Therapeutics and Clinical Risk Management*, 16, 75–85. https://doi.org/10.2147/TCRM.S206883

Geng, J., Huang, D., & De la Torre, F. (2022). DensePose from WiFi. In *Proceedings of ACM Conference (Conference'17)* (Vol. 1, Issue 1). Association for Computing Machinery. http://arxiv.org/abs/2301.00250

Hill, S. W., Mong, S., & Vo, Q. (2022). Three-dimensional motion analysis for occupational therapy upper extremity assessment and rehabilitation: A scoping review. *The Open Journal of Occupational Therapy*, 10(4), 1–14. https://doi.org/10.15453/2168-6408.1901

Hospodarskyy, A. J., & Tsvyakh, A. I. (2020). An application of artificial intelligence for telerehabilitation of patients with injuries of the lower extremities. *Health Systems and Policy Research*, 7(4), ISSN 2254-9137. Available online: www.hsprj.com/health-maintanance/an-application-of-artificial-intelligence-for-telerehabilitation-of-patients-with-injuries-of-the-lower-extremities.pdf

Individual Sensors. Available online: www.shimmersensing.com/products/individual-sensors/ (accessed on 4 September 2022).

Kaku, A., Parnandi, A., Venkatesan, A., Pandit, N., Schambra, H., & Fernandez-Granda, C. (2020). Towards data-driven stroke rehabilitation via wearable sensors and deep learning. In *Machine Learning for Healthcare Conference* (pp. 143–171). Proceedings of Machine Learning Research. https://doi.org/10.48550/arXiv.2004.08297

Karakostas, A., Meditskos, G., Stavropoulos, T. G., Kompatsiaris, I., & Tsolaki, M. (2015). A sensor-based framework to support clinicians in dementia assessment: The results of a pilot study. In *Ambient Intelligence-Software and Applications: 6th International Symposium on Ambient Intelligence (ISAmI 2015)* (pp. 213–221). Springer International Publishing. https://doi.org/10.1007/978-3-319-19695-4_22

Kast, C., Krenn, M., Aramphianlert, W., Hofer, C., Aszmann, O. C., & Mayr, W. (2017). Modular multi-channel real-time bio-signal acquisition system. In *International Conference on Advancements of Medicine and Health Care through Technology; 12th–15th October 2016, Cluj-Napoca, Romania: MEDITECH 2016* (pp. 95–98). Springer International Publishing. https://doi.org/10.1007/978-3-319-52875-5_21

Kato, P. M. (2010). Video games in health care: Closing the gap. *Review of General Psychology*, 14(2), 113–121. https://doi.org/10.1037/a0019441

Khanghah, A. B., Fernie, G., & Fekr, A. R. (2023). Design and validation of vision-based exercise biofeedback for tele-rehabilitation. *Sensors*, 23(3), 1206. https://doi.org/10.3390/s23031206

Khera, P., & Kumar, N. (2020). Role of machine learning in gait analysis: A review. *Journal of Medical Engineering & Technology*, 44(8), 441–467. https://doi.org/10.1080/03091902.2020.1796205

Kidziński, Ł., Yang, B., Hicks, J. L., Rajagopal, A., Delp, S. L., & Schwartz, M. H. (2020). Deep neural networks enable quantitative movement analysis using single-camera videos. *Nature Communications*, 11(1), 1–10. https://doi.org/10.1038/s41467-020-17807-z

Kim, I., Bhagat, Y. A., Homer, J., & Lobo, R. (2016). Multimodal analog front end for wearable bio-sensors. *IEEE Sensors Journal*, 16(24), 8784–8791. https://doi.org/10.1109/JSEN.2016.2624645

Knippenberg, E., Verbrugghe, J., Lamers, I., Palmaers, S., Timmermans, A., & Spooren, A. (2017). Markerless motion capture systems as training device in neurological rehabilitation: A systematic review of their use, application, target population and efficacy. *Journal of Neuroengineering and Rehabilitation*, 14(1), 61. https://doi.org/10.1186/s12984-017-0270-x

Kolanovic, M., & Krishnamachari, R. (2017). Big data and AI strategies: Machine learning and alternative data approach to investing. *JP Morgan Global Quantitative & Derivatives Strategy Report*, May. Available online: https://cpb-us-e2.wpmucdn.com/faculty.sites.uci.edu/dist/2/51/files/2018/05/JPM-2017-MachineLearningInvestments.pdf

Komaris, D. S., Pérez-Valero, E., Jordan, L., Barton, J., Hennessy, L., O'flynn, B., & Tedesco, S. (2019). Predicting three-dimensional ground reaction forces in running by using artificial neural networks and lower body kinematics. *IEEE Access*, 7, 156779–156786. https://doi.org/10.1109/ACCESS.2019.2949699

Kozlovszky, M., Kovacs, L., & Karoczkai, K. (2015). Cardiovascular and diabetes focused remote patient monitoring. In *VI Latin American Congress on Biomedical Engineering CLAIB 2014, Paraná, Argentina 29, 30 & 31 October 2014* (pp. 568–571). Springer International Publishing. https://doi.org/10.1007/978-3-319-13117-7_141

Li, X., & Sun, Y. (2017). NCMB-button: A wearable non-contact system for long-term multiple biopotential monitoring. 2017 *IEEE/ACM International Conference on Connected Health: Applications, Systems and Engineering Technologies (CHASE)*, Philadelphia, PA (pp. 348–355). https://doi.org/10.1109/CHASE.2017.118

Lin, W.-T. M., Lin, B.-S., Lee, I.-J., & Lee, S.-H. (2022). Development of a smartphone-based mHealth platform for telerehabilitation. *IEEE Transactions on Neural Systems and Rehabilitation Engineering*, 30, 2682–2691. https://doi.org.10.1109/TNSRE.2022.3204148

Liu, S. H., Wang, J. J., & Tan, T. H. (2019). A portable and wireless multi-channel acquisition system for physiological signal measurements. *Sensors*, 19(23), 5314. https://doi.org/10.3390/s19235314

Lohse, K., Shirzad, N., Verster, A., Hodges, N., & Van Der Loos, H. F. M. (2013). Video games and rehabilitation: Using design principles to enhance engagement in physical therapy. *Journal of Neurologic Physical Therapy*, 37(4), 166–175. https://doi.org/10.1097/NPT.0000000000000017

Lucisano, J. Y., Routh, T. L., Lin, J. T., & Gough, D. A. (2016). Glucose monitoring in individuals with diabetes using a long-term implanted sensor/telemetry system and model. *IEEE Transactions on Biomedical Engineering*, 64(9), 1982–1993. https://doi.org/10.1109/TBME.2016.2521261

Malasinghe, L. P., Ramzan, N., & Dahal, K. (2019). Remote patient monitoring: A comprehensive study. *Journal of Ambient Intelligence and Humanized Computing*, 10, 57–76. https://doi.org/10.1007/s12652-017-0650-1

Mazzetta, I., Gentile, P., Pessione, M., Suppa, A., Zampogna, A., Bianchini, E., & Irrera, F. (2018). Stand-alone wearable system for ubiquitous real-time monitoring of muscle activation potentials. *Sensors*, 18(6), 1748. https://doi.org/10.3390/s18061748

Meng, L., Zhang, A., Chen, C., Wang, X., Jiang, X., Tao, L., . . . & Chen, W. (2021). Exploration of human activity recognition using a single sensor for stroke survivors and able-bodied people. *Sensors*, 21(3), 799. https://doi.org/10.3390/s21030799

Menon, K. U., Hemachandran, D., & Abhishek, T. K. (2013). A survey on non-invasive blood glucose monitoring using NIR. In *2013 International Conference on Communication and Signal Processing* (pp. 1069–1072). IEEE Xplore. https://doi.org/10.1109/ICCSP.2013.6577057

Michell, A., Besomi, M., Seron, P., Voigt, M., Cubillos, R., Parada-Hernández, F., Urrejola, O., Ferreira-Pacheco, T. B., De Oliveira-Silva, D., Bianca Aily, J., Moreno-Collazos, J. E., Pinzón-Ríos, I. D., Aguirre-Aguirre, C. L., Hinman, R. S., Bennell, K. L., & Russell, T. G. (2022). Implementation of physiotherapy telerehabilitation before and post Covid-19 outbreak: A comparative narrative between South American countries and Australia. *Salud Pública de México*, 64, S31–S39. https://doi.org/10.21149/13160

Mukhopadhyay, S. C., Suryadevara, N. K., & Nag, A. (2022). Wearable sensors for healthcare: Fabrication to application. *Sensors*, 22(14), 5137. https://doi.org/10.3390/s22145137

Mulfari, D., la Placa, D., Rovito, C., Celesti, A., & Villari, M. (2022). Deep learning applications in telerehabilitation speech therapy scenarios. *Computers in Biology and Medicine*, 148. https://doi.org/10.1016/j.compbiomed.2022.105864

Mundt, M., Koeppe, A., Bamer, F., David, S., & Markert, B. (2020). Artificial neural networks in motion analysis—applications of unsupervised and heuristic feature selection techniques. *Sensors (Switzerland)*, 20(16), 1–15. https://doi.org/10.3390/s20164581

Nakano, N., Sakura, T., Ueda, K., Omura, L., Kimura, A., Iino, Y., Fukashiro, S., & Yoshioka, S. (2020). Evaluation of 3D markerless motion capture accuracy using OpenPose with multiple video cameras. *Frontiers in Sports and Active Living*, 2(May), 1–9. https://doi.org/10.3389/fspor.2020.00050

Nasrabadi, A. M., Eslaminia, A. R., Bakhshayesh, P. R., Ejtehadi, M., Alibiglou, L., & Behzadipour, S. (2022). A new scheme for the development of IMU-based activity recognition systems for telerehabilitation. *Medical Engineering and Physics*, 108, 103876. https://doi.org/10.1016/j.medengphy.2022.103876

National Institutes of Health (NIH), Department of Health and Human Services. (2018). Available online at: https://grants.nih.gov/grants/guide/pa-files/PAR-14-028.html (accessed on 03 December 2022).

Needham, L., Evans, M., Wade, L., Cosker, D. P., McGuigan, M. P., Bilzon, J. L., & Colyer, S. L. (2022). The development and evaluation of a fully automated markerless motion capture workflow. *Journal of Biomechanics*, 144, 111338. https://doi.org/10.1016/j.jbiomech.2022.111338

Noor, T., & Tantawy, H. (2019). The internet of medical things (IoMT) towards intelligent healthcare systems. *Journal of Ambient Intelligence and Humanized Computing*, 10(8), 2955–2969. https://doi.org/10.1007/s12652-019-01286-1

Nuara, A., Fabbri-Destro, M., Scalona, E., & Lenzi, S. E. (2022). Telerehabilitation in response to constrained physical distance: An opportunity to rethink neurorehabilitative routines. *Journal of Neurology*, 269(1003). https://doi.org/10.1007/s00415-021-10397-w

O'Brien, M. K., Shawen, N., Mummidisetty, C. K., Kaur, S., Bo, X., Poellabauer, C., Kording, K., & Jayaraman, A. (2017). Activity recognition for persons with stroke using mobile phone technology: Toward improved performance in a home setting. *Journal of Medical Internet Research*, 19(5), e184. https://doi.org/10.2196/jmir.7385

Otoom, A. F., Abdallah, E. E., Kilani, Y., Kefaye, A., & Ashour, M. (2015). Effective diagnosis and monitoring of heart disease. *International Journal of Software Engineering and Its Applications*, 9(1), 143–156. Available online: www.earticle.net/Article/A239338

Palumbo, A., Calabrese, B., Ielpo, N., Demeco, A., Ammendolia, A., & Corchiola, D. (2020). Cloud-based biomedical system for remote monitoring of ALS patients. In *2020 IEEE International Conference on Bioinformatics and Biomedicine (BIBM)* (pp. 1469–1476). IEEE Xplore. https://doi.org/10.1109/BIBM49941.2020.9313485

Palumbo, A., Vizza, P., Calabrese, B., & Ielpo, N. (2021). Biopotential signal monitoring systems in rehabilitation: A review. *Sensors*, 21(21), 7172. https://doi.org/10.3390/s21217172

Palumbo, A., Vizza, P., Veltri, P., Gambardella, A., Pucci, F., & Sturniolo, M. (2009). Design of an electronic device for brain computer interface applications. In *2009 IEEE International Workshop on Medical Measurements and Applications* (pp. 99–103). IEEE Xplore. https://doi.org/10.1109/MEMEA.2009.5167963

Paoli, R., Fernández-Luque, F. J., Doménech, G., Martínez, F., Zapata, J., & Ruiz, R. (2012). A system for ubiquitous fall monitoring at home via a wireless sensor network and a wearable mote. *Expert Systems with Applications*, 39(5), 5566–5575. https://doi.org/10.1016/j.eswa.2011.11.061

Park, E., Lee, K., Han, T., & Nam, H. S. (2020). Automatic grading of stroke symptoms for rapid assessment using optimized machine learning and 4-limb kinematics: Clinical validation study. *Journal of Medical Internet Research*, 22(9), e20641. https://doi.org/10.2196/20641

Pastora-Bernal, J. M., Estebanez-Pérez, M. J., Molina-Torres, G., García-López, F. J., Sobrino-Sánchez, R., & Martín-Valero, R. (2021). Telerehabilitation intervention in patients with COVID-19 after hospital discharge to improve functional capacity and quality of life. Study protocol for a multicenter randomized clinical trial. *International Journal of Environmental Research and Public Health*, 18(6), 2924. https://doi.org/10.3390/ijerph18062924

Peretti, A., Amenta, F., Tayebati, S. K., Nittari, G., & Mahdi, S. S. (2017). Telerehabilitation: Review of the state-of-the-art and areas of application. *JMIR Rehabilitation and Assistive Technologies*, *4*(2), 1–9. https://doi.org/10.2196/rehab.7511

Pinheiro, E. C., Postolache, O. A., & Girão, P. S. (2013). Dual architecture platform for unobtrusive wheelchair user monitoring. In *2013 IEEE International Symposium on Medical Measurements and Applications (MeMeA)* (pp. 124–129). IEEE Xplore. https://doi.org/10.1109/MeMeA.2013.6549623

Plazas-Molano, A. C., Duarte-González, M. E., Blanco-Díaz, C. F., & Jaramillo-Isaza, S. (2020). Exploring the facial and neurological activation due to predetermined visual stimulus using kinect and emotiv sensors. *Communications in Computer and Information Science*, *1274 CCIS*, 268–280. https://doi.org/10.1007/978-3-030-61834-6_23

Postolache, O. A., Mukhopadhyay, S. C., Jayasundera, K. P., & Swain, A. K. (Eds.). (2016). *Sensors for Everyday Life: Healthcare Settings*, vol. 22. Cham: Springer. https://doi.org/10.1007/978-3-319-47319-2

Pueo, B., & Jimenez-Olmedo, J. M. (2017). Application of motion capture technology for sport performance analysis. *Retos*, 2041(32), 241–247. https://doi.org/10.47197/retos.v0i32.59831

Qureshi, F., & Krishnan, S. (2018). Wearable hardware design for the internet of medical things (IoMT). *Sensors*, 18(11), 3812. https://doi.org/10.3390/s18113812

Ramesh, M. V., Anand, S., & Rekha, P. (2012). A mobile software for health professionals to monitor remote patients. In *2012 Ninth International Conference on Wireless and Optical Communications Networks (WOCN)* (pp. 1–4). IEEE Xplore. https://doi.org/10.1109/WOCN.2012.6251346

Ramírez-Sanz, J. M., Garrido-Labrador, J. L., Olivares-Gil, A., García-Bustillo, Á., Arnaiz-González, Á., Díez-Pastor, J.-F., Jahouh, M., González-Santos, J., González-Bernal, J. J., Allende-Río, M., Valiñas-Sieiro, F., Trejo-Gabriel-Galan, J. M., & Cubo, E. (2023). A low-cost system using a big-data deep-learning framework for assessing physical telerehabilitation: A proof-of-concept. *Healthcare*, 11(4), 507. https://doi.org/10.3390/healthcare11040507

Razfar, N., Kashef, R., & Mohammadi, F. (2021). A comprehensive overview on IoT-based smart stroke rehabilitation using the advances of wearable technology. In *2021 IEEE 23rd Int Conf on High Performance Computing & Communications; 7th Int Conf on*

Data Science & Systems; 19th Int Conf on Smart City; 7th Int Conf on Dependability in Sensor, Cloud & Big Data Systems & Application (HPCC/DSS/SmartCity/DependSys) (pp. 1359–1366). IEEE Xplore. https://doi.org/10.1109/HPCC/DSS/SmartCity/DependSys52609.2021.00173

Rehman, H., Kamal, A. K., Morris, P. B., Sayani, S., Merchant, A. T., & Virani, S. S. (2017). Mobile health (mHealth) technology for the management of hypertension and hyperlipidemia: Slow start but loads of potential. *Current Atherosclerosis Reports*, 19(3). https://doi.org/10.1007/s11883-017-0649-y

Rosique, F., Losilla, F., & Navarro, P. J. (2021). Applying vision-based pose estimation in a telerehabilitation application. *Applied Sciences*, 11(19), 1–10. https://doi.org/10.3390/app11197448

Ruotsalainen, P., & Blobel, B. (2022). Transformed health ecosystems—challenges for security, privacy, and trust. *Frontiers in Medicine*, 9(March), 1–10. https://doi.org/10.3389/fmed.2022.827253

Sannino, G., De Falco, I., & De Pietro, G. (2015). A supervised approach to automatically extract a set of rules to support fall detection in an mHealth system. *Applied Soft Computing*, 34, 205–216. https://doi.org/10.1016/j.asoc.2015.05.022

Sarker, V. K., Jiang, M., Gia, T. N., Anzanpour, A., Rahmani, A. M., & Liljeberg, P. (2017). Portable multipurpose bio-signal acquisition and wireless streaming device for wearables. In *2017 IEEE Sensors Applications Symposium (SAS)* (pp. 1–6). IEEE Xplore. https://doi.org/10.1109/SAS.2017.7894057

Sarma Dhulipala, V. R., Devadas, P., & Tejo Murthy, P. H. S. (2016). Mobile phone sensing mechanism for stress relaxation using sensor networks: A survey. *Wireless Personal Communications*, 86, 1013–1022. https://doi.org/10.1007/s11277-015-3187-7

Senapati, B., Kumar, M. G. L., & Ray, K. B. (2017). High resolution reconfigurable bio-potential processor for portable biomedical application. In *2017 Devices for Integrated Circuit (DevIC)* (pp. 517–521). IEEE Xplore. https://doi.org/10.1109/DEVIC.2017.8069269

Seo, N. J., Arun Kumar, J., Hur, P., Crocher, V., Motawar, B., & Lakshminarayanan, K. (2016). Usability evaluation of low-cost virtual reality hand and arm rehabilitation games. *Journal of Rehabilitation Research and Development*, 53(3), 321–334. https://doi.org/10.1682/JRRD.2015.03.0045

Seron, P., Oliveros, M., Gutierrez-Arias, R., Fuentes-Aspe, R., Torres-Castro, R. C., Merino-Osorio, C., Nahuelhual, P., Inostroza, J., Jalil, Y., Solano, R., Marzuca-Nassr, G. N., Aguilera-Eguía, R., Lavados-Romo, P., Soto-Rodríguez, F. J., Sabelle, C., Villarroel-Silva, G., Gomolán, P., Huaiquilaf, S., & Sanchez, P. (2021). Effectiveness of telerehabilitation in physical therapy: A rapid overview. *Physical Therapy*, 101(6), 1–18. https://doi.org/10.1093/ptj/pzab053

Seshadri, D. R., Li, R. T., Voos, J. E., Rowbottom, J. R., Alfes, C. M., Zorman, C. A., & Drummond, C. K. (2019). Wearable sensors for monitoring the physiological and biochemical profile of the athlete. *NPJ Digital Medicine*, 2(1), 72. https://doi.org/10.1038/s41746-019-0150-9

Shem, K., Irgens, I., & Alexander, M. (2022). Getting started: Mechanisms of telerehabilitation. In *Telerehabilitation* (pp. 5–20). Elsevier. https://doi.org/10.1016/B978-0-323-82486-6.00002-2

Smith, P. (2012). Serious games 101. *Rta.Nato.Int*, 1–12. Available online: www.sto.nato.int/publications/STO%20Educational%20Notes/STO-EN-MSG-115/EN-MSG-115-04.pdf

Stetter, B. J., Ringhof, S., Krafft, F. C., Sell, S., & Stein, T. (2019). Estimation of knee joint forces in sport movements using wearable sensors and machine learning. *Sensors (Switzerland)*, 19(17), 1–12. https://doi.org/10.3390/s19173690

Szydło, T., & Konieczny, M. (2015). Mobile devices in the open and universal system for remote patient monitoring. *IFAC-PapersOnLine*, 48(4), 296–301. https://doi.org/10.1016/j.ifacol.2015.07.050

Tan, T. H., Gochoo, M., Chen, Y. F., Hu, J. J., Chiang, J. Y., Chang, C. S., . . . & Hsu, J. C. (2017). Ubiquitous emergency medical service system based on wireless biosensors, traffic information, and wireless communication technologies: Development and evaluation. *Sensors*, 17(1), 202. https://doi.org/10.3390/s17010202

Taylor, M. J. D., & Griffin, M. (2015). The use of gaming technology for rehabilitation in people with multiple sclerosis. *Multiple Sclerosis Journal*, 21(4), 355–371. https://doi.org/10.1177/1352458514563593

Tran, L., & Cha, H. K. (2021). An ultra-low-power neural signal acquisition analog front-end IC. *Microelectronics Journal*, 107, 104950. https://doi.org/10.1016/j.mejo.2021.104950

Tran, T., Chang, L. C., Almubark, I., Bochniewicz, E. M., Shu, L., Lum, P. S., & Dromerick, A. (2018). Robust classification of functional and nonfunctional arm movement after stroke using a single wrist-worn sensor device. In *2018 IEEE International Conference on Big Data (Big Data)* (pp. 5457–5459). IEEE Xplore. https://doi.org/10.1109/BigData.2018.8622553

Vellata, C., Belli, S., Balsamo, F., Giordano, A., Colombo, R., & Maggioni, G. (2021). Effectiveness of telerehabilitation on motor impairments, non-motor symptoms and compliance in patients with Parkinson's disease: A systematic review. *Frontiers in Neurology*, 12(August). https://doi.org/10.3389/fneur.2021.627999

Vieira, A. G. D. S., Pinto, A. C. P. N., Garcia, B. M. S. P., Eid, R. A. C., Mól, C. G., & Nawa, R. K. (2022). Telerehabilitation improves physical function and reduces dyspnoea in people with COVID-19 and post-COVID-19 conditions: A systematic review. *Journal of Physiotherapy*, 68(2), 90–98. https://doi.org/10.1016/j.jphys.2022.03.011

Vijayan, V., Connolly, J. P., Condell, J., McKelvey, N., & Gardiner, P. (2021). Review of wearable devices and data collection considerations for connected health. *Sensors*, 21(16), 5589. https://doi.org/10.3390/s21165589

Vishnu, S., Jino Ramson, S. R., & Jegan, R. (2020). Internet of Medical Things (IoMT)-An overview. In *ICDCS 2020 5th International Conference on Devices, Circuits and Systems*, pp. 101–104. https://doi.org/10.1109/ICDCSyst49879.2020.00036

Wade, L., Needham, L., McGuigan, P., & Bilzon, J. (2022). Applications and limitations of current markerless motion capture methods for clinical gait biomechanics. *PeerJ*, 10, 1–27. https://doi.org/10.7717/peerj.12995

Wang, L., Ali, Y., Nazir, S., & Niazi, M. (2020). ISA evaluation framework for security of internet of health things system using AHP-TOPSIS methods. *IEEE Access*, 8, 152316–152332. https://doi.org/10.1109/ACCESS.2020.3017221

Wang, Z., & Oates, T. (2015). Imaging time-series to improve classification and imputation. In *Twenty-Fourth International Joint Conference on Artificial Intelligence*. https://doi.org/10.24963/ijcai.2015/50

Wei, W., McElroy, C., & Dey, S. (2019). Towards on-demand virtual physical therapist: Machine learning-based patient action understanding, assessment and task recommendation. *IEEE Transactions on Neural Systems and Rehabilitation Engineering*, 27, 1824–1835. https://doi.org/10.1109/TNSRE.2019.2933706

World Health Organization. (2013). *Guidelines on Health-Related Rehabilitation (Rehabilitation Guidelines)*. Available online: www.who.int/disabilities/care/rehabilitation_guidelines_concept.pdf

World Health Organization. (2017). *World Bank and WHO: Half the World Lacks Access to Essential Health Services, 100 Million Still Pushed into Extreme Poverty Because of Health Expenses*. Available online: www.who.int/news/item/13-12-2017-world-bank-and-who-half-the-world-lacks-access-to-essential-health-services-100-million-still-pushed-into-extreme-poverty-because-of-health-expenses

World Health Organization. (2018). mHealth: Use of appropriate digital technologies for public health: Report by the director-general. World Health Organization. *World Health Organization*, 10(1). https://doi.org/10.2337/dc11-0366.4

Yu, L., Lu, Y., Zhu, X. L., & Feng, L. (2012). Research advances on technology of internet of things in medical domain. *Jisuanji Yingyong Yanjiu*, 29(1), 1–7. https://doi.org/10.3969/j.issn.1001-3695.2012.01.001

Yuce, M. R., & Dissanayake, T. (2013). Easy-to-swallow antenna and propagation. *IEEE Microwave Magazine*, 14(4), 74–82. https://doi.org/10.1109/MMM.2013.2261630

Zhang, G., Rao, Y., Wang, C., Zhou, W., & Ji, X. (2021). A deep learning method for video-based action recognition. *IET Image Processing*, 15(14), 3498–3511. https://doi.org/10.1049/ipr2.12303

Zhao, S., Liu, J., Gong, Z., Lei, Y., OuYang, X., Chan, C. C., & Ruan, S. (2020). Wearable physiological monitoring system based on electrocardiography and electromyography for upper limb rehabilitation training. *Sensors*, 20(17), 4861. https://doi.org/10.3390/s20174861

Index